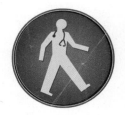

Resident Readiness

General Surgery

Notice

Medicine is an ever-changing science. As new research and clinical experience broaden our knowledge, changes in treatment and drug therapy are required. The authors and the publisher of this work have checked with sources believed to be reliable in their efforts to provide information that is complete and generally in accord with the standards accepted at the time of publication. However, in view of the possibility of human error or changes in medical sciences, neither the authors nor the publisher nor any other party who has been involved in the preparation or publication of this work warrants that the information contained herein is in every respect accurate or complete, and they disclaim all responsibility for any errors or omissions or for the results obtained from use of the information contained in this work. Readers are encouraged to confirm the information contained herein with other sources. For example and in particular, readers are advised to check the product information sheet included in the package of each drug they plan to administer to be certain that the information contained in this work is accurate and that changes have not been made in the recommended dose or in the contraindications for administration. This recommendation is of particular importance in connection with new or infrequently used drugs.

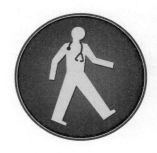

Resident Readiness
General Surgery

Debra L. Klamen, MD, MHPE

Associate Dean for Education
 and Curriculum
Professor and Chair
Department of Medical Education
Southern Illinois University School
 of Medicine
Springfield, Illinois

Alden H. Harken, MD

Professor and Chair
Department of Surgery
University of California,
 San Francisco—East Bay
Oakland, California

Brian C. George, MD

Resident, General Surgery
Department of Surgery
Massachusetts General Hospital
Boston, Massachusetts

Debra A. DaRosa, PhD

Professor of Surgery
Vice Chair for Education
Department of Surgery
Northwestern University Feinberg
 School of Medicine
Chicago, Illinois

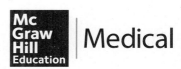

New York   Athens   Chicago   San Francisco   London   Madrid
Mexico City   Milan   New Delhi   Singapore   Sydney   Toronto

Resident Readiness: General Surgery

Copyright © 2014 by McGraw-Hill Education. All rights reserved. Printed in the United States of America. Except as permitted under the United States Copyright Act of 1976, no part of this publication may be reproduced or distributed in any form or by any means, or stored in a data base or retrieval system, without the prior written permission of the publisher.

1 2 3 4 5 6 7 8 9 0   DOC/DOC   18 17 16 15 14 13

ISBN 978-0-07-177319-5
MHID 0-07-177319-3

This book was set in Minion Pro by Thomson Digital.
The editors were Catherine A. Johnson and Cindy Yoo.
The production supervisor was Richard Ruzycka.
Project management was provided by Shaminder Pal Singh, Thomson Digital.
The designer was Eve Siegel; the cover designer was Anthony Landi.
RR Donnelley was the printer and binder.

This book is printed on acid-free paper.

Cataloging-in-Publication Data is on file with the Library of Congress.

McGraw-Hill Education books are available at special quantity discounts to use as premiums and sales promotions or for use in corporate training programs. To contact a representative, please visit the Contact Us pages at www.mhprofessional.com.

This book is dedicated to all my friends, family, co-workers and colleagues who have enriched my life and allowed me to follow my passion. Special thanks to my husband Phil who encouraged me, and to my mom Bonnie Klamen and late father Sam Klamen who raised me to try.—Debra L. Klamen

To the surgical residents in the UCSF-East Bay Department of Surgery whose dedication to their patients and professional commitment to continued learning are an inspirational indicator of the great good health of American Surgery.—Alden H. Harken

For Autumn.—Brian C. George

CONTENTS

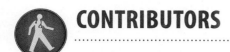

CONTRIBUTORS

Joel T. Adler, MD
Resident, General Surgery
Massachusetts General Hospital
Boston, Massachusetts
Chapter 19

Hasan B. Alam, MD
Section Head, General Surgery
Norman W. Thompson Professor of Surgery
University of Michigan Health System
Ann Arbor, Michigan
Chapter 56

Peter Angelos, MD, PhD, FACS
Linda Kohler Anderson Professor of Surgery and Surgical Ethics
Chief, Endocrine Surgery
Associate Director
MacLean Center for Clinical Medical Ethics
The University of Chicago
Chicago, Illinois
Chapters 51, 52, 53

Anne-Marie Boller, MD
Associate Professor of Surgery
Northwestern University
Feinberg School of Medicine
Chicago, Illinois
Chapter 39

Marie Crandall, MD, MPH
Associate Professor
Department of Surgery
Northwestern University
Feinberg School of Medicine
Chicago, Illinois
Chapters 7, 8, 11, 35, 37, 41, 42

Debra A. DaRosa, PhD
Professor of Surgery
Vice Chair for Education
Department of Surgery
Northwestern University Feinberg School of Medicine
Chicago, Illinois
Chapters 1, 2, 51, 52, 53

Amy Robin Deipolyi, MD, PhD
Clinical and Research Fellow
Graduate Assistant in Vascular Imaging and Intervention
Department of Radiology
Massachusetts General Hospital
Boston, Massachusetts
Chapter 25

Shawn P. Fagan, MD, FACS
Assistant Professor
Department of Surgery
Division of Burns
Massachusetts General Hospital
Boston, Massachusetts
Chapter 21

Eric N. Feins, MD
Surgical Resident
Department of Surgery
Massachusetts General Hospital
Boston, Massachusetts
Chapters 17, 36

Brian C. George, MD
Resident, General Surgery
Department of Surgery
Massachusetts General Hospital
Boston, Massachusetts
Chapters 1, 2, 3, 9, 10, 12, 15, 16, 22, 26, 27, 30, 31, 32, 33, 40, 49, 50, 56

Jeremy Goverman, MD, FACS
Assistant Surgeon
Division of Burns
Massachusetts General Hospital
Harvard Medical School
Boston, Massachusetts
Chapter 21

Ashley Hardy, MD
Resident
Department of General Surgery
Northwestern University
Feinberg School of Medicine
Chicago, Illinois
Chapters 7, 37

Alden H. Harken, MD
Professor and Chair
Department of Surgery
University of California, San Francisco—East Bay
Oakland, California
Chapters 1, 2, 3, 10, 12, 15, 16, 26, 27, 28, 29, 30, 31, 32, 33, 40, 49

Alexander T. Hawkins, MD, MPH
Resident, General Surgery
Massachusetts General Hospital
Boston, Massachusetts
Chapters 13, 14, 25

Amanda V. Hayman, MD, MPH
Fellow
Division of Colon and Rectal Surgery Mayo Clinic
Rochester, Minnesota
Chapter 4

Xavier Jimenez, MD
Assistant Professor
Department of Psychiatry
Neurological Institute, The Cleveland Clinic Foundation
Cleveland, Ohio
Chapter 54

Haytham M.A. Kaafarani, MD, MPH
Instructor in Surgery
Harvard Medical School
Division of Trauma
Emergency Surgery and Surgical Critical Care
Massachusetts General Hospital
Boston, Massachusetts
Chapter 56

Teresa S. Kim, MD
Resident
Department of Surgery
Massachusetts General Hospital
Boston, Massachusetts
Chapter 5

John Maa, MD, FACS
Assistant Professor
Division of General Surgery
University of California, San Francisco
San Francisco, California
Chapter 55

Michael F. McGee, MD
Assistant Professor of Surgery
Department of Surgery
Northwestern University
Feinberg School of Medicine
Chicago, Illinois
Chapters 22, 50

Emily Miraflor, MD
Surgical Resident
Department of Surgery
University of California, San Francisco—East Bay
Oakland, California
Chapter 16

Jahan Mohebali, MD
General Surgery Resident
Massachusetts General Hospital
Cardiac Surgery Research Fellow
Brigham and Women's Hospital
Boston, Massachusetts
Chapters 34, 44, 48, 59

Shamim H. Nejad, MD
Director
Burns and Trauma Psychiatry
Psychiatry Consultation Service
Massachusetts General Hospital
Assistant Professor
Harvard Medical School
Boston, Massachusetts
Chapters 20, 24, 54

Virendra I. Patel, MD, MPH
Assistant Professor of Surgery
Harvard Medical School
Division of Vascular and Endovascular Surgery
Massachusetts General Hospital
Boston, Massachusetts
Chapter 19

Allan B. Peetz, MD
Fellow
Acute Care Surgery and Surgical Critical Care
Brigham and Women's Hospital
Boston, Massachusetts
Chapter 35

Roy Phitayakorn, MD, MHPE (MEd)
Director
Surgical Education Research
Massachusetts General Hospital
Instructor, Surgery
Harvard Medical School
Boston, Massachusetts
Chapters 6, 46, 47, 58

Nadia Quijije, MD
Psychiatrist
Department of Psychiatry
Massachusetts General Hospital
Boston, Massachusetts
Chapter 20

Aisha Shaheen, MD, MHA
Resident
General Surgery Residency Program
Department of Surgery
Montefiore Medical Center
Albert Einstein College of Medicine
Bronx, New York
Chapters 8, 11, 42

Selma Marie Siddiqui, MD
Resident
Department of Surgery
St. Joseph Hospital
Chicago, Illinois
Chapter 41

Justin B. Smith, MD
Staff Psychiatrist
Western State Hospital
Staunton, Virginia
Chapter 24

Joel M. Sternbach, MD, MBA
Resident
Department of General Surgery
Northwestern Memorial Hospital
Chicago, Illinois
Chapter 39

Mamta Swaroop, MD, FACS
Assistant Professor of Surgery
Northwestern University
Feinberg School of Medicine
Chicago, Illinois
Chapters 18, 38, 43, 45, 57

Abigail K. Tarbox, MD
Critical Care Surgeon
Jesse Brown VA Medical Center
Assistant Professor of Surgery
Department of Trauma and Critical Care
Northwestern University
Feinberg School of Medicine
Chicago, Illinois
Chapters 18, 38

Ezra N. Teitelbaum, MD
Surgery Resident
Department of Surgery
Northwestern University
Feinberg School of Medicine
Chicago, Illinois
Chapter 23

Anthony Visioni, MD
Resident, General Surgery
Univevrsity Hospitals Case Medical Center
Cleveland, Ohio
Chapter 6

Michael W. Wandling, MD
Resident
Department of Surgery
Northwestern University
Feinbrg School of Medicine
Chicago, Illinois
Chapters 45, 57

Molly A. Wasserman, MD
Resident, General Surgery
Northwestern University
McGraw Medical Center
Chicago, Illinois
Chapter 43

Louise Y. Yeung, MD
Surgical Resident
Department of Surgery
University of California, San Francisco—East Bay
Oakland, California
Chapter 16

ACKNOWLEDGMENTS

The idea for this series came from watching a dedicated educator Dr. David Rogers create and implement a successful residency readiness course. So successful was this course that it was adopted across Southern Illinois University Medical School's fourth year curriculum. It has been a joy working with my co-authors, especially Brian George, a devoted educator himself. He assembled a great group of case writers without whom this book would not exist. I am, as always, greatly indebted to my editor, Catherine Johnson, who believed in me and this series right from the very beginning, championing it on to production. I appreciate McGraw-Hill's continued support as well. Finally, I deeply appreciate the continued support of my colleagues at SIU, which gave me the freedom to work on this book as I needed to. Most of all, I appreciate the support of my family, Phil, Wes, Boss, Aleksei, and Zory—I couldn't have done it without you!

Debra L. Klamen

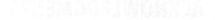

Section I.
Introduction

Welcome

Brian C. George, MD, Alden H. Harken, MD, and Debra A. DaRosa, PhD

We are excited for you! You are about to embark on an exhilarating journey that will be filled with fear, awe, pride, fatigue, reward, and fun. It will, in all likelihood, be a transformative experience that you will look back on with warm nostalgia. While we hope you too are excited about starting your residency, we also recognize that it may seem a bit daunting. You have, no doubt, heard a lot of fanciful stories about the surgical intern year, and you've watched some hardy souls weather the experience. But attending an opera or watching a boxing match is a whole lot different from singing or slugging it out in one.

When Columbus set sail for the New World, his destination on the map was blank. In between Spain and the edge of the world, some helpful cartographers penciled in storms and sea monsters. Like Columbus, you too are sailing into unfamiliar territory. And in surgery the storms and monsters are real enough. But while all people need to captain their own ships and embark on their own journeys, in this case the map is not totally blank. This book is just one of many resources to help guide your forward motion.

We have written this book with the goal of helping you, the soon-to-be-new intern, to develop a deeper understanding of all the "basics"—and nothing more. We have worked hard to keep this book as focused, succinct, and clinically relevant as possible. For example, the book does not include any information about how to manage pancreatic cancer, because as an intern you are never actually going to do that anyway. It does have chapters on how to replete electrolytes, how to triage multiple simultaneous admissions and/or consults, and what your role should be during a trauma. Indeed, we have focused on those areas where you might be expected to already know what to do (even if, like many new interns, you don't). In some cases we simply explain the potential significance of various symptoms and signs, so that you will know when you should call for help.

But how did we come up with the final list of topics we wanted to cover? We started with the "prerequisite" knowledge that an expert panel at the American College of Surgeons (ACS) felt that all medical students should know prior to starting their internship. The list is long—too long. It includes a lot of topics that are already understood by 99% of medical students or not actually that useful in everyday practice. We didn't want to include any of those topics, as that would be a waste of your time and needlessly decrease the signal-to-noise ratio. In order to help sort it out we therefore conducted a survey of "real live interns" during their fourth month of internship, while they could still remember what it was like on their first day. Using a structured instrument we determined which topics the interns wished they had known more about before they started their internships. We analyzed and ranked those responses, added our own 2 cents, and came up with the book you are now reading. While we cannot guide you all the way to your ultimate destination, we feel confident that this book will provide you with a map that will get your voyage safely underway.

This introduction would not be complete without extending a hearty thank you to all of the authors who helped put this book together. We hope that you, the reader, will appreciate their selfless efforts as much as we do.

As a final note, we also hope you will write to us and share your comments and suggestions. Not only would it be fun to hear your reaction to our hard work, but it would also help us make improvements for the next edition. You can reach us by e-mailing rrsurgery@briangeorge.com—we welcome your feedback!

How to Read this Book

Brian C. George, MD, Alden H. Harken, MD, and Debra A. DaRosa, PhD

The chapters in this book follow the same format and include multiple elements, all specifically designed to maximize your learning. Most chapters start with a case written in the second person. We expect these cases will help make the discussion more tangible and will emphasize the relevance of each topic to your new job. After the case, there is a set of questions designed to help you assess your own knowledge on the given topic. Well-established learning theory suggests that you should try to answer those questions before moving on, as doing so will help you retain what you are about to read. The answers to those questions can be found in the text of the case discussion that follows. After the case discussion you will find a set of questions and answers. Again, these are designed to help you assess your own knowledge, and to provide some repetition (as you probably know, repetition is the mother of all learning, and repetition is the mother of all learning). The last part of each case-based chapter includes a list of the most important tips to remember. If you learn nothing else from each chapter, you should try and remember the tips. A couple of days prior to starting your internship you could even flip through the book and review just these bullet points—they are incredibly high yield and can serve as a brief overview of the entire book.

The chapters are organized into sections:

1. Introduction
2. Handling Patients in the ED
3. Handling Inpatients
4. Handling Patients in Clinic

With the exception of Section I, each section is organized around one type of patient care. It should be emphasized that while each case takes place in a specific setting, the chapter as a whole will often discuss topics that are more broadly applicable. We trust that the reader who is using this book as a reference will, with the help of the index, be able to find those topics that are of most interest. For the reader using this as preparation for internship, the sequence of chapters has been organized to be read from start to finish.

General Advice

Brian C. George, MD and
Alden H. Harken, MD

As you complete the final stages of medical school it is now time to turn your thoughts to that next stage: internship and residency. This chapter will introduce you to some common issues faced in that stage and give you some basic guiding principles.

A CASE OF THE JITTERS

We were all nervous when we started our internships. In fact, it would be frightening if you *weren't* nervous—those are the interns who are dangerous! But you should also have some confidence not only in yourself but also in your co-residents, your attendings, and the system. You are not alone, and nobody expects you to know everything your first day. They *do* expect you to care about your patients and to do everything in your power to "do the right thing." Often that means asking for help. Contrary to what you might think, an intern who asks for help is held in much higher esteem than the one who avoids calling (whether out of embarrassment, an inappropriate concern for the feelings of the supervisor, ignorance, or just plain laziness). The worst thing that somebody might think about you if you call is that you don't know what you are talking about. And, well, there is some truth to that. Sorry. But the sooner you come to accept the limitations in your knowledge, the faster you will learn and the better you will be for your patients. Of course, there will come a point where you do need to start working through things on your own, but the first day of internship is not that time. Until then, try and revel in the excitement and awe that you are about to become a surgeon. You deserve to be proud. Just not too proud.

GETTING TO KNOW YOUR PATIENTS

This is the fun of medicine. Patients are people with wonderful stories. A patient with lung or pancreatic cancer who has a daughter about to graduate from law school will likely respond very differently to "standard therapy" compared with a Norwegian bachelor farmer whose immediate future is completely encompassed by the snowy winter of his discontent. Clinical medicine is not like physics, where when you drop a brick out of the window, you expect it to go down every time. In medicine it is frankly surprising when 2 patients with an identical diagnosis respond to "conventional therapy" in the same manner.

Patients' symptoms are their perceptions, and perceptions are more important than reality. You have a role in helping to shape their perceptions, especially if you work to understand and care about what they think. Patients want to trust and love you. This trust in surgical therapy is a formidable tool. The more a patient understands about his or her disease, the more the patient can participate in getting better. Recovery is faster when the patient helps.

Similarly, the more the patient understands about his or her therapy (including its side effects and potential complications), the more effective that therapy is (this principle is not in the textbooks). You can be your patients' interpreter as they work to understand what is going on. This is the fun of surgery—and medicine.

SIMPLE RULES FROM THE TRENCHES

Some of your job as an intern is only indirectly related to patient care. While the rules below don't tell you how to operate better, they will help you to be a more effective team member and colleague. These elements are important for any medical specialty, but especially in surgery where the stakes are that much higher.

Get along with the nurses. The nurses know more than you do about the codes, routines, and rituals of making the wards run smoothly. In the beginning they often know more than you do about how to treat the most commonly encountered problems. They may not know as much about pheochromocytomas and intermediate filaments, but about the stuff that matters, they know a lot. Acknowledge that, ask politely, and they will take you under their wings and teach you a ton.

Stay in the loop. In the beginning, you may not feel like a real part of the team. If you are persistent and reliable, however, soon your residents will trust you with more important jobs.

Talk to your patients. Chatting with the patient is one of the places where you can soar to the top of the team. As an intern, you have the opportunity to place the patient's chief complaint into the context of the rest of his or her life. Talk to your patients about everything (including their disease and therapy) and they will love you for it. You can serve a real purpose as a listener and translator for the patient and his or her family. While it isn't appropriate to do this in the middle of morning rounds, you can often have these conversations in the afternoon as you check on your patients.

Say "Thank you." When you are lost (and you will be), the most effective answer to many questions includes a "Thank you." Like enthusiasm, gratitude is an invaluable tool on the wards.

Say "Thank you," revisited. Thank you can also be used to avoid making a bad situation worse. In general, most clinical questions can be answered with a "yes," "no," "I don't know," or "thank you." The "thank you" is for those times when all the other answers seem wrong. This takes practice and can initially feel awkward. For example, let's say you were told to do something by your senior resident but were later called by the attending who was not happy with this action. She asks, "Is that what you always do in this situation?" There are no good answers to this question, only answers that are less bad. If you say no, then you are going to ultimately get cornered and end up having to throw your senior resident under the bus (always a terrible idea). If you answer yes, you are needlessly sabotaging yourself. The best option is to simply say, "Thank you for the feedback, I'll make sure it doesn't happen again." This usually works to diffuse the situation, and demonstrates humility, an interest in learning, and concern for the patient.

Be punctual. Type A people don't like to wait, and most surgeons are nothing if not type A.

Be clean. You must look, act, and smell like a doctor. You owe at least that much to your patients and your colleagues.

TIME MANAGEMENT AND EFFICIENCY

It is the rare intern who is intuitively efficient. For most of us it involves reflection and practice. The most important thing you can do to be more efficient is to be constantly analyzing your behavior, looking for opportunities to shave off a second here or a minute there. If you do that enough times, those seconds and minutes accumulate and pretty soon you are "in the flow," where you make it look easy to handle everything that comes your way.

Of course, there are some helpful tips that you don't need to reinvent:

Notes should be succinct. Most surgeons move their lips when they read—so keep it short and to the point.

If you aren't busy, you are wasting time. There is always something that can be done, and if you aren't busy, you aren't thinking far enough ahead. Pro-actively anticipating future tasks will help smooth the workload.

Understand the difference between urgent and important. While many tasks are urgent, not all of them are important. The difference is easy to see when, for example, you get a page to renew an order for restraints while you are having a conversation with the attending about the course of a sick patient. But there are many other times when deciding which task to do first will be more difficult. Try and step back and assess what things are truly important, and prioritize them.

Write it down. You might have heard the saying "there are two kinds of interns—those who write it down and those who forget." Writing things down and periodically reviewing your list of tasks can help you continuously prioritize all the tasks you need to do and organize yourself to accomplish them in the most efficient manner possible.

Combine trips. If you are going to the ICU to do a postoperative check, you can check on the other patients while you are there and avoid a separate trip later in the day.

TEAMWORK

Surgery is a team sport. Yet as a new surgical intern, you may feel that you are not a crucial part of the team. Even if you are incredibly smart, you are unlikely to be making critical management decisions. So what does that leave? A lot, actually:

Keep a positive attitude. If you are enthusiastic and interested, your residents will enjoy having you around, and they will work to keep you involved and satisfied. Enthusiasm also covers a multitude of the inevitable sins. A dazzlingly intelligent but morose complainer is better suited for a residency in the morgue. Remember, your resident is likely following 15 sick patients, gets paid less than $5 an hour, and hasn't slept more than 5 hours in the last 3 days. Simple things such as smiling and saying thank you (when someone teaches, helps, or notices you) go an incredibly long way and are rewarded.

Work hard. This internship is an apprenticeship. If you work hard, you will get a realistic idea of what it means to be a resident (and a practicing surgeon).

Embrace the scut. Medical school is over, welcome to being a doctor. While we would all like a secretary, one is not going to be provided during your internship. And your residents do a lot of their own scut work without you even knowing about it. So if you feel that scut work is beneath you, perhaps you should think about another profession.

Help out. If your residents look busy, they probably are. So, if you ask how you can help and they are too busy even to answer you, asking again probably won't yield much. Always leap at the opportunity to grab admission/discharge forms, track down lab results, and retrieve bags of blood from the blood bank. The team will recognize your positive attitude and reward your contributions.

TAKING CARE OF YOUR HEALTH

Let me be honest: I (BCG) struggle with this issue-1 didn't see a dentist for the first 3 years of residency, which is frankly disgusting. The standard advice is to exercise, eat healthy, and sleep as much as you can, but it is hard to do when you work >80 hours a week. I sympathize. But there are still some things you can do that don't take that much time.

Eat healthy. I love fat and protein, especially when I'm stressed, which is pretty much all the time in the hospital. But hopefully your cafeteria has some decently healthy food, or you can bring some from home. I would always rather have the bacon cheeseburger than the turkey sandwich without mayo, but I try and remind myself that I don't need to eat every meal for enjoyment. One of the biggest drawbacks to eating healthy is, ironically, cost. I know you will be an underpaid resident, but suck it up. Someday you'll be making 6 figures and you can pay off whatever debt you accumulate from getting those fresh vegetables on your salad.

Walk the stairs. I have a rule that I'll walk anything less than 5 flights, and more if I'm not really busy. This is free exercise because waiting for an elevator is usually about the same amount of time anyway. Plus, research has demonstrated the significant positive benefits of even nonsustained aerobic exercise like this. Win–win.

Be disciplined with your sleep. When I first started internship, I would come home post call and "hang out," sometimes the whole day. Even when I wasn't post call, similar things would happen in the evening, and I wouldn't get to bed until midnight or 1 AM. But I quickly learned how self-destructive it can be to not pay attention to my "sleep budget." I know I need 7 hours to be rested. If I ignore those needs, my cognitive performance starts to deteriorate. Plus I just feel bad. And my GERD acts up, I get migraines, etc. So, I finally learned that I need to set a bedtime for myself and enforce it strictly. This can be particularly difficult if you have a partner with whom you are trying to spend time. But remember that you aren't very fun to be around when you are exhausted anyway, and even less so when you develop major depression or an anxiety disorder (both incredibly common among residents). Residency is a marathon, not a sprint. Take the long view, and take care of your sleep.

Prioritize your loved ones. Time is short, and there are many other competing demands. Bills need paying, dinner needs cooking, and the list goes on. But one of the most sustaining and healthful uses of your time is to spend it with those you love, whether a spouse, significant other, family, or friends. While relationships are the most significant determinant of human well-being, be careful not to cast the net too wide. Your sister's college roommate is in town? Forget it, you don't have time. Your second cousin once removed? Too bad, you can catch up after residency. I know it sounds harsh, but spending time with them means you are spending less time with those who matter most.

HAVE FUN!

This is the most exciting, gratifying, and fun profession you could ever hope for, and it is light-years better than whatever is second best. While there are challenges, the rewards continue to motivate us on our journey. We hope you enjoy yours as much as we have enjoyed ours. Bon voyage!

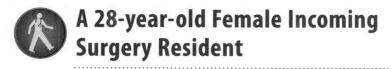

A 28-year-old Female Incoming Surgery Resident

Amanda V. Hayman, MD, MPH

Jennie, a 28-year-old fourth-year medical student, is thrilled—she just matched into the surgical residency of her choice. However, she is also apprehensive; her live-in boyfriend has agreed to move with her across the country, but she is worried if she will be able to maintain their relationship given the rigors of her chosen profession. She is also worried that, even if the relationship succeeds and they get married, will she be able to balance residency with raising a family? She's unsure how to begin planning for this and doesn't know of any role model to whom to turn.

1. **What people could serve as resources for Jennie to discuss her concerns?**
2. **What expectations should Jennie set with her boyfriend about how her residency will affect their relationship?**
3. **What obstacles (prenatal, perinatal, and postnatal) will she face if she wants to have a baby during residency?**
4. **Name some healthy and unhealthy coping mechanisms for stress during residency.**

WORK–LIFE BALANCE

Answers

> *You can have it all, just not all at once.*
> Motto of the Association of Women Surgeons

The responsibilities of a surgical resident are impressive and can be overwhelming. One of the biggest challenges is that the hours are unpredictable and inflexible. There are few jobs that require 14-hour shifts, 12 days in a row, including holidays and weekends. Sick days and personal days are pretty much nonexistent, except for extreme circumstances; it's hard to take any time off when you know your team and your sick patients are depending on you. As a physician, maintaining the health and safety of your patients is paramount, occasionally at the expense of your own. This commitment to duty means many missed family dinners, friends' weddings, and other important milestones. These time demands frequently detrimentally impact interpersonal relationships. Therefore, it is important for the surgical resident to have a robust set of tools for the recognition and management of work–life conflicts.

On the bright side, the surgical world is changing and is, overall, much more humane today. Thanks to work-hour restrictions, residents are finding time for social outlets, meeting significant others, and starting families. There are many more female surgical attendings today, some of whom are also married with children. However, the relentlessness of resident work responsibilities will consume a much greater proportion of time, and for a much longer duration, than arguably anything else a medical student has faced thus far. Think of it as a transition from running the 100-yd dash to a marathon. While it may be possible to put off personal responsibilities during a tough medical student rotation or 2, life cannot be managed that way for the 5 to 7 years of a surgery residency. Therefore, it is imperative to be aware before starting residency about the dilemmas one will face and to have some idea about how to manage them.

Six Tips for Managing Your Personal Life While in Residency

1. **Prioritize your loved ones.** Those who support us have to sacrifice a lot on our behalf. We are absent from our parents' houses at many holidays, and, when we are there, we are likely napping. Our girlfriends and boyfriends tolerate us showing up late at restaurants or missing friends' weddings. Therefore, we owe it to them to show them our appreciation. On days off, make a date night. Call your mother.

   Don't forget birthdays or anniversaries. Above all, remember we chose this life; your family and friends didn't. They may want to hear an interesting anecdote or 2, but they don't want to hear how miserable you are. Put on a good face—and don't forget to ask about their lives, too!

2. **Get organized.** Use an online calendar, such as Google Calendar, to organize your work and personal responsibilities. Automate all your bill payments. Use an online money management system such as Mint.com to track your budgets and account balances. Set up reminders for conference presentations, American Board of Surgery In-training Exams (ABSITEs), and birthdays.

3. **Manage (or outsource) your household chores.** It's hard to stomach spending your 1 day off a week scrubbing a toilet. If your budget can handle it, look into getting a bimonthly cleaning service. Or cut your jobs into smaller sections: do 1 load of laundry during the week. Drop your car off and have them change the oil *and* get it smog tested. Think of your time in terms of how much per hour you are worth: if outsourcing an activity would cost you less than $20 an hour, perhaps your time is worth more than that.

4. **Stay active.** Physical activity is not only important for health but also a great way to blow off frustration and stress. It's also a much healthier coping mechanism than going to the bar after work every night. Try hitting the gym first. Bike to work if you can. Take the stairs on rounds.

5. **Don't procrastinate.** As a resident, you will have more responsibilities than just patient care; you will have to read for conferences, prepare for cases, present at morbidity and mortality, and perhaps present even at Grand Rounds or other department-wide conferences, not to mention excelling on the ABSITE. Therefore, give yourself a reading plan and stick to it; get a textbook you like (popular ones include Greenfield, Cameron, and Sabiston) and make yourself read a chapter a month. Your ABSITE performances and your poise on the podium go far in establishing your reputation with the department attendings.

6. **Know when to ask for help.** The pressures on a resident can feel overwhelming, and a poor patient outcome or being yelled at by an attending having a bad day can trigger an emotional crisis when you are exhausted and angry. Some residents cope by "kicking the can down the road," that is, abusing or blaming friends, family, or colleagues. Most "problem residents" are not mean or insensitive; they are likely depressed and overwhelmed. Many may be scared at appearing weak by showing emotion after the death of a patient to whom they were particularly attached or by a family crisis. Residency doesn't slow down for grief, which can be an extremely isolating, and dangerous, situation. Alcohol, and even drug, use and abuse are often prevalent in these situations and should trigger an immediate, confidential discussion with an employee assistance program or program director. For less serious issues, residents should have a cadre of people they feel comfortable turning to for professional issues, such as one of their chief residents, junior attendings, or their academic mentors. Having a more senior person in your corner can go very far, both for career development and during the periodic academic review process.

FAMILY PLANNING

Most residents begin their training in their mid-twenties and finish in the early to mid-thirties, which is the traditional time to start a family. Therefore, many residents will face the decision regarding how to best time this. Starting a family during surgical residency requires impeccable planning and comes with a large and new collection of demands on your time and energy. If the resident is female, it will also pose additional demands, both physical and emotional.

At times, a resident may feel that it is impossible to be both a successful parent and a surgical resident. Without a doubt, it is very challenging to balance being a successful physician, spouse, and parent. Part of the answer may be that, while it is impossible to be perfect at all 3 roles, one can strive to be "good enough" every day. Below are some practical tips to help.

Eight Tips for Being a Successful Parent and Surgical Resident

1. **Plan early (aka "When is the right time?").** One of the first challenges is trying to plan an inherently unpredictable event (conception) within the rigid time constraints of residency. Many residencies offer the opportunity to spend 1 or 2 years dedicated to research, and many surgical residents choose to start their families then. The more flexible and manageable hours of this time are better suited to having a child, especially if the mother is the resident. However, this may not be an option for everyone. If not, consider waiting until after intern year, traditionally a call-heavy period. You should also consider avoiding your fifth year, a very heavy operative year that is fundamental to your surgical education. The fifth year is also the time where you may need to travel for fellowship interviews. If this is not possible, try to avoid being off during call-heavy months. Also, the sooner you tell your program director, the better he or she will be able to plan, which will reduce stress on your colleagues and your bosses, which can only be to your advantage.

2. **Build good will.** If you know you plan to have a child, especially during clinical time, be aware that you may inadvertently be burdening other residents with extra call responsibility. This may not be appreciated, especially by residents without children or partners, or by those who chose to delay childbearing because of their professional demands. Therefore, waiting until later in your residency, once you have established a relationship of being hard-working, reliable, and a team player, can allow you to "cash in" when you need time off. Make sure you have always been the one to take up someone's offer to switch calls or cover for other residents.

3. **Have a good support system (aka emergency backup).** There will be many times when you literally will just not be able to be there for your child, whether you are in the trauma bay actively resuscitating a patient, or have to stay late to finish a difficult colon resection. You need to have a child care partner who will understand the vagaries of our profession and who will be able to be there when you cannot. This point is perhaps the most important to stress; although we are accustomed to delayed gratification, some spouses may not want or be able to be. Make sure that you have very open conversations with your partner prior to delivery so that expectations are clear about what you will and won't be able to do. Also, be aware that, even though you are tired, once you are a parent you will need to put aside your own needs when you get home and focus on those of your child and partner. You may have to wait until the baby is down before you read that chapter on pancreatic cancer. Above all, make sure your partner knows how much you value his or her contributions to the family. Tell him or her daily, and help out whenever you can.

This does not mean you need to marry a stay-at-home mom (or dad). You don't necessarily need to be married at all. Many residents get quite a bit of help from their parents or neighbors. Or, if a partner has a decent income, do what many dual-doctor families do: hire help. Nannies are frequently the most convenient (albeit most expensive) child care option outside of the family. Regardless, it is essential to have reliable regular and backup child care.

4. **Be flexible.** You and your partner may not be able to get pregnant at the ideal time. It might happen before you are ready or later than you planned. Just remember that there is truly no good time to have a child during residency. You may have to reorganize your call or rotation schedules. Also, don't get discouraged. It may not happen in the time frame you wanted, but will usually still happen.

5. **Organize your priorities.** Once you have a child, he or she will take up the majority of your leisure time, what little of it you had. Gone are the days of coming home from a long day in the hospital and sitting in front of the TV with a beer, thumbing through surgical journals. You'll need to prepare mac and cheese, give baths, and read *Goodnight Moon* for the 120th time. Your time for reading for conferences will often have to wait until the last kiss goodnight or mean getting up an hour earlier in the morning. It will also be important to know when to delegate; this is an especially difficult dilemma with new work-hour restrictions; all good surgical residents loathe the thought of being referred to as "shift workers." However, many of us have workaholic bents and need to force ourselves to pass off the 6 PM "appy in the ER" to the covering resident if we have a steaming spouse and a screaming child waiting for us.

6. **Know when to let go.** You will not be able to be involved in the day-to-day activities of your child and trying to will create undue stress for both you and your caregiver. Create a plan with your caregiver regarding updates, phone pictures, and, above all, establish care guidelines in a written, signed contract. Find alternative ways of touching base: Skype in at bedtime from your phone, record your voice reading a favorite bedtime story, or ask your spouse to bring the baby to hang out with you in the call room.

7. **Have a mentor.** This is perhaps the most important point. Find a surgeon early on who is respected in his or her career *and* who makes time for family life. This doesn't have to be a woman, just someone who can give you tips about your career path and sometimes the much-needed perspective that, like most things, residency will eventually end.

8. **Know the rules for maternity leave.** Rules will depend on your institution, but most programs will allow 6 weeks maternity leave. Per the American Board of Surgery (ABS), no resident can take more than 4 weeks off

in any academic year, with the exception of maternity leave, in which the resident can take 6 weeks. Be aware, however, that this includes *all* time off in a year, including vacation, interviews, and conference time. Per the ABS, "For documented medical problems or maternity leave, the ABS will accept [a minimum of] 46 weeks of training in *one* of the first three years of residency and [a minimum of] 46 weeks of training in *one* of the last two years, for a total of [not less than] 142 weeks in the first three years and 94 weeks in the last two years. Unused vacation or leave time cannot be applied to reduce the amount of full-time experience required per year without prior written permission from the ABS. Such requests may only be made by the program director." Most programs will pay for 4 weeks of vacation and then may allow some sick time. After that, most will pay short-term disability at 80%. Know the updated rules: http://www.absurgery.org/default.jsp?policygsleave, but also check with your GME office.

TIPS TO REMEMBER

- Find a personal and academic mentor early on in surgery residency.
- Recognize unhealthy coping skills, such as poor anger management or excessive alcohol use.
- Good communication and a good work ethic can help ease some of the logistical issues regarding maternity leave as a resident.
- Prioritizing family and friends is essential to maintaining good relationships while in residency.

COMPREHENSION QUESTIONS

1. What challenges are *unique* to residency, which make life management more difficult?
     A. Difficult personalities
     B. Large amount of responsibility
     C. Little to no flexibility regarding personal time
     D. Not paid much

2. Which of the following people could serve as a mentor for Bill, a surgical resident interested in vascular surgery?
     A. The general surgery program director
     B. A junior vascular surgery attending
     C. A chief surgical resident who did research in neointimal hyperplasia
     D. All of the above

3. What are warning signs that residents may be overwhelmed and at risk of burnout?

    A. Forgetting their mother's birthdays

    B. Frequently not showing up at get-togethers with friends because they are "too tired"

    C. Blaming the nurse practitioner when an attending gets mad at the resident for forgetting to place an important order

    D. Routinely late in paying rent and credit card bills

    E. All of the above

4. Which of the following is not a good coping strategy for stress?

    A. Training for a marathon

    B. Averaging 3 to 4 six packs of beer a week

    C. Talking to a medical school friend at another residency on a weekly basis

    D. Scheduling a monthly date night with your significant other

    E. Taking your dog for a walk

5. Which of the following is not an ABS-approved option for maternity leave(s) by a resident?

    A. Taking 4 weeks as an intern plus 2 weeks' vacation

    B. Taking 5 weeks as a PGY4 plus 1 week away for fellowship interviews

    C. Taking 6 weeks as a PGY2 and 6 weeks as a PGY5

    D. Taking 6 weeks as a PGY1 and 6 weeks as a PGY3

Answers

1. **C.** It is important to remember that many other jobs have a lot of responsibility, pay poorly, and may involve difficult personalities, but most have more flexibility in regards to time off.

2. **D.** Mentors may come in many forms, and the most helpful mentor may not always be the most senior or well-known member of the field.

3. **E.** Overwhelmed residents may display unhappiness as disorganization, self-isolation, and quick tempers.

4. **B.** Although the occasional beer may be appropriate for stress relief, averaging 3 to 4 drinks a night is not. All the other options are excellent options for managing stress.

5. **D.** The ABS allows only one 6-week medical/maternity leave in the first 3 years and one in the last 2 years. The total time off any year can never exceed 4 weeks for regular leave or 6 weeks for medical/maternity leave.

How to Write a Note—Fast!

Teresa S. Kim, MD

KNOW YOUR PURPOSE; DEVELOP A SYSTEM; STICK TO IT

Surgical internship demands efficiency and neurotic attention to detail, 2 often opposing *modi operandi*. As the workhorse of the inpatient surgical team, you will need to perfect both. Toward this goal, we recommend you do the following:

Develop a system. Develop a system—for patient care, daily rounds, whatever—and stick to it. If you follow your system, you will be able to work more efficiently, organize the chaos of the day, prioritize tasks and information, catch things you otherwise would have missed, and, most importantly, keep your head on your shoulders when others around you are panicking, for example, in the middle of a chaotic code. You will become a better doctor, and your patients and colleagues will benefit.

In this chapter, we provide 1 example of a systematic approach to patient encounters and note writing. Patient assessment and oral and written communication are grouped together because all 3 processes are integrally related. A written note is simply the end result of organized and thoughtful patient assessment.

Understand that the purpose of a note is to communicate pertinent data, impressions, and plans with other members of the care team. A note is not just useless paperwork. Nor is it an arena to show off esoteric medical knowledge. Your notes will become a vital line of communication to other residents, attendings, nurses, and consults, and your handiwork will either facilitate or hinder patient care. You must learn how to write a useful note quickly for every situation that arises: admissions, consults, daily rounds, postoperative checks, acute events, and procedures. You do not need to adopt the exact approaches and templates presented in this chapter. But you must remember your purpose. And you must make and stick to a system to stay organized, thorough, and efficient.

GENERAL APPROACH

Whether admitting a patient from clinic, fielding a new consult, or assessing an unstable postoperative patient, our general approach is the following:

1. Right now, before you start internship:

   A. Program your brain:

      i. Ingrain the basic H+P and SOAP formats. Make it second nature. Be able to ascertain, process, and present complicated patient histories in minutes, in the right order, with all the right information. Soon, you will need to do this countless times per day under far less favorable conditions than medical school (picture your pager going off every 30 seconds, impatient colleagues, difficult families, crashing patients, etc). To get it right, every time, you need to learn and stick to a system.

    B. Make yourself some templates:

        i. Make yourself some skeleton note templates (see examples, Figures 5-1 to 5-4) and store in a readily accessible e-mail or computer location.

2. Preencounter:

    A. Prioritize:

        i. As soon as possible after hearing about a patient, eyeball the patient to determine if she or he is sick or not sick and how much time you have to review the medical records/take care of more urgent issues before seeing him/her.

    B. Note preparation:

        i. If the patient is not sick and you have the luxury of time, use your general H+P template to start a preliminary note on the patient, copying and pasting in any pertinent information from the medical records (name, age/sex, medical record no., PMH, medications, allergies, recent labs, and imaging).

        ii. Print and bring with you **to confirm** any information in your note and fill in the blanks. *Note*: **Do not post information in your note that you, yourself, have not yet confirmed with your patient—this is unethical and dangerous.** If you must include an unconfirmed piece of data (ie, a medication list obtained from the electronic medical record of an obtunded patient), then you should clearly note the source and the fact that the data have not been confirmed.

3. During the encounter:

    A. Once-over:

        i. The moment you walk into the room, make note of general patient observations and vital signs. Address any abnormalities immediately—for example, hypotension, hypoxia, and somnolence—and if severe, alert your senior. If no acute issues jump out at you, jot down vitals and move on. Include vital signs in every note—they are essential objective data.

    B. The CC:

        i. Before mashing on a belly, make absolutely certain you understand what is ailing your patient, that is, the **primary** issue that drove him/her to the hospital, and the primary focus of everything you do henceforth.

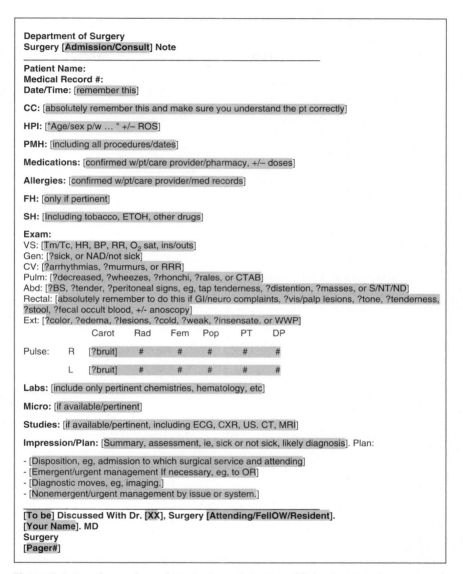

Figure 5-1. Sample template: admission/consult H+P. Highlighted areas indicate tips and fields to be filled in by the writer.

```
Surgery Progress Note
_____
Patient Name:
Medical Record #:
Date/Time: [remember this]

CC: [Any o/n issues, any current complaints, e/o bowel function or dysfunction, eg, flatus vs. n/v.]

O:
VS: [Tm/Tc, HR, BP, RR, O₂ sat, ins/outs including urine and drain outputs]
Gen: [?sick, or NAD/not sick, MS If issues w/delirium or sedation]
CV: [?arrhythmias, or RRR]
Pulm: [?decreased, ?wheezes, ?rhonchi, ?rales, or CTAB]
Abd: [?BS, ?tender, ?peritoneal signs, eg, tap tenderness, ?distention, ?masses, ?incision/wound
Issues, or S/NT/ND w/incision clean/dry/intact]
Ext: [?edema, ?cold, ?pulses, or WWP]
Labs/Imaging: [service dependent]

A/P: [Age/sex POD# s/p procedure or HD# with issue … now improving/stable/worsening with any new
issues….] Plan:
- [If new issues, ddx/plan.]
- (If resolving issues, continued management. eg, course of abx.]
- [If routine postoperative pathway, can be concise.]
- [Disposition, especially if anticipating transfer to different level of care, or discharge to home or rehab.]
_____
[Your Name], MD
Surgery
[Pager#]
```

Figure 5-2. Sample template: SOAP note. Highlighted areas indicate tips and fields to be filled in by the writer.

```
Surgery Progress Note
_____
Patient Name:
Medical Record #:
Date/Time: [remember this]

Procedure: [be specific, eg, "Right internal jugular vein central venous catheter placement"]

Indication: [be precise/concise, eg, "Shock, need for central venous access for treatment and
hemodynamic monitoring"]

Details:
[- informed consent obtained from pt/health care proxy
- positioning, prepping/draping, anesthesia
- major steps of procedure, including anatomic site and type/size/location of any tubes/lines/drains
- disposition/recommendations, eg, any complications, any pending imaging, eg, CXR after subclavian
or internal jugular venous line placement prior to catheter use
- discussed with/supervised by which attending/senior resident.]
_____
[Your Name], MD
Surgery
[Pager#]
```

Figure 5-3. Sample template: procedure note. Highlighted areas indicate tips and fields to be filled in by the writer.

Brief Operative Note

Patient Name:
Medical Record #:
Date/Time: [remember this]

Preoperative Dx:
Postoperative Ox:

Procedure:

Surgeon: Assistant:

Anesthesia:

Findings: [anything pertinent to postoperative care, eg, extent of whatever resection, necrotic organs, fecal, peritonitis, unexpected findings, intraoperative imaging, new anatomy of any reconstructions]

Specimens:

Ins/outs: [IVF, blood products, EBL, UOP]

Drains: [eg, Foley, chest tubes, intra/extra peritoneal abdominal drains; note type, no., anatomic site]

Complications:

Condition/Disposition: [eg, "stable to PACU" vs "intubated on pressors to ICU"]

[Your Name], MD
Surgery
[Pager#]

Figure 5-4. Sample template: brief operative note. Highlighted areas indicate tips and fields to be filled in by the writer.

    C. Everything else:

        i. Fill in the blanks. Follow your system to avoid missing any key history or exam findings. Formulate a quick impression in your head. Offer to the patient/family/primary team to return and explain impressions/plans once you discuss with your higher-ups.

4. Post encounter:

    A. Fill in gaps:

        i. At a computer, pull up your skeleton note, fill in information acquired from the patient, and fill in any gaps by quickly perusing online medical records, calling care providers or pharmacies, and reviewing lab/culture/imaging data.

    B. Process the information:

        i. Jot down your impressions. (Sick or not sick? DDx? One or multiple active issues?)

        ii. Jot down any key diagnostic or management moves you would make.

    iii. Jot down any questions for your senior/fellow/attending, lest you forget to ask (eg, are we going to the OR/should I hold tonight's Coumadin dose?).

    iv. A wise adage: There are interns who write things down, and there are interns who forget.

C. Discuss:

    i. After taking a **minute** to collect your thoughts, page your senior and present the case in a concise, organized manner. Follow your H+P or abridged SOAP format, depending on the context. Remember to stick to your system, the same way every time. The alternative—presenting data out of order and forgetting key details—generates verbal diarrhea, which confuses your listener, guarantees you getting interrupted and flustered, and hinders patient care.

    ii. Write down the plan dictated by your senior, and remember to amend both your note and your to-do list with any additional impressions and plans dictated by your attending.

D. Execute:

    i. Carry out the plan.

    ii. By now, your note should already be written. Print, sign, and place in the chart as promptly as possible, that is, in real time for daily progress notes and postoperative checks, and within several hours to half a day for admissions/consults. *Note*: Patient care always comes first. In the worse case scenario, when you are between bedsides of unstable patients and unable to write a complete admission or consult note, jot a "brief note" in the chart (date/time, 1-liner about the patient, and brief plan) and remember to write the full note as soon as time allows.

ADMISSION NOTE SPECIFICS

Purpose: To organize myriad data into a comprehensive *and* concise H+P that highlights your patient's primary problem and provides all necessary baseline data and proposed plans. This note should help focus and guide your team and consultants.

Essentials:

1. As mentioned before, make sure you understand your patient's chief complaint.

2. Confirm and document all medications, doses, and allergies. While tedious, this is helpful for consultants and essential to writing appropriate admission orders.

3. Tailor the exam to the chief complaint, but remember to check and document baseline vitals, mental status, cardiopulmonary exam, and pulses, as

any of these things can deteriorate perioperatively or over the course of an acute illness and are difficult to monitor if you have no knowledge of the patient's baseline.

4. Guided by insight from your senior/fellow/attending, write a clear assessment of the patient's condition and cause of chief complaint, and lay out a comprehensive plan by organ system or issue (see Figure 5-1). *Note*: Do not document anything that you are unsure about and have not clarified with your senior. Assumptions lead to confusion and, in the worse case, patient harm.

CONSULT NOTE SPECIFICS

Purpose: To identify and address the specific reason for consultation with pertinent data, impressions, and management recommendations. Stay focused.
    Essentials:

1. Absolutely speak with the primary team to clarify their exact question/reason for consultation. If the intern is unclear, go up the chain. If you are unclear, you waste a lot of people's time. Document the reason for consultation (in addition to or in lieu of CC) in your note.

2. Document the date/time of consult.

3. Clarify and document from whom and to whom (ie, from/to which service and attending) the consult is being requested.

4. Focus your history and exam on the reason for consultation. You are not the patient's primary doctor. *Caveat*: If you encounter an unstable patient, be a doctor, alert the primary team immediately, and help stabilize the patient as appropriate.

5. Communicate a very **specific** assessment and plan to the primary team, in person and in writing. Include:

    A. Your team's impression of the problem/question being asked

    B. Specific management recommendations, including what exam findings/vital signs/labs/imaging to monitor and how often, diet/NPO status, IV fluids, medications, surgery, and other procedures

    C. Threshold to call, and whom to call, with any questions or concerns

6. Remember to document with whom you discussed the plan on both your and the primary team's note.

DAILY PROGRESS NOTE SPECIFICS

Purpose: To provide a concise and thoughtful daily update of inpatient progress and anticipated disposition. *Remember*: These notes are a major avenue of communication with attendings and consults and are useless if late, illegible, inaccurate, or lacking in explanations for any new plans.

Essentials:

1. Pare down the H+P to a SOAP approach/note in real time (see Figure 5-2).

2. Develop and stick to a system that enables you to write your notes/drop in the charts on rounds. Get help when possible (thank you, medical students).

3. Learn to differentiate sick from not sick, and pathway versus nonpathway progress (eg, mild postoperative nausea on POD #0 vs nausea/vomiting on POD #3 s/p laparoscopic colectomy).

4. Learn and only include essential data (markers of progress, eg, flatus vs nonpathway complaints/exam findings).

5. Remember to include at least a quick impression and plan to explain to later-morning rounders (attendings and consultants) why you are enacting the plans listed in your note.

POSTOPERATIVE CHECK SPECIFICS

Purpose: To identify and document any acute, postoperative, life-threatening complications, any active issues requiring timely management, and baseline patient condition—this is particularly important when new issues arise over the ensuing 12 to 24 hours.

Essentials:

1. As for daily progress notes, pare down the H+P to a SOAP approach/ note in real time (write/drop your note in the chart while assessing your patient), learn how to determine sick versus not sick, and learn/document only essential data.

2. Pay particular attention to harbingers of sickness (eg, pulmonary issues, unexpected hemodynamic instability, chest pain, focal neurologic deficits) and address as appropriate.

3. Check for, document, and manage common postoperative issues (eg, pain, nausea, oliguria, wound/drain issues).

4. Remember to follow up on all pending postoperative labs, imaging, and bedside reassessments if necessary. Document any abnormal findings or changes in the original plan.

ACUTE EVENT SPECIFICS

Purpose: To document all/only essential information in a timely manner without compromising patient care.

Essentials:

1. Obvious events that require documentation include death, cardiopulmonary arrest, unresponsiveness, and hemodynamic or neurologic instability

requiring transfer to the ICU. Less obvious events that still require documentation include any new symptom or change in exam that prompts unplanned labs/imaging/studies/procedures/transfers.

2. Stick to your SOAP system for structure amidst chaos. While approaching the patient's bedside, run through Figure 5-2, tailored to this setting:

A. Note the date and time.

B. S: What did the patient or provider complain of?

C. O: What are the current vitals and trend since the patient was last well? What is the patient's current exam and trend since last well? (It can be helpful for you or another person to grab the chart to check recent notes/labs/imaging.)

D. A/P: What postoperative/hospital day s/p what procedure/illness is this patient? What is my quick impression and plan? (It can be as simple as sick; stabilize airway, breathing, circulation [ABCs]; call senior.)

E. Use this system to organize your thoughts, actions, communications with seniors, and, lastly, your event note.

3. Remember priorities. First, take care of your patient. Then, jot your note in the chart, formatted as above. Timing is situation dependent. You will ideally complete this task within several hours of the event, when either your patient is improving or another doctor has relieved you, at least temporarily.

PROCEDURE NOTE SPECIFICS

Purpose: To immediately document any invasive procedure you perform, to inform other members of the care team about procedural details, postprocedure management, and any potential postprocedure complications. For OR cases, the brief operative note provides useful information when an acute postoperative issue arises prior to completion of the full operative note.

Essentials:

1. Develop a basic approach to any procedure, and develop a general procedure note template that you can apply to different procedures (see Figure 5-3). To belabor the point, develop a system and stick to it. If you always review and document procedure indications, you will be less likely to insert a chest tube on the incorrect side. If you always review and document from whom consent was obtained, you will be less likely to forget to consent the patient.

2. Read about common intern/junior-level procedures (eg, arterial/central venous catheter placement, chest tube placement/removal, abscess incision and drainage, laceration repair). Reading will facilitate both hands-on

learning and obligatory note writing. Reading will also remind you of post-procedure studies and potential complications to watch for.

3. Document with whom you discussed the procedure and who supervised, if relevant.

4. After cases in the OR, jot down a brief operative note in the chart (see Figure 5-4). If you were not involved in the case but are entering orders/writing the note at the close of the case, make sure to clarify with the resident in the case *all* the following information:

   A. Objective: procedure(s) performed, findings, unexpected procedures or findings, blood loss, drain placement, intraoperative complications

   B. Management plan: pathway versus special considerations regarding postoperative analgesia, pulmonary toilet, hemodynamic monitoring and goals, diet, incision/wound care, drain care, IV fluids, postoperative labs, transfusion threshold, DVT prophylaxis, postoperative antibiotics, postoperative glucose management if diabetic, postoperative steroids if relevant, disposition, for example, to floor versus ICU

SUMMARY

Know the purpose of every task you undertake. Develop a systematic approach. Stick to it. For patient assessment and note writing, boost your efficiency with templates, but always remember to use your brain. Godspeed.

Section II.
Handling Patients in the ED

Admissions

Anthony Visioni, MD and
Roy Phitayakorn, MD, MHPE (MEd)

IS THIS SCUT WORK OR WHAT?

The bread and butter procedures in general surgery include hernias, appendectomies, and laparoscopic cholecystectomies. However, one of the most important bread and butter procedures for a surgical intern is actually the admission of the patient. Do not be mistaken into thinking this is "scut work" or a mindless task. Admissions are an opportunity to learn the most important lesson a surgeon can learn—whom to operate on and why.

Each surgical admission should be approached in a systematic manner. Particular regard should be given to triage, time management, communication, entering orders, and avoiding common mistakes.

TRIAGE

Choosing which patient to see first is not necessarily based on the order the pages came in or on the disease the patient has. It is the severity of each patient's condition that dictates the order in which he or she is seen. In other words, patients are triaged.

It is helpful to know the most common diagnoses for each rotation you are on and how to work them up. However, when triaging patients, knowing the management of every surgical disease is not as important as being able to recognize several important signs of a severely ill person. These signs include fever, hypotension, and tachycardia. It goes without saying that a patient with unstable vitals needs urgent attention. However, surgery patients are the most fickle patients in the hospital. They will look good one minute and be on their way down the next. It is the ability to pick up the subtleties that make the difference. For example, an elderly patient with a heart rate of 90 does not fall into the textbook definition of tachycardia. However, when considering that the patient is on a β-blocker and his baseline heart rate is 50, this person can be considered to have a relative tachycardia and may be quite sick. Triaging patients is a skill that will improve with time, but only if it is practiced with attention to detail.

Occasionally, people have no major abnormalities of their vital signs, but there is other information that affects their priority. There are 3 "trigger words" that should raise a patient's level of triage regardless of the vital signs. Peritonitis, free air, and ischemia should never be neglected.

Patients with the physical exam finding of peritonitis (diagnosis symptom, not a diagnosis!) are the exclusive domain of the surgeon. These patients demand prompt surgical evaluation if not immediate surgical intervention. It is important to remember that a normal computed tomographic (CT) scan in a person with a clinical exam of peritonitis is not reassuring. These patients are sick regardless of what the radiograph shows.

The same can be said for patients with free air. This is essentially synonymous with a gastrointestinal perforation, and demands a surgeon guiding the care of this patient. Patients with free air may have a relatively benign exam and stable vitals; however, they should be assumed to have the potential to worsen quickly until proven otherwise.

Ischemia is also a time-dependent condition. While more frequently seen on vascular services in the form of limb ischemia, visceral ischemia is a potentially fatal condition that needs urgent intervention. While limb ischemia is a fairly straightforward diagnosis to make, ischemic intra-abdominal organs can be subtle. Do not delay in calling a chief resident or attending because you are unsure of the diagnosis at any point, but especially when ischemia is a concern.

TIME MANAGEMENT

So, you've decided what order to see your patients, but how do you fit 5 admissions in before evening rounds? The key to effective time management is to develop a systematic approach and refine it throughout your first few years of residency. Chief residents and attendings can use shortcuts and pattern recognition because of years of experience. For the novice, it is more effective to use a system in which you only see a patient once and do it right, rather than to do it quickly and miss information or findings. The following paragraph will describe what we have found to be the most effective approach during our intern years. Your system will likely be somewhat different, but we hope that our approach gives you a framework from which to start.

Our first step when evaluating a patient is to realize that you are just one of many people who have interviewed this patient so far and the patient is likely in a fair amount of pain. Therefore, start with a polite introduction and state why you were asked to see the patient. Then follow the same progression of questions for every patient: history of present illness, past medical/surgical history, current medications, allergies, social history, family history, and review of systems, and then proceed to the exam. Finally, review the labs and then radiology. It is not important in what order you gather the information (eg, for some patients you may want to start by looking at the labs and imaging), what is important is that it is done the same way every time. This system ensures no missed points that may be crucial to the care of the patient.

You notice that we did not mention note writing while interviewing the patient. While it sounds counterintuitive, we believe that writing your note after obtaining all the information, and not during, will be quicker in the beginning. When you are talking with patients, they may not always want to go by your preconceived script. This is not a problem, and by letting patients tell their story in their own way they will often tell it faster. Waiting to write the note lets you focus on the patient and even perform some aspects of the physical exam during the interview. Also, by writing the note at the end of the interview and data gathering, you can synthesize it into a concise, but thorough note that will be the most beneficial to the next person who reads it. Notes written during the interview often don't have a coherent "story line" and are less clear to the next reader.

The last step when seeing a potential surgical admission is to decide if any requests should be made for further imaging or testing or should you be calling your chief resident ASAP to book the next operating room. This step requires you to create an effective differential diagnosis and decide what further information (if any) is needed to clarify the differential. You will often make mistakes at this last step in the beginning, but it is important that you always take a stab at it—in that way you learn from each mistake and improve your admissions system.

COMMUNICATION

Clear communication is extremely important in hospitals, and miscommunication is a proven major cause of medical errors. The first moment of communication in the admission process is when you find out there is a patient to be seen. This information can come from your chief resident, attending, a call from the ED, or even the nurse on the floor. Regardless of where the information comes from, there are several questions to be answered for sure. First, you need to make sure you have the right patient, typically the name, medical record number, and location. This is also the time to ask a few pointed questions to help with the triage of this patient. You should not grill the person for every aspect of this patient's history and physical examination—that's your job to find out. What you should do is ask for the vitals and general condition of the patient. Finally, it is important and good professional behavior to let this person know generally how long it will be before you see the patient.

Communication is also important when you talk to your chief resident about the patient you have just seen. In general, you should try to talk to your chief after each patient you see. This "check-in" will prevent you from mixing up information and also ensures that each patient's care is initiated in a timely manner. When speaking with your chief, the key to a good patient presentation is to incorporate the important points in a clear logical manner. Invariably, there will be questions about the history, physical, labs, etc. Answer the questions confidently, but never under any circumstances lie or bend the truth—"I don't know" is the best answer if, in fact, you don't. Lastly, briefly present what your plan would be—this provides you an opportunity to get feedback.

After your presentation the chief or attending will outline the final plan of care for the patient; make sure you are clear on this. Asking questions to clarify a plan of care is not a sign of weakness, especially when it is for the benefit of the patient. It can also be an opportunity for you to learn, especially when the plan differs from your own attempt.

Similarly, communication is key when conveying the plan of care to the primary and covering teams in the form of a handoff. Patient handoffs are fraught with chances for medical errors. Therefore, as in all aspects of the admissions process, a systematic approach is necessary. Briefly, inform the covering team about the history of present illness, significant medical history that impacts the covering team's care, allergies, medications, and what needs to be done. All of these points should be covered clearly and ideally written in some form of patient list.

Another important place for communication in the admissions process is between you and the nursing staff. Rarely do interns forget to talk to their chiefs, but talking to the nurses is often overlooked to the detriment of the patient. Interns should not rely solely on orders to convey information to the nursing staff. If there are important aspects of patient care that must be accomplished, then direct person-to-person communication is the best way to ensure that no mistakes are made. For admissions from the ED, one approach is to write an order asking the nurse to call you when the patient arrives on the floor.

Finally, as an intern you will often be the most visual face of a surgery service. This means that you will often have to inform patients and their families of the plan of care and patients' progress. When admitting a patient, it is extremely important that the patient and family are made aware of the reasons for admission and the plans for the patient. Patients and families will often have questions, and you may not know all the answers. In that circumstance it is unacceptable to "fake it." People can be very understanding for an intern who says, "I'm not sure, but I will find out for you."

ORDERS

Again, a systematic, consistent approach to order entry will ensure that no orders are forgotten. This system includes actually writing the orders and then performing a medication reconciliation. There are many approaches to writing admission orders, but the mnemonic ADCVANDAML CALL-HO (pronounced "ADC Van Daml Call-HO") has proven quite useful to many:

Admit: indicates which ward the patient is admitted to and under which attending.

Diagnosis: the patient's diagnosis.

Condition: the general acuity of the patient (eg, stable, guarded, critical).

Vitals: how often you want nurses to perform vital signs (if you write "per routine/protocol," know what that means for each ward).

Allergies: the patient's known allergies, including the reactions that occur.

Nursing: these are specific orders to nursing staff for patient care (eg, dressing changes, tube management).

Diet: what the patient is allowed to eat. Be specific. Nothing (ie, NPO) is a diet.

Activity: what the patient is allowed to do and also what the nursing staff will encourage the patient to do (eg, ambulate 3 times per day).

Medications: inpatient medications the patient needs. Include prn medications for possible symptoms the patient may experience (eg, Zofran for nausea, Dilaudid for pain, Colace for constipation).

Labs/radiology: think critically about what labs the patient needs. For example, does the patient really need a daily CBC with differential or will a standard CBC suffice?

CALL-HO: this set of orders tells the nurses when to notify you. Typically these are abnormalities of vital signs, but also include patient-specific details (eg, hoarseness or expanding neck mass after thyroid surgery).

Following a simple mnemonic each time you write admission orders can provide a clear plan of care and prevent many calls to correct omissions. This technique is still useful in the age of the electronic medical record (EMR). While the EMR often provides order sets or checkboxes, even the most detailed admission order sets were designed for a disease and not a patient—there is no "Mr. Smith order set." You should therefore systematically check your work (ie, run through this or some other mnemonic) before finalizing the orders.

Anther important aspect of admission ordering that is often overlooked is medication reconciliation. This process clarifies the patient's home medications and determines what should be continued or held on admission. This process should extend beyond simply finding out the names and dosages of medications; it should also include why the patient is taking these medications. Does the patient with prn Xanax take her pills once per week or 3 times per day? If the answer is 3 times a day, then this patient will likely go into benzodiazepene withdrawal if the medication is withheld. Is the patient on metoprolol taking it for high blood pressure, coronary artery disease, or atrial fibrillation? Each answer has different implications for this medication and the care of the patient. Unfortunately, it is the rare patient who will remember every medication, dosage, and reason for the prescription. Using a patient's old medical records, clinical notes, or discharge summaries will provide useful insight. When in doubt, ask a family member to bring in the actual bottles of medications the patient takes at home. If even that doesn't work, you can call the patient's pharmacy or PCP's office.

AVOIDING COMMON ADMISSION MISTAKES

While the admission process may seem daunting, there are several common pitfalls that can be easily avoided. The first is to recognize when you need help. This is not a question of being weak or a challenge to your ego, but rather a matter of patient safety. There will be times when there are too many admissions to be seen in a reasonable amount of time or there are too many sick patients. These are the times to tell your chief that you need some backup. Interns need to keep their chiefs informed of pertinent or unexpected events, such as changes in a patient's condition or concerning lab/radiology results. Another common pitfall is not following up on a test; every physician who orders a test is responsible for checking the result. For surgeons this includes looking at the radiology images themselves, not just reports. Finally, some patients are anything but routine. These patients need everyone to be clear about how to proceed, and that includes the nursing staff. When good communication exists between nurses and interns, it is to the benefit of the patient and the intern.

GO GET 'EM

To take the most benefit from each admission you have to be an active participant. While a good intern will gather information thoroughly, present it concisely, and execute the plan conscientiously, a great resident will be thinking, "What would I do if I were in charge?" With each new admission you should see the patient, make a plan, listen to the attending, and keep score. The pursuit of the perfect score is what keeps surgeons operating and helping one patient at a time.

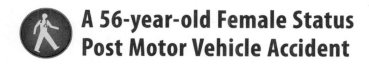# A 56-year-old Female Status Post Motor Vehicle Accident

Ashley Hardy, MD and Marie Crandall, MD, MPH

While on your night float rotation, you and other members of the surgical team are called to the emergency department (ED) in response to the activation of the trauma team. As the patient is being wheeled into the trauma bay, the paramedics inform you that the patient is a 56-year-old female who was a restrained driver in a motor vehicle crash (MVC). She rear-ended a stopped car going at a speed of approximately 45 mph. There was no loss of consciousness at the scene and the patient appears alert. The paramedics report that the patient has obvious deformities of her proximal upper right arm and distal left thigh. You hear your senior resident announce that she is going to begin the primary survey.

1. Why was it appropriate to initiate a trauma activation in this patient?

2. What is your role during this trauma? Where should you stand?

3. What is the goal of the trauma primary survey?

TRAUMA PRIMARY SURVEY

Answers

1. Per CDC guidelines, the trauma team should be activated if 1 or more specific anatomic, physiologic, and mechanistic criteria are met as illustrated by Table 7-1. The patient in this scenario meets criteria for trauma team activation given her involvement in a high-speed MVC and likelihood of her having at least 2 proximal long bone fractures.

2. Although minor variations may exist from institution to institution, the trauma team at most academic medical centers consists of a team leader, an airway specialist, primary and secondary surveyors, and ED nurses. Note that depending on the nature of the injury, other specialized staff (ie, orthopedic surgery or neurosurgery) may also be present. It is imperative that members of the trauma team are aware of their roles to ensure that the best care possible is given to the traumatically injured patient. Trauma team members and their respective job

Table 7-1. Anatomic, Physiologic, Mechanistic, and Other High-risk Criteria for Trauma Activation

Category	Criteria
Anatomic	Penetrating injuries to the head, neck, torso, and extremities above the knee and elbow
	Open or depressed skull fracture
	Chest wall deformity
	≥2 proximal, long bone fractures
	Amputation above the wrist or ankle
	Crushed, mangled, or pulseless extremity
	Unstable pelvic fracture
	Paralysis or any spinal cord injury
Physiologic	GCS ≤13
	SBP <90 mm Hg
	RR <10 or >29 breaths/min
Mechanistic	Fall >20 ft
	High-speed MVC with:
	• Significant intrusion of the car into the passenger compartment(s), >12 in into the passenger compartment and >18 in into any site
	• Ejection
	• Death within the same compartment
	• Pedestrian who is thrown, run over, or hit by a car at a speed >20 mph
	Motorcycle collision at a speed >20 mph
Other high-risk situations	Extremes of age (older adults and young children)
	Patients with bleeding disorders or on anticoagulant therapy
	Pregnant patients, particularly if >20 weeks' gestation
	Burn injuries
	Hypothermia

Adapted from the Centers for Disease Control and Prevention. 2011 Guidelines for Field Triage of Injured Patients.

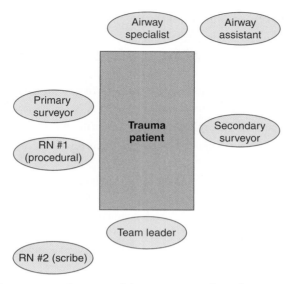

Figure 7-1. Trauma team. Diagram of the various members that comprise the trauma team and their position with respect to the traumatically injured patient.

descriptions are listed below and a diagram of their position with respect to the patient is illustrated in Figure 7-1:

Team leader (trauma surgery attending or the senior surgical resident until the attending arrives):

- Obtains history from Emergency Medical System (EMS) staff
- Directs team members on how and when to perform their respective tasks
- Orders the administration of drugs, fluids, or blood products
- Performs or assists with any lifesaving procedures
- Determines the patient's disposition (ie, additional imaging, OR, ICU)
- Discusses the patient's status with the family members

Airway specialist (2 people—anesthesiologist, ED attending, or senior residents of either specialty with 1 person serving as an assistant):

- Controls the airway, ensuring patency
- Performs any airway interventions, excluding the performance of a surgical airway
- Maintains cervical spine stabilization

Primary surveyor (surgical resident):

- Performs the primary survey, relaying all pertinent findings to the team
- May perform the secondary survey, relaying all pertinent findings to the team
- Performs or assists in the performance of any lifesaving procedures at the direction of the team leader

Secondary surveyor (surgical resident or intern—this is you!):

- Assists with the "exposure" aspect of the primary survey (see below) and applies warm blankets
- May perform the secondary survey, relaying all pertinent findings to the team
- Performs or assists in the performance of any lifesaving procedures at the direction of the team leader

ED nurses (usually 2, with 1 person performing procedures and 1 serving as a recorder):

ED nurse #1 (procedural). Obtains vital signs:

- Establishes peripheral intravenous (IV) access for the administration of drugs, fluids, or blood products
- Inserts indwelling devices (ie, nasogastric or orogastric tubes and urinary catheters) at the direction of the team leader

ED nurse #2 (scribe). Records all vital and physical exam findings obtained from the primary survey:

- Lists in chronological order any interventions performed on the patient

Note that, as a new intern, you should position yourself next to the patient, most likely next to the primary surveyor or on the patient's left. You should expect to aid with removing clothing and getting warm blankets. You may also be called on to perform all or part of the secondary survey, perform the FAST exam, or generally be another set of hands. As you become more experienced, you may be able to move into the role of primary surveyor, especially for those trauma activations that are less acute.

3. The goal of the trauma primary survey is to identify and immediately treat any life-threatening injuries. This is in contrast to the secondary survey, the purpose of which is to ensure that no other major injuries were missed and to identify any additional, non–life-threatening injuries.

The primary survey is best accomplished in a team-oriented, standardized fashion in order to ensure the best possible outcome for the patient. The mnemonic ABCDE (**A**irway, **B**reathing, **C**irculation, **D**isability, and **E**xposure/**E**nvironment) is useful in helping one remember the order in which the primary survey should be carried out. Note that these steps should be repeated any time there is a change in the patient's status.

The first priority should always be the airway, with the assessment focused on determining if the patient's airway is patent or not and, if so, determining whether or not the patient can maintain an intact airway. This can be initially assessed by simply asking the patient a question such as "What is your name?" If the patient is able to speak in a clear voice, the airway is intact. However, if there is no response, speech is garbled, or it takes considerable effort to speak, intervention is required. This may simply consist of a chin lift, jaw thrust maneuver to open up the airway, suctioning if the airway is occluded by blood or vomitus, or removal of any foreign bodies. In some cases, however, placement of an endotracheal tube (ETT) is indicated. If orotracheal or nasotracheal intubation is not possible, then a surgical airway (ie, cricothyroidotomy) may be necessary. During the airway assessment, inline stabilization of the cervical spine should be maintained until a cervical injury has been ruled out.

Next, the patient's breathing or the ability to ventilate should be assessed. An inspection of the chest and neck may identify the presence of penetrating injuries, bruising, tracheal deviation (ie, from a tension pneumothorax), and abnormal chest wall movements (ie, from a flail chest). Auscultation may reveal the absence of breath sounds or asymmetry (ie, as a result of a pneumothorax). Life-threatening injuries to the chest should be addressed at this point prior to moving on with the remainder of the survey. This is particularly the case if the patient has a suspected tension pneumothorax, in which treatment entails immediate needle decompression followed by tube thoracostomy placement.

The patient's circulation should then be evaluated as hemorrhage is the most common cause of preventable postinjury deaths. This is assessed by looking for any evidence of external hemorrhage, palpating central pulses (most commonly the carotids or femorals), obtaining a blood pressure and heart rate, and taking note of any distended neck veins or muffled heart sounds (both of which are highly concerning for cardiac tamponade). Any external bleeding should be controlled by applying direct pressure. Cardiac tamponade should be treated immediately by a pericardiocentesis or pericardial window. In general, hypovolemia should be treated with aggressive fluid resuscitation after the establishment of 2 large-bore (14- or 16-gauge) IV catheters.

The disability of a patient can be determined by performing a quick evaluation of the pupils and by making an assessment of mental status and gross motor function in all 4 extremities. Examine the pupils for any discrepancies in size, symmetry, and reactiveness to light. Use the Glasgow Coma Scale (GCS) to quantify the degree of neurologic abnormalities and to determine if the level warrants emergent intubation (ie, if the GCS is less than 8; see Table 7-2).

Finally, the patient's body should be completely exposed by removing all clothing. This facilitates the full head-to-toe examination that should be carried out during the secondary survey in order to look for any previously missed

Table 7-2. Glasgow Coma Scale

Eye response	
Spontaneous	4
Opens in response to command	3
Opens in response to pain	2
None	1
Verbal response	
Oriented	5
Confused	4
Inappropriate words	3
Incomprehensible sounds	2
None	1
Motor response	
Obeys commands	6
Localizes to pain	5
Withdraws from pain	4
Flexion to pain or decorticate	3
Extension to pain or decerebrate	2
None	1
Maximum score	**15**

injuries. At this time, the patient's back should also be examined for any signs of spinal injury in the form of tenderness or bony step-offs, and the axillae and perineum evaluated for any traumatic wounds. Be sure to cover the patient with warm blankets and be sure to maintain cervical spine stabilization when logrolling the patient to assess the back.

TIPS TO REMEMBER

- The goal of the trauma primary survey is to identify and treat any life-threatening injuries.
- As a trauma team member, make sure you are aware of who your leader is and what your role is during a trauma activation.
- When performing the primary survey, use the mnemonic ABCDE to help you remember the order in which the patient should be assessed.

- The ABCDE steps of the primary survey should be repeated with any change in patient status.
- Use the GCS to determine a patient's level of consciousness and any neurologic changes that might warrant an emergent intervention.

COMPREHENSION QUESTIONS

1. While in the midst of exposing the patient during the primary survey, one of the ED nurses announces that the patient's SBP has dropped from 120 mm Hg on arrival to 70 mm Hg. The trauma team leader orders the initiation of a 2 L fluid bolus. In addition to this, the next step should be which of the following?

    A. Pericardiocentesis as you weren't sure if the heart sounds were normal during the initial assessment.

    B. Take the patient to the CT scanner to determine the source of the hypotension.

    C. Repeat the steps of the primary survey, starting with a reassessment of the patient's airway.

    D. Proceed with the secondary survey.

2. A patient is brought to the trauma bay after sustaining a fall from the roof of his 2-story home. When a deep sternal rub is applied to the patient, he extends his arms and legs. He lacks any eye or verbal response. What is the patient's GCS score?

    A. 4

    B. 8

    C. 9

    D. 12

3. Which scenario meets criteria for trauma team activation?

    A. A patient who "twists" her ankle after falling from a chair in her kitchen.

    B. A patient who was hit by an oncoming car driving at a speed of 25 mph.

    C. A patient who is rear-ended in a parking garage by a car driving at speed of 10 mph.

    D. None of these scenarios meet criteria for trauma team activation.

Answers

1. **C.** With any change in a patient's status, you should quickly repeat the ABCDEs of the primary survey before moving on with the rest of the assessment (secondary survey). It was okay for the trauma team leader to order a fluid bolus as this can be done concurrently with the primary survey. Pericardiocentesis is seldom performed without a high index of suspicion, such as a positive FAST or high-risk mechanism, like a stab wound to the chest. Even then it is used only as an

emergent bridge to definitive therapy, which would be thoracotomy or sternotomy with cardiac repair. Finally, the patient in this scenario is too unstable to undergo a CT scan. Furthermore, determining the source of the patient's hypotension may not require the use of CT imaging.

2. **A**. The absence of eye (1) or verbal responses (1) paired with decerebrate posturing (2) would give the patient a GCS score of 4.

3. **B**. This scenario meets criteria for trauma team activation because of the speed of >20 mph.

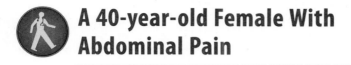

A 40-year-old Female With Abdominal Pain

Aisha Shaheen, MD, MHA and Marie Crandall, MD, MPH

Ms. Bradford is a 40-year-old female with no past medical history who presents to the emergency room with abdominal pain. She describes the pain as a dull ache that began after eating a heavy meal a few hours earlier. She has difficulty in pinpointing the exact location of the pain, although she states the pain seems centered on the midepigastric region. She incidentally notes pain around her right scapula. She has no other complaints.

On exam her vitals are unremarkable. She has minimal tenderness to deep palpation in the RUQ and no Murphy sign. You suspect a disease that causes visceral pain.

1. **What 3 processes cause visceral pain in abdominal organs?**

2. **Based on the location of her pain, is this pain most likely to be caused by foregut, midgut, or hindgut disease?**

3. **What factors in this clinical scenario suggest that the source of her pain is visceral?**

4. **Why is this pain unlikely to represent acute cholecystitis?**

ABDOMINAL PAIN OVERVIEW

Answers

1. Pain can be divided into 2 pathways: visceral pain and somatic pain. Visceral pain is the pain from afferent nerve fibers located in the abdominal organs. These fibers respond only to inflammation, ischemia, and distension. The signals from these nerves are perceived as dull, achy pain, in the midline and difficult to localize precisely.

   Somatic pain, in contrast, is derived from somatic afferent fibers that are found in tissues such as skin, muscles, bones, and connective tissue. Somatic sensory afferent nerve signals are perceived as pain that is sharp and well localized. In the abdomen, somatic pain is caused by irritation of the nociceptive nerves in the parietal peritoneum. This can be caused by direct extension of inflammation from the visceral wall into the parietal peritoneum as occurs with acute cholecystitis or acute appendicitis. Somatic pain in the abdomen can also be caused by anything that irritates the peritoneum, including pus, blood, or gastrointestinal contents—or palpation of the inflamed tissue by the examiner. Unlike visceral pain, somatic pain can "lateralize" (ie, be perceived distinctly off the midline axis).

2. Visceral pain tends to be referred to areas corresponding to the embryonic origin of the affected organ. The abdominal viscera receive sensory fibers from the sympathetic chain, from T5 down to L3. Visceral pain is perceived as poorly localized pain in the corresponding dermatomal distribution. For example, foregut structures (the stomach, duodenum, biliary tree, liver, and pancreas) are innervated mainly by T5-T8. As a result, foregut pain is perceived as originating in the T5-T8 dermatome (which is the epigastrium). Biliary colic—pain that originates from distension of the gallbladder—is one such foregut process that causes visceral pain that is referred to this region. Visceral pain from midgut structures (small bowel, appendix, and proximal two thirds of the colon) results in pain in the mid-abdomen and periumbilical areas that correspond to the dermatomal distribution of T9-T11. Appendicitis is an example of a midgut process causing periumbilical pain (as long as it hasn't advanced enough to cause peritoneal inflammation and hence somatic pain in the RLQ!). The distal third of the transverse colon down to the rectum are hindgut structures, innervated mainly by T12 to L3, with visceral pain from this area felt in the hypogastrium, or lower abdomen. "Gas pain" (due to distension of the colon) is the classic example (Figure 8-1).

3. For Ms. Bradford, factors associated with visceral pain include the dull quality, the patient's difficulty in localizing her pain, and the lack of significant findings on exam. Her complaint of right scapular pain is also interesting as it likely represents referred pain, a phenomenon associated only with visceral pain. Referred pain is pain perceived at a site remote from the location of the affected organ. It occurs when visceral sensory neurons converge in the spinal cord with

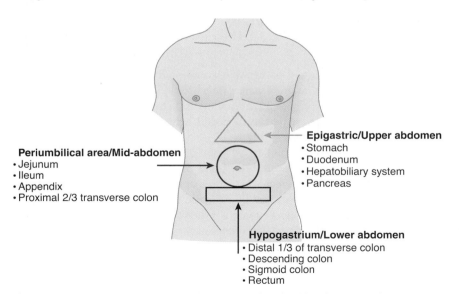

Periumbilical area/Mid-abdomen
• Jejunum
• Ileum
• Appendix
• Proximal 2/3 transverse colon

Epigastric/Upper abdomen
• Stomach
• Duodenum
• Hepatobiliary system
• Pancreas

Hypogastrium/Lower abdomen
• Distal 1/3 of transverse colon
• Descending colon
• Sigmoid colon
• Rectum

Figure 8-1. The perceived locations of foregut, midgut, and hindgut visceral pain.

nerve pathways that carry information from the somatic system. As a result of this convergence the vague visceral pain is "referred" as pain that is well localized to the sites innervated by these somatic nerves.

4. Whenever you approach a patient with abdominal pain, an understanding of the perception of pain can help you narrow your differential. Ms. Bradford's history of postprandial pain in combination with what sounds like foregut visceral pain suggests she is suffering from biliary colic. Biliary colic is a classic example of visceral pain. The pain is caused by transient outflow obstruction within the gallbladder or cystic duct that causes a buildup in pressure within the gallbladder. That buildup of pressure and the subsequent distension cause visceral pain. As described above, only distension, ischemia, and inflammation cause pain in the hollow abdominal viscera.

It is useful to compare the pain associated with biliary colic with that of cholecystitis. If this was cholecystitis, the inflammation of the gallbladder and hence the peritoneum would have caused the patient to feel somatic pain, that is, sharp, lateralizing, and localized pain. That same inflammation is also the cause of the focal tenderness as seen, for example, with a positive Murphy sign.

TIPS TO REMEMBER

● Visceral pain is dull, diffuse, and poorly localized and can be referred to distant sites.

● Somatic pain in the abdomen involves irritation of the somatic parietal peritoneal nerves. It is sharp and well localized.

● Foregut structures cause visceral pain in the epigastrium, midgut structures in the periumbilical area, and hindgut structures in the hypogastrium.

COMPREHENSION QUESTIONS

1. Which of the following types of pain is *not* associated with visceral pain?
    A. Dull
    B. Diffuse
    C. Lateralizing
    D. Referred

2. Visceral pain from a midgut structure such as the appendix causes pain in which of the following areas?
    A. Epigastrium
    B. Periumbilical area
    C. Hypogastrium
    D. Right lower quadrant

3. A Murphy sign is _____ pain.
     A. Somatic
     B. Visceral

Answers

1. **C**. Visceral pain is dull and diffuse, and causes referred pain. Somatic pain, in contrast, is well localized and can lateralize to 1 side or the other.

2. **B**. The appendix is a midgut structure and, as such, its *visceral* pain is felt in the periumbilical or middle abdominal area. RLQ pain is somatic pain associated with inflammation of the peritoneum overlying the appendix.

3. **A**. Inflammation of the peritoneum results in somatic pain because the peritoneum is innervated by somatic afferents. A Murphy sign results from palpation of the inflamed peritoneum overlying the gallbladder.

A 42-year-old Man With Severe Right Upper Quadrant Pain

Brian C. George, MD

Mr. Johnson is a 42-year-old engineer complaining of constant severe right upper quadrant (RUQ) abdominal pain that began gradually about 36 hours ago. He reports subjective fevers and chills, is currently experiencing moderate nausea, and had 1 episode of nonbilious nonbloody emesis. He denies jaundice, reports normal urine and stool color, and incidentally notes a 10-lb weight loss in the last 6 months due to voluntary changes in his diet. He does describe at least 6 previous episodes of postprandial epigastric pain that always resolved within 2 to 4 hours. He notes that the previous pain was different from the current pain in that it is now "more on the right."

On physical exam, his vitals are T: 102.3, HR: 110, BP: 150/90, R: 16, and O_2: 99% on RA. Abdominal exam reveals mild tenderness in the epigastrium, moderate tenderness in the RUQ, and a positive Murphy sign. Abdomen is otherwise soft and nontender. The remainder of exam is normal. You suspect cholecystitis.

1. List several diseases that cause RUQ pain.

2. Which of those diseases commonly cause RUQ tenderness?

3. What distinguishes a positive Murphy sign from simple RUQ tenderness?

4. In the case above, can you pick out the 3 clinical features that most strongly support the diagnosis of acute cholecystitis?

5. If this patient has an elevated serum bilirubin, what do you need to look for?

6. Assume that his lab values were consistent with acute cholecystitis. If an ultrasound was equivocal, what would you do next?

RUQ PAIN

Answers

1. All RUQ pain is not cholecystitis—although it will sometimes seem like it. While other causes *are* less common, the differential for RUQ pain is still moderately broad. To generate the differential, one approach is to think anatomically:

   - Stomach/duodenum: peptic ulcer disease
   - Biliary collecting system: biliary obstruction (eg, from a stone or a pancreatic mass)
   - Pancreas: pancreatitis
   - Liver: hepatitis
   - Gallbladder: plain ol' biliary colic, acute cholecystitis

Biliary colic can sometimes be confusing because, like acute cholecystitis, it is also caused by gallstones. Biliary colic, however, is not an inflammatory process—hence the reason that it does not have an "-itis" in the name. Instead, it is caused by a gallstone *transiently* obstructing outflow from the gallbladder. This is perceived as visceral pain that refers to the epigastrium. If, on the other hand, the stone gets stuck and the obstruction therefore persists, the resulting stasis and increased pressure eventually lead to cholecystitis and associated somatic pain in the RUQ.

2. Focal abdominal tenderness is usually caused by an inflammatory process that will involve the peritoneum. When that peritoneum is irritated by your palpation, the patient feels somatic pain, that is, pain localized to where you are palpating. We call that *focal* peritonitis. So, to rephrase this question: which of the above diseases commonly cause *focal* RUQ peritonitis? Clearly, acute cholecystitis is one culprit. Hepatitis can also cause some adjacent peritoneal inflammation. As described above, biliary colic is an obstructive and not an inflammatory condition, and hence causes visceral pain but no focal peritonitis.

3. A positive Murphy sign is *cessation of inspiration* when the examiner's hand comes in contact with the gallbladder. It is a physical exam maneuver that elicits somatic pain in the RUQ. It is performed by asking the patient to inspire while the examiner's hand is placed inferior and deep to the liver edge, in a position where one would expect to find the gallbladder. With inspiration the abdominal contents are pushed down by the diaphragm that causes the gallbladder to move toward the examiner's hand. If there is inflammation of the peritoneum overlying the gallbladder, the peritoneal somatic afferents will be stimulated when the examiner's hand "touches" the gallbladder. This stimulation is perceived as sharp, localized somatic pain that causes the patient to abruptly halt inspiration.

4. The key feature of cholecystitis is the inflammatory process. It is this inflammation that causes the 3 findings that together are highly suggestive of acute cholecystitis (see Figure 9-1):

   - Pain in the RUQ (*not* in the midline—remember that focal peritoneal inflammation causes localized *somatic* pain)
   - Tenderness in the RUQ (again, due to focal peritonitis)
   - Fevers and/or leukocytosis and/or elevated CRP (*more* evidence of inflammation!)

If you look back at the other diseases on the differential, only hepatitis would regularly cause RUQ somatic pain, RUQ tenderness, and systemic signs of inflammation. Fortunately, hepatitis is easily distinguished from cholecystitis by history and by routine laboratory studies—it isn't usually associated with a

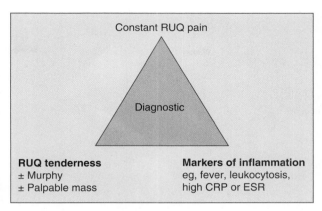

Figure 9-1. The diagnosis of acute cholecystitis can be made if a patient has all three elements of the so-called diagnostic triangle. (Figure adapted from Indar AA, Beckingham IJ. Acute cholecystitis. *BMJ*. 2002;325(7365):639–643.)

significant leukocytosis, and the transaminases are markedly elevated. About one third of the time you cannot make a diagnosis on clinical information alone. In those circumstances imaging can help.

5. Biliary obstruction—by ultrasound, ERCP, or MRCP. Clinically this patient has acute cholecystitis, and since 90% of acute cholecystitis is caused by gallstones, it is a fair assumption that he is at risk for dropping a stone into the common bile duct. If it gets hung up somewhere, it causes hyperbilirubinemia and can lead to an infection of the biliary tree (aka cholangitis). If it goes far enough down, it can also obstruct the pancreatic outflow and lead to pancreatitis. In other words, gallstones can cause 3 distinct disease entities, 2 of which are associated with hyperbilirubinemia.

6. First, what does it mean to be "equivocal?" Or stated differently, what features are consistent with acute cholecystitis? We can divide ultrasound findings into 2 categories: causes of cholecystitis and effects of cholecystitis. The causes of cholecystitis that we look for on ultrasound would most commonly include gallstones, but might also include a mass either within or adjacent to the neck of the gallbladder (ie, cancer). Effects of cholecystitis that we might look for on ultrasound are the natural sequelae of inflammation, namely, a thickened gallbladder wall and pericholecystic fluid (both due to edema), as well as a so-called sonographic Murphy sign. See Figure 9-2.

While ultrasound is good, it is far from perfect. Sometimes you might suspect cholecystitis based on clinical features, but the story isn't a slam dunk and the ultrasound doesn't reveal any stones. What do you do? One option is to get a HIDA scan.

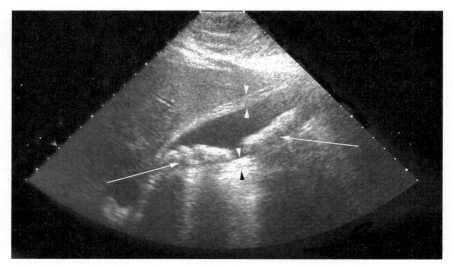

Figure 9-2. In this ultrasound image we can clearly see hyperechoic masses as well as the shadowing indicated by the large arrow. (Reproduced with permission from Brunicardi FC, Andersen DK, Billiar TR, et al. *Schwartz's Principles of Surgery.* 9th ed. New York: McGraw-Hill; 2010 [Figure 32-14].)

A HIDA scan is a nuclear scan in which bile is tagged with a mildly radioactive tracer. Because bile is normally sequestered in the gallbladder until a meal, the gallbladder should be filled with the radioactive bile and therefore clearly seen on the scan. If, on the other hand, the gallbladder is not seen, this indicates that it is "nonfilling," that is, it has an inflow and therefore almost certainly an outflow obstruction. As we know from above, outflow obstruction is one of the key steps in the pathophysiology of acute cholecystitis, and therefore an absent gallbladder on HIDA scan is strongly suggestive of the disease.

TIPS TO REMEMBER

● Acute cholecystitis is a clinical diagnosis that can often be made on the basis of RUQ pain, RUQ tenderness, and systemic signs of inflammation.

● A positive Murphy sign is cessation of inspiration with deep palpation of the RUQ.

● Besides biliary colic and acute cholecystitis, gallstones in the biliary tree can also cause cholangitis or gallstone pancreatitis.

● Don't forget the HIDA scan if the diagnosis remains uncertain after labs and an ultrasound.

COMPREHENSION QUESTIONS

1. Which of the following findings is *not* needed to make the diagnosis of acute cholecystitis?
   A. RUQ pain
   B. RUQ tenderness
   C. Gallstones on ultrasound
   D. Systemic signs of infection (fever, leukocytosis, etc)

2. A patient has an elevated white count, elevated bilirubin, and stones seen on a RUQ ultrasound. What other lab do you need to order?
   A. Alkaline phosphatase
   B. Lipase
   C. AST
   D. CRP

3. A 40-year-old obese female presents to the ED with RUQ pain and tenderness but a normal white count and no fevers. A RUQ ultrasound is somewhat limited by the patient's body habitus, but from what the ultrasonographer could see the patient didn't have any stones or any signs of inflammation. What is the next step?
   A. Book the OR and obtain the patient's consent for a laparoscopic cholecystectomy.
   B. Send her home with precautions to return if she develops a fever.
   C. Admit her and begin IV antibiotics.
   D. Obtain a HIDA scan.

Answers

1. **C.** If a patient has all 3 features of the "diagnostic triangle," ultrasound is not needed.

2. **B.** The patient almost certainly has a stone that is obstructing biliary outflow. The only question that remains is whether or not it is also obstructing pancreatic outflow, and therefore if the patient's pain might be due to (gallstone) pancreatitis.

3. **D.** This is the perfect indication for a HIDA scan—a decent story but not all 3 features of the "diagnostic triangle."

A 23-year-old Student With Periumbilical Pain That Has Migrated to Her RLQ

Brian C. George, MD and Alden H. Harken, MD

Megan O'Flaherty is a 23-year-old graduate student with a 36-hour history of periumbilical pain that has migrated to her RLQ. She states that she has felt febrile and is nauseated but denies vomiting or diarrhea. She is sexually active with a single partner and her last menstrual period was 2 weeks ago.

She denies prior hospitalizations and her only medications are birth control pills.

On physical examination, her vital signs are:

Temperature: 38.5°C

Blood pressure: 130/80

Heart rate: 80 (regular)

Respirations: 18

Finger oximetry: 98.5% (room air)

Abdominal examination reveals RLQ tenderness without rebound and hypoactive bowel sounds. Pelvic examination reveals right adnexal tenderness without cervical discharge or motion tenderness. Rectal examination confirms RLQ tenderness and brown, soft, guaiac-negative stool.

Your working diagnosis is: acute abdomen, rule out appendicitis.

1. What findings support the diagnosis of appendicitis?

2. What confirmatory laboratory tests are indicated?

3. Are any imaging studies indicated?

4. What is the next therapeutic step?

5. What are the next steps if, at surgery, you find a normal appendix?

6. What if the RLQ pain developed over days and weeks instead of hours?

RLQ PAIN

Answers

1. Ms. O'Flaherty has clearly read the textbook chapter on appendicitis. Her pain developed over 36 hours and began with visceral (appendiceal) irritation that she perceived as midline discomfort. As her appendiceal inflammation became

transmural, she stimulated somatic peritoneal nerves sufficient to cause RLQ pain but not sufficient to cause rebound. "Rebound" can be elicited by pressing very gently on the RLQ and then releasing the pressure. When the inflamed visceral and parietal peritoneum rub against each other, this causes discomfort. If the patient winces during this procedure, he or she has an inflamed peritoneal surface.

As with all patients, the history and physical examination can help you narrow the differential. For example, if this patient had recently eaten at an unfamiliar ethnic restaurant and now had raging diarrhea, you would think more of gastroenteritis. If she had a cervical discharge and exquisite tenderness with cervical motion (chandelier sign), you would think of pelvic inflammatory disease (PID).

2. (A) Obtain a CBC with differential. The Surviving Sepsis Campaign defines a "septic state" as WBC less than 4000 or greater than 12,000. We obtain a hemoglobin, hematocrit, and platelets probably because it is part of the "CBC package" (and, because "we have always done it that way").

   (B) A normal menstrual period 2 weeks ago does not preclude pregnancy. A serum HCG is an exquisitely sensitive test and should be obtained.

3. Calculating an Alvarado score (which does not, unfortunately, include C-reactive protein) can help you decide whether you need additional confirmatory data or if you can take the patient directly to the OR (Table 10-1).

   A French group (Pouget-Baudry et al) took patients with an Alvarado score of ≥6 directly to the OR and found 3 of 174 "negative" appendices. This group safely "watched" patients with <4 points. A Dutch group (Ünlü et al) evaluated routine diagnostic imaging in patients with appendicitis and reported diagnostic accuracy of ultrasound 71% and CT scan 95%.

4. Take the patient to the operating room with the preoperative diagnosis of "acute abdomen," not "appendicitis." Give antibiotics to cover colonic gram-negatives

Table 10-1. Calculation of an Alvarado Score

	Points
Abdominal pain that migrates to RLQ	2
Anorexia	1
Nausea or vomiting	1
RLQ tenderness	1
Temperature >37.5°C	1
WBC >10,000	2

From Alvarado A. A practical score for the early diagnosis of acute appendicitis. *Ann Emerg Med.* 1986;15(5):557–564.

and anaerobes (such as ciprofloxacin and Flagyl, or cefotetan), and prepare for a laparoscopic RLQ exploration.

5. Darn—but, in young females (this is the highest-risk group) it is permissible to bat 80%. After viewing a perfectly healthy appendix, you should fall back upon a routine series of exploratory steps:

   A. If the right adnexa is socked in with inflammation, the diagnosis is PID and should be treated with IV antibiotics.

   B. In young women, a large ovarian cyst is most likely to contain old blood (chocolate cysts) and is unlikely to harbor cancer. If you want to be conscientious, you may ultrasound the cyst looking for solid tissue (indicative of cancer). If you suspect ovarian cancer (usually in the middle of the night), this is not an emergency, and it is permissible to close and obtain GYN consultation. When a cyst reaches 6 to 8 cm, there is a risk of torsion, and this ovary should be "pexed" to the pelvic side wall.

   C. If halfway down the Fallopian tube you see a walnut-sized bulge, you must suspect an ectopic pregnancy. The appropriate response is to make a linear incision in the tube and scoop out the ectopic fetus (do not perform a salpingectomy). Then close loosely with absorbable sutures.

   D. When the GYN organs also appear healthy, redirect your attention to the terminal ileum (TI). In 2% of patients, 2 ft proximal to the TI, a Meckel diverticulum will become inflamed (rule of 2s). A narrow-neck Meckel diverticulum with thick tissue in the fundus (ectopic gastric mucosa) should be resected (either staple the neck or sleeve resection of the ileum). A wide-based diverticulum with no ectopic tissue may be safely left alone.

   E. Inspect the terminal ileum for boggy, edematous, "creeping" mesenteric fat involvement indicative of Crohn disease. In the absence of intestinal obstruction (which Megan doesn't have), don't poke a skunk—leave this alone. If this inflammatory process does not appear to involve the base of the appendix, however, remove the appendix.

   F. Having interrogated the "usual suspects," you should remove the appendix—but there is 1 remaining "curve ball." If you find a tan mass at the base of the appendix, you must suspect a carcinoid tumor. Carcinoids may exist anywhere in the GI tract from mouth to anus, but 60% present in the appendix. Most are benign. When the tumor reaches 2 cm in diameter, especially if it appears to invade the mesoappendix, it is considered malignant, obligating a right hemicolectomy.

6. Some stoic patients will tough it out through a bout of appendicitis and even appendiceal rupture. They present with chronic RLQ discomfort, and your first step is a CT scan looking for loculated "drainable" pus that is accessible by interventional radiology. A RLQ phlegmon with no abscess is treated with

IV antibiotics. The issue of late "interval" appendectomy is controversial and hospital specific.

TIPS TO REMEMBER

- The location of pain and tenderness helps you narrow the differential dramatically—focal tenderness suggests local inflammation of the peritoneum.
- The Alvarado score can be used to gauge the probability that a patient has acute appendicitis. If less than 4, acute appendicitis is unlikely and observation is a reasonable approach. If greater than 6, then acute appendicitis is very likely. For borderline cases or unusual presentations, imaging can be helpful.
- The differential for RLQ pain includes acute appendicitis, inflammatory bowel disease, Meckel diverticulum, ectopic pregnancy, ovarian cyst and/or torsion, PID, or cancer (eg, carcinoid).

COMPREHENSION QUESTIONS

1. What does focal tenderness in the RUQ represent?
    A. Acute cholecystitis
    B. A high-riding appendix
    C. Visceral inflammation
    D. Peritoneal inflammation

2. Do you need further imaging for a 19-year-old male patient with anorexia, nausea, vomiting, diarrhea, diffuse periumbilical abdominal pain, and a white count of 13?
    A. Yes, because the Alvarado score is 7
    B. Yes, because the Alvarado score is 4
    C. No, because the Alvarado score is 7
    D. No, because the Alvarado score is 4

3. What *is not* on the differential for RLQ pain?
    A. Meckel diverticulitis
    B. Viral enteritis
    C. Crohn disease
    D. Ovarian cyst
    E. PID
    F. Ectopic pregnancy
    G. Cancer

Answers

1. **D**. Focal abdominal tenderness represents focal peritoneal inflammation. While this could be secondary to either acute cholecystitis or a high-riding appendix, further testing would be needed. Visceral "tenderness," as opposed to visceral pain, is not commonly encountered because visceral pain is not elicited by examination maneuvers—this principle underlies the phrase "pain out of proportion to exam."

2. **D**. His Alvarado score is 4, which suggests he does not have acute appendicitis. It would be reasonable to watch the patient for progression versus resolution of his symptoms. To calculate the Alvarado score of 4, you score anorexia as 1 point, nausea and vomiting as 1 point, and a WBC >10,000 as 2 points.

3. **B**. Viral enteritis is not transmural and therefore does not cause localized peritoneal inflammation that would result in RLQ tenderness. The other items are worth memorizing for use when you are called to evaluate a patient with RLQ pain.

SUGGESTED READINGS

McGowan DR, Sims HM, Zia K, Uheba M, Shaikh IA. The value of biochemical markers in predicting a perforation in acute appendicitis. *ANZ J Surg.* 2013;83(1–2):79–83.

Pouget-Baudry Y, Mucci S, Eyssartier E, et al. The use of the Alvarado score in the management of right lower quadrant abdominal pain in the adult. *J Visc Surg.* 2010;147:e40–e44.

Ünlü C, De Castro SMM, Tuynman JB, Wüst AF, Steller EP, Van Wagensveld BA. Evaluating routine diagnostic imaging in acute appendicitis. *Int J Surg.* 2009;7(5):451–455.

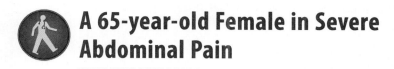

A 65-year-old Female in Severe Abdominal Pain

Aisha Shaheen, MD, MHA and Marie Crandall, MD, MPH

The emergency department house staff pages you to see Ms. Panosian, a 65-year-old female, who is complaining of severe, unremitting abdominal pain. Ms. Panosian tells you the pain is sharp and diffuse and began a couple of days ago. Eating makes her pain worse. Her vitals are:

Temperature 100.8

BP: 140/90

HR: 118

RR: 24

O_2 (%): 95% on RA

When you first see her, she appears very uncomfortable, but her vocalized complaints seem out of proportion to her physical exam findings. A digital rectal exam is positive for occult blood.

You initiate your diagnostic workup. Labs are notable for a WBC of 24,000 and a lactic acid of 4.4. Her ABG shows an early metabolic acidosis. While reviewing the chart, you noticed her EKG shows atrial fibrillation.

You go back to see the patient who tells you she is on chronic anticoagulation medication but ran out last week and has not refilled her prescription. You reexamine her and she now has generalized peritonitis.

You suspect ischemic bowel.

1. Describe the physical findings associated with generalized peritonitis.

2. Based on the presence of generalized peritonitis alone, would you say that Ms. Panosian has early or late ischemic bowel?

3. What is the most appropriate next step?

4. List 3 other surgical causes of generalized peritonitis.

5. List 3 nonsurgical causes of generalized peritonitis.

6. You inform your senior resident about Ms. Panosian and she instructs you to "optimize" the patient for the operating room and begin empiric antibiotic coverage. What organisms should be covered?

ACUTE ABDOMEN

Answers

1. Generalized peritonitis is inflammation of the parietal peritoneum. It can result from any inflammatory or infectious disease process that occurs in the abdomen including rupture of a hollow viscus and spillage of gastrointestinal contents, bile, blood, or bacteria.

   As with all processes that involve the peritoneum, the pain in generalized peritonitis is constant and sharp. It is also associated with reflexive contraction of the abdominal wall and, on physical exam, "board-like" rigidity. Even lightly tapping on the abdominal wall will usually elicit pain. The patient will sometimes report that, on the trip to the hospital, every bump in the road was excruciating.

2. Ischemic bowel initially results in visceral pain—the visceral afferents of the bowel are exquisitely sensitive to ischemia. In this early phase there is no inflammation of the peritoneum and therefore no somatic pain or any signs of peritonitis. The lack of peritonitis explains the classic teaching that patients with early ischemic bowel have "pain out of proportion to physical exam."

   If the ischemia is not reversed, however, transmural inflammation and eventually necrosis will ensue. Even if the bowel doesn't perforate, the inflammation irritates the peritoneum and therefore causes peritonitis localized to the area of the abdomen in which the bowel is ischemic. When the bowel perforates, bowel contents are spilled into the abdominal cavity, leading to generalized peritonitis. Given the progression of Ms. Panosian's exam, she has most likely perforated and this is therefore relatively "late" ischemic bowel.

3. Generalized peritonitis often represents an "acute" abdomen, meaning urgent surgical intervention is mandatory. As such, when an intern or junior level resident is consulted on a patient with this finding, the information should be relayed to a senior resident in an expeditious manner. This is best done by performing a quick but thorough history and physical exam and then letting the senior resident know you have a patient who may require emergent surgery. In the meantime, standard labs should be ordered (at a minimum CBC, chemistries [BMP], venous blood gas [VBG], and coags).

4. A variety of disease processes, both surgical and nonsurgical, can cause generalized peritonitis. Surgical causes include the rupture of any hollow viscus (eg, ruptured appendicitis, perforated peptic ulcer, or perforated diverticulitis) as well as any process that results in intraperitoneal blood (eg, traumatic hemorrhage). Less common surgical causes include ruptured ectopic pregnancy or a large segment of infarcted and inflamed bowel.

5. Nonsurgical causes of generalized peritonitis can be divided into 4 major categories: drugs/toxins, endocrine/metabolic, hematologic, and inflammatory/infectious (see Table 11-1).

Table 11-1. Nonsurgical Causes of Generalized Peritonitis

Drugs/toxins	• Black widow spider bite
	• Lead poisoning
	• Narcotic withdrawal
Endocrine/metabolic	• Diabetic ketoacidosis
	• Adrenal insufficiency
	• Hypercalcemia/hyperthyroidism
Hematologic	• Acute intermittent porphryia
	• Familial Mediterranean fever
	• Sickle cell disease
Inflammatory/infectious	• Amebiasis
	• Gastroenteritis
	• Pancreatitis
	• Pelvic inflammatory disease
	• Inflammatory bowel disease
	• Radiation proctitis

6. Once generalized peritonitis is diagnosed and the underlying cause is identified as being surgical in nature, the patient should be expeditiously prepared for the operating room. This preparation involves correction of any electrolyte disturbances, IV hydration, and appropriate antibiotic coverage. The antibiotic regiment should be started immediately on diagnosis and should initially be broad enough to cover the most likely causative agents. For the gastrointestinal tract the major involved pathogens are likely to be gram-negative enteric organisms (*E coli*, *Klebsiella*) and anaerobes (*B. fragilis*). Appropriate coverage can be obtained with the combination therapy of a third- or fourth-generation cephalosporin (ceftriaxone, cefepime) or a fluoroquinolone (ciprofloxacin or levofloxacin) + metronidazole (Flagyl). Single-agent therapy with a β-lactam (Zosyn) or carbapenem (imipenem-cilastatin) is another alternative. After culture results have been obtained, the antibiotic regimen can be tailored to cover the organisms identified.

TIPS TO REMEMBER

● Generalized peritonitis, or an "acute" abdomen, mandates urgent surgical evaluation.

- A variety of surgical diseases including ischemia, infection, obstruction, and perforation can result in generalized peritonitis.
- Key exam findings for generalized peritonitis include sharp pain, abdominal distension, and peritoneal signs such as guarding, rigidity, and rebound tenderness.
- Drugs/toxins, metabolic/endocrine disorders, hematologic diseases, and inflammatory/infectious processes can all present similar to generalized peritonitis but should be treated medically.
- Patients with surgical causes of generalized peritonitis should be hydrated and started on empiric antibiotic coverage for anaerobes and gram-negative bacteria.
- Junior residents should inform their seniors of any patient with generalized peritonitis sooner rather than later!

COMPREHENSION QUESTIONS

1. Why isn't "early" ischemic bowel associated with generalized peritonitis?
    A. It hasn't involved enough bowel.
    B. The parietal peritoneum is not inflamed.
    C. The visceral and parietal peritoneum are not inflamed.

2. Which of the following processes can mimic generalized peritonitis?
    A. Myocardial infarction
    B. Pneumonia
    C. Pregnancy
    D. Sickle cell disease

3. What organisms should be covered in the empiric antibiotic therapy for generalized peritonitis?
    A. Anaerobes + gram-positive rods
    B. Anaerobes + gram-negative enteric bacteria
    C. Aerobic organisms only
    D. Anaerobic organisms only

Answers

1. **B.** Generalized peritonitis indicates that the parietal peritoneum is diffusely irritated. In early ischemic bowel there is neither transmural inflammation nor perforation, and the somatic afferents of the parietal peritoneum are not yet activated. There is of course significant visceral pain even while there is no tenderness.

2. **D**. An acute sickle cell crisis can present with a diffuse abdominal pain that may be difficult to distinguish from a surgical disorder causing generalized peritonitis.

3. **B**. Empiric antibiotic coverage for generalized peritonitis should cover the major GI pathogens, including primarily anaerobes and gram-negative enteric bacteria.

A Patient in the ER With a Blood Pressure of 60/– and a Heart Rate of 140

Alden H. Harken, MD and Brian C. George, MD

A new patient arrives by private vehicle to the ER. The nurse runs over from triage and says to you: "Doctor, this patient doesn't look so good."

You bring him back to the trauma bay and check his vital signs: his blood pressure is 60/— and his heart rate is 140.

1. Is this patient in shock?

2. What is the first thing you would do to treat his hypotension?

SHOCK

Answers

1. Given the information in the case, we can't actually tell. Remember, "shock" is not just "looking bad" and is not just a low blood pressure. And shock is not just decreased peripheral perfusion. And shock is not just reduced systemic oxygen delivery. Ultimately, shock is decreased end-organ tissue respiration. Stated differently, "shock" is suboptimal oxygen consumption and carbon dioxide excretion at the cellular level.

   The most practical method of diagnosing shock is to look at end-organ function. The organs most sensitive to hypoperfusion are the brain and the kidneys. A confused or anxious patient should be a source of concern, just as oliguria should trigger you to investigate further. Perfusion of the skin and extremities can also be sensitive indicators of shock, as the body preferentially shunts blood to the core when cardiac output is compromised. This is why surgeons will often feel the big toe as a quick and dirty measure of cardiac output. Other organ systems can of course also be hypoperfused, but evidence of, for example, cardiac or hepatic dysfunction is usually a late sign.

   Another method of diagnosing shock is to look for systemic signs of decreased end-organ tissue respiration. This is most easily done by measuring the pH of the blood. While arterial blood gases are traditionally used, venous blood gases can also be of huge practical clinical value when a patient is really sick. Venous gases reflect arterial acid/base status with useful precision. Just add 0.05 to the venous pH and you will get the arterial pH. Subtract 5 from the arterial P_{CO_2} and you get arterial P_{CO_2}. So you don't need to repeatedly stick the artery (see Table 12-1).

Table 12-1. How to Interpret Venous Blood Gases

When the Venous pH Is	The Arterial pH Will Be
7.25	7.30
7.40	7.45
7.52	7.57
When the Venous Pco_2 Is	**The Arterial Pco_2 Will Be**
60	55
40	35
25	20

A little bit like sorting your socks, some surgeons are more comfortable "classifying" shock—all the while acknowledging that it is the cardiovascular response to a stressor (blood loss/myocardial ischemia) that dictates the danger. Class I (fully compensated) shock is how a young healthy patient presents following a 2-U (750 mL) bleed. This young person can vasoconstrict, diverting blood flow away from his extremities in a manner that preserves completely normal coronary and carotid flow. The problem, of course, is that the same 2-U bleed in a Supreme Court justice may prove lethal.

On the other end of the clinical spectrum, class IV shock represents a near-death state that is seen with severe blood loss (eg, 6 U, or 2000 mL). If the patient is still alive, there will almost certainly be severe organ dysfunction, including coma and/or stroke, renal failure, and myocardial ischemia (see Table 12-2).

2. "Shock" may be treated in a logically sequential fashion that is the same for all patients. So, when a chubby, cigar-chomping, sixtyish personal injury lawyer presents hypotensive with a big GI bleed, or with crushing chest pain, or with a sigmoid perforation, you should activate the following steps in order:

A. **Optimize volume status**: Give the patient volume until an increase in the right-sided central venous pressure (CVP) and/or left-sided pulmonary capillary wedge pressure (PCWP) confers no additional benefit to either blood pressure or cardiac output. This is strictly Starling law. It doesn't make any difference how good the engine is, if there is no gas in the tank. You want your patient's ventricles working at the top of this Starling curve (Figure 12-1). In the absence of a Swan catheter it can sometimes be difficult to precisely measure the cardiac output—in those cases, you can also target a CVP of 8 to 12.

Table 12-2. Classification of Shock

Parameter	Class			
	I	**II**	**III**	**IV**
Blood loss (mL)	<750	750–1500	1500–2000	>2000
Blood loss (%)	<15	15–30	30–40	>40
Pulse rate (beats/min)	<100	100–120	120–140	>140
Blood pressure	Normal	Normal	Decreased	Decreased
Pulse pressure (mm Hg)	Normal or increased	Decreased	Decreased	Decreased
Respiratory rate (breaths/min)	14–20	20–30	30–40	>35
Urine output (mL/h)	>30	20–30	5–15	Negligible
Mental status	Slightly anxious	Mildly anxious	Anxious, confused	Confused, lethargic
Fluid replacement	Crystalloid	Crystalloid	Crystalloid and blood	Crystalloid and blood

Modified from Committee on Trauma, American College of Surgeons. *ATLS: Advanced Trauma Life Support Program for Doctors.* 8th ed. Chicago: American College of Surgeons; 2008:61.

B. **Augment cardiac performance**: If the blood pressure, cardiac output, and tissue perfusion remain inadequate despite optimal volume resuscitation, your patient has a pump problem (cardiogenic shock). You should infuse cardiac inotropic drugs up to the point of toxicity (typically ventricular ectopy). Start with dobutamine 5 µg/kg/min or epinephrine 0.05 µg/kg/min, and go up.

C. **Assess for peripheral vascular collapse**: Occasionally, a patient will present with a surprisingly high cardiac output (warm big toe) and a paradoxically low blood pressure. This unusual loss of peripheral vascular autoregulatory control is associated typically, but not always, with sepsis. In this instance, you should infuse norepinephrine 0.4 µg/kg/min or vasopressin (ADH) 0.04 U/min to achieve the desired blood pressure. But remember you are playing with Ohm's law. As you increase systemic resistance, you will most likely reduce cardiac output.

To illustrate these concepts, let's examine 3 patients who come in with the exact same heart rate and blood pressure.

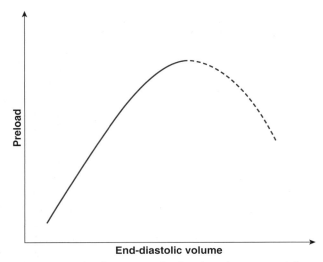

Figure 12-1. The relationship between preload and cardiac output. There is a point at which there is too much preload and cardiac output actually falls—this is what is happening when a patient develops heart failure from volume overload.

Case 1: Hypovolemic Shock

A sixtyish man just arrived with stab wounds in the RUQ and just below his left nipple. He is covered in blood. Blood pressure is 60/— and heart rate 140. The guy says his name is Duncan. He states that he's a king. He was visiting his friend's castle when his host came into his bedroom in the middle of the night and stabbed him.

You aren't terribly sure of the accuracy of this patient's story, but the fact that he can tell you one means that he is perfusing his brain.

You start 2 large-bore IVs and complete your primary survey. Following 500 mL of crystalloid, your patient is still hypotensive. You should follow the goal-directed therapy (GDT) protocol (first outlined by Rivers et al) for patients in septic shock. Continue infusing crystalloid up to a CVP of 12 mm Hg. This patient suffered an isolated liver laceration, and with fluid resuscitation, he became hemodynamically stable. Two days later he was able to return to the castle—where he was able to make peace with his despondent host.

Case 2: Cardiogenic Shock

Another pudgy, pale, sixtyish male arrives, stating his name is Polonius. He claims to be the Lord Chamberlain of Elsinore and his story is that he was standing behind a hanging tapestry, "minding my own business" (an activity that, in most trauma centers, is a robust predictor of trouble) when, for no apparent reason, a young man enters the room and stabs him right through the tapestry with a sword. This patient's blood pressure is also 60/—, with a heart rate of 140. You are reassured that this patient is also talking and therefore perfusing his brain. You start 2 large-bore IVs and complete your primary survey. The patient has a single RUQ laceration and after 500 mL LR × 3, his blood pressure has increased to 80/50 with a heart rate of 120. Again, following GDT protocol, you place a central venous line, and it is already 16 cm H_2O. So, his tank is full. He has a pump problem. Castle life, for a favored courtier, has permitted a high-fat diet and open access to the wine cellar—so, he has ample reason for both an ischemic and an alcoholic cardiomyopathy. You start dobutamine 5 µg/kg/min, acknowledging that the β_2 vasodilation may actively drop his blood pressure, but hoping that the β_1 inotropic stimulation will more than compensate. This patient had both a hypovolemic and a cardiogenic component to his initial "shock" presentation. He also resolves his liver laceration and you are able to shepherd him through his inadequate cardiovascular response to this massive stress. He returns to Elsinore in time to provide his son some sage advice as he departs for college.

Case 3: Peripheral Vascular Collapse Shock

You are cleaning things up when another patient arrives. Unlike the first 2, this patient is a young, healthy-appearing athlete. He says his name is Laertes, and he claims he was pierced in the RUQ by a poisoned sword during a duel. To your surprise, his blood pressure is also 60/— and heart rate 140, and during your otherwise negative primary survey, you are surprised that his feet are warm. Wow, he is perfusing both his brain and his feet with a systolic of 60 mm Hg! Using the same logically sequential (GDT) therapeutic response to shock, you infuse 500 mL LR × 2 and this patient's blood pressure does increase to 90/— with a heart rate of 130. Again, using goal-directed principles, you place a central venous line. The CVP is still 3 cm H_2O. After 4 more 500 mL boluses of LR this patient's blood pressure is 80/50 with a heart rate of 100 beats/min. This guy has received a lot of fluid; so following GDT guidelines, you obtain a mixed venous oxygen saturation through the central line. Venous O_2 saturation is 80%! Using mixed venous O_2 saturation as a surrogate for cardiac output, you reason that this patient must have a colossal cardiac output because he is extracting relatively little oxygen peripherally. The poison (like endotoxin) on the venomous sword must be a potent vasodilator. You infuse norepinephrine 0.4 µg/kg/min or vasopressin 0.04 U/min until your patient's systolic pressure clears 100 mm Hg systolic. Two days later, he has metabolized the poison and is hemodynamically stable again. He returns to the castle, makes amends with his old friend, and both of them conspire to ". . . outwit the divinity that shapes our ends."

A savvy surgical resident, using GDT strategies, could have capably resuscitated many of the victims of Shakespeare's tragedies, transforming these "tragedies" into much more comfortable "histories."

TIPS TO REMEMBER

- All shock will respond to logically sequential GDT principles:
  - First optimize volume.
  - If you're still in trouble, infuse cardiotonic drugs.
  - If you're still in trouble, search for a septic focus and document a high mixed venous O_2 saturation prior to infusing vasoconstrictive drugs.
- The Surviving Sepsis Campaign has focused a lot of high-octane light on septic shock recovery. In the absence of an obvious septic focus, most shock is still hypovolemic, cardiogenic, or both.
- Infusing a vasoconstrictive agent is a form of instant gratification. Remember, though, that you are playing with Ohm's law. An increase in systemic vascular resistance does increase the blood pressure while it invariably decreases cardiac output.

COMPREHENSION QUESTIONS

1. For a previously healthy young trauma patient involved in a high-speed motor vehicle crash, which of the following findings enables you to diagnose shock?
   A. Venous blood gas of 7.25/45/100
   B. Blood pressure of 75/55
   C. Heart rate of 170
   D. Lethargy

2. How much volume should you give a patient whom you suspect is in shock?
   A. Enough to normalize the blood pressure
   B. 2 L
   C. Until oxygenation is compromised due to pulmonary edema
   D. Until there is no additional effect on blood pressure or cardiac output

3. A trauma patient remains hypotensive despite adequate volume resuscitation. Adding pressors will do which of the following?
   A. Increase end-organ perfusion
   B. Decrease end-organ perfusion

Answers

1. **A**. If we convert the VBG to an ABG, we can see that this patient has a metabolic acidosis. This reflects anaerobic metabolism, that is, end-organ hypoperfusion. Lethargy, while sensitive for cerebral hypoperfusion, is not specific—it could also be due to head trauma. Blood pressure and heart rate alone are not diagnostic unless they are associated with end-organ hypoperfusion.

2. **D**. You give volume until you are convinced the patient is at the peak of the Starling curve, based on blood pressure and/or cardiac output. Sometimes you will be able to normalize the blood pressure with volume alone, but you can imagine a scenario with a septic patient who cannot constrict his arterioles and might therefore remain hypotensive even if you've given him 50 L (and caused him to go into congestive heart failure).

3. **B**. It is counterintuitive, but this patient is not hypotensive for lack of arterial vasoconstriction. The patient is hypotensive because the heart cannot produce enough output. Increasing the afterload with pressors will reduce the already inadequate cardiac output by increasing the systemic vascular resistance that, in turn, decreases the stroke volume. The only time pressors might be indicated for a patient in shock is if there is peripheral vascular collapse from, say, sepsis or anaphylaxis.

SUGGESTED READING

Rivers E, Nguyen B, Havstad S, et al. Early goal-directed therapy in the treatment of severe sepsis and septic shock. *N Engl J Med.* 2001;345(19):1368–1377.

A 67-year-old Man With Mental Status Changes and a Suspected Diverticular Abscess

Alexander T. Hawkins, MD, MPH

You are called to the emergency department to see a 67-year-old male for a suspected diverticular abscess. The EM resident tells you that "he's starting to look sick" and you go immediately to see him. Vitals reveal a temperature of 102.7°F (39.3°C), pulse 102, blood pressure 90/50, a respiratory rate of 22, and an oxygen saturation of 96%. Physical exam reveals a somnolent male who grimaces when you palpate his abdomen. The nurse reports a clear mental status 1 hour prior. Stat labs reveal normal electrolytes and a leukocytosis of 17,000 WBC.

1. **Does this patient meet the diagnostic criteria for systemic inflammatory response syndrome (SIRS)?**
2. **Does he meet the diagnostic criteria for sepsis?**
3. **What features distinguish sepsis from severe sepsis?**
4. **What features distinguish severe sepsis from septic shock?**
5. **How would you obtain source control for this patient?**
6. **Name 3 other evidence-based interventions, besides source control, that you would do for this patient.**

SEPSIS

Sepsis is a clinical syndrome characterized by a massive inflammatory response to infection. Over 650,000 cases of sepsis are diagnosed each year in the United States. Mortality is high and estimates range from 20% to 50% with rates increasing proportional to the severity of sepsis. Sepsis is thought to result from an overreaction of the immune response—a massive and uncontrolled release of proinflammatory mediators that leads to cardiovascular collapse and tissue injury. In its most severe form, sepsis can lead to multiorgan dysfunction syndrome (MODS) and subsequent death.

As sepsis is a clinical entity with a full spectrum of stages, much work has been done to codify and define its features.

Answers

1. SIRS is the clinical syndrome that results from a dysregulated inflammatory response to an insult. It is nonspecific and can be caused by ischemia, inflammation, trauma, infection, or a combination of several insults.

This patient has SIRS. To establish the diagnosis of SIRS, 2 of the following criteria must be met:

- High or low WBC (>12,000 cells/mm³, <4000 cells/mm³, or >10% bands)
- High or low temperature (>38.5°C or <35°C)
- Heart rate >90
- Respiratory rate >20 (or $Paco_2$ <32 mm Hg)

2. Sepsis is the clinical syndrome that results from the body's abnormal inflammatory reaction to infection. Very simply:

Sepsis = SIRS + documented infection

This patient, in the absence of a documented infection, does not therefore have sepsis. Keep in mind that sepsis and bacteremia (bacteria in the bloodstream) are 2 different things. Patients can be bacteremic without being septic if they don't meet diagnostic criteria for SIRS.

3. Severe sepsis is defined by sepsis plus organ dysfunction (see Figure 13-1). This can be:

- Areas of mottled skin
- Capillary refill ≥3 seconds
- UOP <0.5 mL/kg for at least 1 hour
- Lactate >2 mmol/L
- Change in mental status
- Platelet count of <100,000 cells/mL or DIC
- Acute lung injury/ARDS

4. Septic shock is severe sepsis *plus* hypotension, which can include the following (see Figure 13-1):

- MAP <60 mm Hg after fluid resuscitation
- Pulmonary capillary wedge pressure between 12 and 20 mm Hg and need for vasopressors

5. From the above definitions, for a patient to have sepsis there must be a source for the infection. This source can take the form of an abscess, infected tissue, perforated bowel, or any other place that bacteria can cause systemic effects. Source control relates to the need to eliminate the source of the original bacterial infection. This can mean percutaneous drainage of an abscess, wide debridement of infected tissue, or laparotomy and repair of a bowel perforation. In the case of our patient, source control means drainage of his abscess— through either open surgery or interventional radiology (IR) placement of a drain.

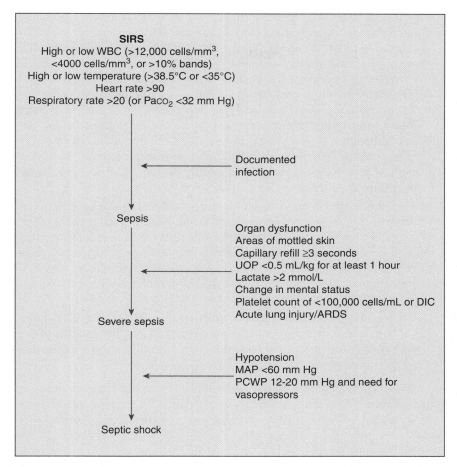

Figure 13-1. The stepwise relationship between SIRS, sepsis, severe sepsis, and septic shock.

A. **Respiratory support**: The patient's airway and ability to breathe should be assessed. Supplementary oxygen and pulse oximetry are mandatory for septic patients. Intubation and mechanical ventilation may be required both for the increased work of breathing that sepsis induces and to protect the airway of a somnolent and encephalopathic patient.

B. **Resuscitation and cardiovascular support**: Sepsis causes end-organ hypoperfusion through abnormal vasodilation (see the chapter on shock). Relative intravascular hypovolemia is common and needs to be addressed early in the course of the illness. This takes the form of central venous line placement followed by "goal-directed therapy." "Goal-directed therapy" employs guidelines to assist in proper resuscitation. Isotonic IV fluids (crystalloid) should be administered in boluses to achieve a central venous pressure (CVP) of between 8 and 12 mm Hg. If the patient remains hypotensive despite "filling up the tank," then vasopressors need to be added to improve vascular tone. Norepinephrine and dopamine are the recommended vasopressors. If the patient remains in septic shock (as indicated by, eg, urine output less than 0.5 mL/kg/h, mixed venous saturation less than 65%, or continued metabolic acidosis), then inotropic support can be used to augment cardiac output. Although it is somewhat controversial, if the mixed venous saturation remains below 70%, then many will also transfuse a patient up to a hematocrit of 30%. Notice that this is essentially the same goal-directed therapy algorithm presented earlier, in the chapter on shock.

C. **Antibiotics**: While source control is critical, antibiotics also have an important role. Your antibiotic choice should be informed by local patterns of bacteria and drug resistance. Choose antibiotics that have a broad spectrum and good penetration. Proper empirical therapies include carbapenems, third- or fourth-generation cephalosporins with additional anaerobic covers, or antipseudomonal penicillins. Vancomycin or linezolid should be employed if there is suspicion of methicillin-resistant *Staphylococcus aureus*.

D. **Other issues**: Adequate glycemic control (less than 180 mg/dL or 10 mmol/L) has been shown to improve mortality in sepsis and is an integral part of supportive care. See the chapter on perioperative insulin for more information on this topic.

Glucocorticoid use has been a major topic of research that has produced equivocal results as to the relative risks and benefits. For patients who are presently hypotensive despite maximum resuscitation, a trial of glucocorticoid steroids is appropriate.

Finally, nutritional support is an important part of the care of the septic patient. Unfortunately, consensus does not exist as to the method and timing of nutritional support.

In summary, a patient with sepsis should be transferred to and cared for in an intensive care unit. Time is of the essence and supportive treatment and antibiotics should be started as soon as you suspect a patient may have sepsis.

TIPS TO REMEMBER

- SIRS = 2 of the following 4:
  - High or low WBC (>12k, <4k, or 10% bands)
  - High or low temperature (>38.5°C or <35°C)
  - Heart rate >90
  - Respiratory rate >20 (or $Paco_2$ <32 mm Hg)

- Sepsis = SIRS + infection.
- Septic shock = severe sepsis + hypotension.
- The pillars of care involve treatment of the infection (source control and antibiotics) and resuscitation (goal-directed fluids and vasopressors).

COMPREHENSION QUESTIONS

1. Which of the following would *not* count toward a diagnosis of SIRS?
   - A. MAP of 55
   - B. Temperature of 102.3°F
   - C. Heart rate of 96
   - D. 12% bands on CBC

2. Which of the following would be an inappropriate **first** step in the treatment of a patient in septic shock?
   - A. 1 L bolus of normal saline
   - B. IV administration of vancomycin, cefepime, and metronidazole
   - C. CT of abdomen to look for an abscess
   - D. 100% O_2 via non-rebreather mask

Answers

1. **A.** The criteria for SIRS include heart rate, temperature, respiratory rate (or $Paco_2$), and elevated or depressed WBC. Hypotension plus SIRS defines septic shock.

2. **C.** Although identification of infection and source control are integral parts of the treatment of the septic patient, they should not delay respiratory support, resuscitation, or administration of antibiotics. The patient should be stabilized in an intensive care unit prior to any radiological procedure.

SUGGESTED READING

Dellinger RP, Levy MM, Carlet JM, et al. Surviving Sepsis Campaign: international guidelines for management of severe sepsis and septic shock. *Crit Care Med*. 2008;36:296–327 [published correction appears in *Crit Care Med*. 2008;36:1394–1396].

A 57-year-old Man With a Chief Complaint of Nausea and Vomiting

Alexander T. Hawkins, MD, MPH

You are asked to see a 57-year-old male in the emergency department with a chief complaint of nausea and vomiting. The patient reports that 1 day prior to presentation he began to experience vague abdominal cramping followed by persistent nausea and vomiting. On questioning, he reports that his last bowel movement was 3 days ago and he has not passed gas for over 24 hours. His past medical history is significant for an exploratory laparotomy and bowel resection for trauma 20 years ago. On examination, his abdomen is distended, tympanic, and diffusely tender.

1. **Name the 3 most common causes of a mechanical small bowel obstruction (SBO).**
2. **How do you diagnose an SBO?**
3. **What is the first decision you have to make in treating an SBO?**
4. **When is nasogastric tube (NGT) placement warranted?**
5. **What size NGT do you want to place and what else do you need to do to place it?**
6. **List the 2 supportive interventions, besides an NGT, that are commonly ordered for a patient with an SBO.**

SMALL BOWEL OBSTRUCTION

An SBO occurs when the normal flow of intestinal contents is interrupted. SBOs can be divided into 2 categories based on their etiology: functional and mechanical.

Functional

A functional SBO refers to obstipation (failure to pass stools or gas) and intolerance of oral intake resulting from a nonmechanical disruption of the normal propulsion of the GI tract. This is synonymous with an ileus. As a surgical intern, you will mostly come across these patients in the immediate postoperative period. Most ileuses will resolve on their own with conservative measures such as IV fluid resuscitation, nasogastric decompression, minimization of narcotics, correction of electrolyte abnormalities, and ambulation. Gum chewing has been shown to stimulate gut motility and is a nice option as one of the few active measures you can employ.

Mechanical

A mechanical SBO refers to intrinsic or extrinsic physical blockage of the GI tract. As a functional SBO rarely requires surgical intervention (and some surgeons say is not even an SBO at all!), we will focus more on the mechanical SBO. Going forward, when we are talking about an SBO, we will be discussing a *mechanical* obstruction.

Answers

1. The most common cause of an SBO is postoperative adhesion (56% of cases). About 1 out of every 5 patients undergoing an abdominal operation will develop an SBO in 4 years. The type of abdominal surgery impacts the risks of SBP. Laparoscopic operations result in much lower rates of SBO than open operations.

   Malignant tumors or strictures of the small bowel can cause intrinsic blockage and are the second most common cause of SBO (30% of cases). Strictures can result from Crohn disease, ischemia, radiation therapy, or drugs (NSAIDs, enteric-coated KCl).

   Hernias cause extrinsic compression and are the third most common cause (10% of all cases). Make sure you check for hernias in any patient you suspect of an SBO. Ventral and inguinal hernias account for most of the cases, but internal hernias also can cause an SBO.

   Other less common causes of SBO in the adult population are intussusception, volvulus, and gallstone ileus.

2. First, you have to suspect it. Patients presenting with SBO will report nausea, vomiting, and obstipation (failure to pass stools or gas). Often they will report a history of previous abdominal operations. Their abdomens will be distended and tympanic. Abdominal pain is usually dull and diffuse. Focal or generalized peritonitis is a danger sign of ischemia and/or perforation.

   Radiological examination should include an upright chest x-ray to rule out free air as well as supine and upright abdominal films (aka KUB) to look for air–fluid levels and dilated loops of bowel (see Figure 14-1A and B).

   Though more time-consuming, a CT of the abdomen and pelvis is the most sensitive diagnostic tool. This study, unlike a KUB, can provide information about the precise location, severity, and etiology of the obstruction. Often times a transition point (a change in caliber between dilated proximal and collapsed distal small bowel loops) can be identified.

3. The biggest challenge in treating an SBO is knowing when to take a patient to the operating room. The real danger of an SBO comes from bowel that has dilated or twisted to the point where its blood supply has been compromised. This can lead to necrosis, perforation, and sepsis. Patients with severe abdominal pain, no prior history of abdominal surgery, or those suspected to have a closed loop obstruction should undergo prompt laparotomy. Unfortunately, most patients fall into more of a gray area and neither physical examination nor CT scan is very accurate in predicting the need for an operation. In these patients, watchful waiting with serial abdominal examinations is an acceptable choice. Increasing abdominal pain or persistent obstruction after 24 to 48 hours is a commonly accepted indication for surgery.

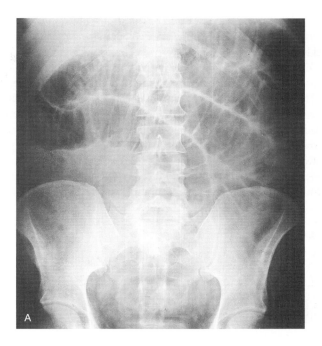

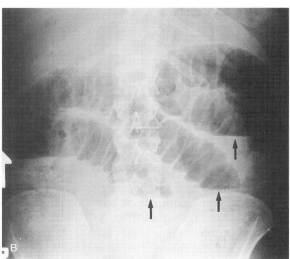

Figure 14-1. (**A**) Supine KUBs with dilated loops of small bowel. (Reproduced with permission from Zinner MJ, Ashley SW. *Maingot's Abdominal Operations*. 11th ed. New York: McGraw-Hill; 2007 [Figure 17-9].) (**B**) Upright KUB with multiple air–fluid levels (arrows). (Reproduced with permission from Zinner MJ, Ashley SW. *Maingot's Abdominal Operations*. 11th ed. New York: McGraw-Hill; 2007 [Figure 17-9].)

4. In a patient with a suspected SBO, an NGT is almost always warranted. An NGT can be both therapeutic and prophylactic. By emptying the GI system, it allows the bowel to decompress, edema to resolve, and, if the obstruction is partial, the bowel to "open up." It is prophylactic in the sense that it drains the stomach and prevents aspiration of vomitus. This is especially important in elderly or altered patients. The only patients who might not need an NGT are those who have only minimal vomiting and are otherwise healthy enough to protect their airways.

If you are on the fence about placing an NGT, you can order a plain film KUB. Dilated bowel or stomach suggests that an NGT would be helpful. Though unpleasant, it is always safer to put one in than have the patient aspirate in the CT scanner.

Placement of an NGT is contraindicated in patients with a suspected basilar skull fracture, severe oropharyngeal trauma, and recent esophageal or gastric surgery.

5. To place an NGT, you will need:

14 to 18 Fr NGT (bigger is less susceptible to clogging)

Water-based lubricant

Tape to secure tube

Foley tip syringe

Safety pin to attach tube to gown

For an awake patient, you should also include:

Topical anesthetic jelly or spray

Cup of water with a straw

With an awake patient, it is imperative that you enlist his participation in placing an NGT. Sit the patient upright and have him extend his head like he is sniffing something in front of him. Measure out the length of the tube you plan to insert by holding the tip of the tube at the xyphoid process and wrapping the tube around the back of the ear and then out to the nostril. Next, explain the procedure thoroughly while you inject topical anesthetic jelly into the nares or spray topical anesthetic into the posterior oropharynx. Topical anesthesia should be administered at least 5 minutes before the start of the procedure.

The insertion takes 2 steps. The first part is placing the NGT in the nasal cavity and advancing it to the back of the oropharynx. Make sure you are inserting the tube into the nostril at a 90° angle to the plane of the face and are not aiming it cranially (see Figure 14-2). The anatomy of the nasopharynx is such that the tube makes a 90° turn as it enters the oropharynx. This first part feels like getting punched in the nose.

It is extremely helpful to stop at this point, reassure the patient, and then have him drink some water. This enlists the muscles of deglutition to help advance the tube into the esophagus. As the patient drinks, advance the tube

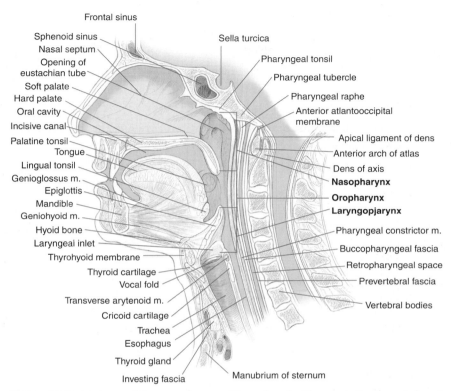

Figure 14-2. Anatomy of the nasopharynx. (Reproduced with permission from Lalwani AK. *Current Diagnosis & Treatment in Otolaryngology—Head & Neck Surgery.* 3rd ed. New York: McGraw-Hill; 2012 [Figure 1-15].)

until you reach your premeasured distance. If the patient starts coughing, you should immediately withdraw the tube back into the oropharynx as you are most likely advancing the tube through the larynx and into the trachea.

Once the tube is in place, tape it securely to the nose. A butterfly bandage (or tape on each side of the nose) that then coils around the NG tube is a typical approach. Secure the tube to the gown with tape and a safety pin so that any tension on the tube will result in pulling of the gown and not the material securing the tube to the nose. Be sure to leave enough slack in the tube so the patient can move his head without dislodging the tube, but not so much that a long loop will get pulled out accidentally.

How to confirm that the tube is in the stomach:

1. Have the patient say "Hello." If the patient is unable to speak, the tube is likely in the trachea and should be withdrawn. Note that this technique can also be used as you are advancing the tube, for similar reasons.

2. Aspirate with the Foley-tipped syringe. Aspiration of gastric contents suggests the tube is in the correct place.

3. Again using the Foley-tipped syringe, instill 20 cm³ of air forcefully into the tube while auscultating in the left upper quadrant. You should hear a "burp" of air over the stomach.

4. Ideal tube positioning should be confirmed with a plain x-ray.

Never instill anything other than air until you are sure the tip of the tube is in the stomach.

6. Patients presenting with an SBO are usually dehydrated due to the edematous bowel losing its normal absorptive function. This, coupled with vomiting, can lead to severe volume depletion with associated electrolyte derangement. Key to both preoperative and nonoperative treatments is adequate fluid resuscitation and electrolyte replacement. A Foley catheter should, in all but the most robust patients, be placed to monitor urine output and subsequent resuscitation.

Following initial resuscitation, a trick for patients with a suspected *partial* SBO is the administration of water-soluble contrast. The hypertonic solution draws fluid into the lumen and theoretically reduces edema. In a number of trials, water-soluble contrast was found to reduce the need for operative intervention.

TIPS TO REMEMBER

- SBO patients are usually hypovolemic and in need of resuscitation—placing a Foley catheter and following the urine output can help guide you.
- SBO patients who do not require immediate surgery should be watched very closely for signs of bowel ischemia.
- Always have an awake patient help you by swallowing during placement of an NGT.
- Never instill anything in an NGT until you are sure it is in the stomach.

COMPREHENSION QUESTIONS

1. Which of the following is *not* something you should specifically look for on physical examination in a patient you suspect of having an SBO?

    A. Rovsing sign (palpation of the left lower quadrant resulting in increased pain in the right lower quadrant)

    B. Abdominal tenderness to palpation

    C. Inguinal or ventral hernia

    D. Abdominal surgical scars

2. Which of the following warrants immediate surgical exploration?
>   A. Patient who has been vomiting for 24 hours
>   B. A patient with dilated loops of small bowel on KUB
>   C. A patient with a closed loop obstruction on CT scan
>   D. A patient with NGT output of 200 cm³/h

3. You attempt to place an NGT and think you hear a puff near the stomach when you instill 20 cm³ of air. What's next?
>   A. Place the NGT on suction and go write orders.
>   B. Get a plain film to ensure proper positioning.
>   C. Instill 50 cm³ of water-soluble contrast to help relieve the partial obstruction.
>   D. Take the tube out and try again.

Answers

1. **A.** Rovsing sign is a test for appendicitis. All of the others are good things to look for in a patient who you suspect has an SBO.

2. **C.** A closed loop obstruction is indication for immediate surgical exploration. All of the others describe patients who may require an operation, but more information is needed.

3. **B.** A plain film is the gold standard when determining NGT placement. In the scenario above, the tip could be in the stomach, but you are not sure.

A 65-year-old Man Status Post Surgery With a HCT of 24%

Alden H. Harken, MD and
Brian C. George, MD

Three days ago, a 65-year-old man underwent a sigmoid resection, end colostomy, and Hartman's for a free diverticular perforation and raging peritonitis. Perioperatively the patient was aggressively fluid-resuscitated and monitored with a CVP, A-line, and Foley. Current vitals are 100/60, HR 110, and CVP 12. He remains intubated on an FiO_2 of 0.6 and ABGs: Po_2 100, Pco_2 35, and pH 7.35. When you arrive in the SICU, this patient's most recent urine output was 20 mL/h. The 6:00 AM labs just returned, and his HCT is 24% and Hgb 8 g%.

1. **Should this patient be transfused with packed red blood cells?**
2. **What else is in banked blood besides hemoglobin?**
3. **What is an appropriate transfusion threshold for a patient who is actively bleeding?**
4. **When should you order a type and screen, and when should you order a type and cross?**

RED BLOOD CELL TRANSFUSIONS

Answers

1. This patient's anemia is most likely dilutional, caused by his body beginning to mobilize all the fluid he received during his perioperative resuscitation 3 days prior. Still, his hemoglobin does seem low and his oliguria most likely represents some element of renal hypoperfusion. The most rapid way to increase this patient's systemic oxygen delivery is to transfuse him with bank blood. But will that improve his overall outcome?

    Goal-directed therapy (Rivers et al; see Chapter 12) protocol mandates that, following initial fluid resuscitation and inotropic support, and if the mixed venous O_2 saturation remains below 70%, then transfuse blood to an Hct of 30%. But the Transfusion Requirements in Critical Care (TRICC) trial (Hébert et al) provides persuasive evidence that permitting patients to float down to an Hbg of 7 g% is safe (if not safer than transfusing at an Hbg threshold of 9 g%).

    In fact, there is no controversy. Both of these beautifully conducted trials were conducted in very different cohorts of patients:

    - GDT patients were all in septic shock and were treated within 6 hours of admission.

- TRICC patients were all documented euvolemic (normal CVP) and were randomized only after 3 days in the ICU.

So, in this case you search hard for evidence of myocardial ischemia (12-lead electrocardiogram) and in the absence of ischemia, your patient is euvolemic and has been in the ICU for 3 days. So, TRICC trumps GDT—don't give blood yet.

2. When you transfuse banked blood, you are infusing much more than oxygen-carrying hemoglobin. There is a nonzero rate of infectious contamination. Also, the white cells in transfused blood are all "primed" to release toxic oxygen metabolites and proteases. Those white cells can also attack the patient, in a process called graft-versus-host disease. Leukodepletion does cut the white count by several orders of magnitude—but not to zero. And hemolyzed RBC membranes are also toxic. In our hospital, it is OK to transfuse blood that has been sitting in the refrigerator for up to 42 days. More like gymnasts than wine, banked blood does not improve with age.

3. The GDT or TRICC trials cannot and should not be generalized to patients who are actively bleeding. In fact, even using the Hgb to determine when to transfuse is a risky proposition. As an example, let's say your patient's Hgb is 13. If you remove half of his blood volume in the next 5 minutes, his Hgb will still be 13—as many red cells were removed as were white cells, platelets, and serum. Eventually equilibration with interstitial fluid will result in a low hematocrit, but not before he is dead. In general, you should aim to replace any ongoing blood loss greater than about 1.5 L—and to do so early, even prophylactically. Oh, and stop the bleeding!

4. Both "type and screen" and "type and cross" result in a determination of the patient's blood type (ie, ABO antigen and Rh[D] antigen). The difference really comes down to the "screen" and the "cross." For a type and *screen*, the patient's blood is *screened* for a standard panel of foreign red blood cell antibodies. It takes about 30 minutes to complete. For a type and *cross*, the blood bank also *cross*-matches the patient's blood against a specific unit of blood to determine if there is any *cross*-reactivity. It takes another 30 minutes in addition to the time required for the type and screen (ie, 1 hour total for both). Unless it is an emergency and you are going to transfuse O negative blood, you must order a type and cross before any transfusion.

Once a type and cross has been performed, the blood bank will set those units of blood aside specifically for that patient. This means they are out of circulation, and can impact the utilization of what is a very precious and limited resource. In order to address this issue most blood banks will not reserve cross-matched blood for longer than 3 days.

These tests are not only used when a patient already needs a transfusion, but also sent as part of the preoperative workup for all but the most trivial elective operations. Ordering these tests will often be your responsibility. But do you order a type and screen or a type and cross? The risk of significant bleeding determines which test is ordered. For low-risk procedures (eg, inguinal hernia repair, small bowel resection), a type and screen is done. On the off chance that blood is needed intraoperatively, this will save 30 minutes. It also enables the blood bank to provide ABO and Rh(D) matched (but uncrossed) blood while the cross-match is being performed. For procedures that have a high risk of bleeding (eg, liver transplant, open aortic aneurysm repair, cardiac surgery), a specific number of units of blood are typed and crossed and set aside for the patient. In that case it is available almost immediately in the more likely event that the patient needs it.

TIPS TO REMEMBER

- Red blood cell transfusions can sometimes be more harmful than helpful.
- The TRICC trial suggests that ICU patients who are euvolemic should be transfused only for an Hgb less than 7.
- The Early Goal-directed Therapy trial suggests that patients who are acutely septic, have been volume resuscitated, are on appropriate inotropic support, and still have a mixed venous oxygen saturation of <70% should be transfused to a goal Hct of 30%.
- Type and cross reserves blood specifically for that patient, but only for a limited time. It should be used for procedures with a significant risk of significant bleeding.

COMPREHENSION QUESTIONS

1. A patient in the ICU has a Hgb of 9.2. It has been slowly drifting down over the past 5 days. She is noted to be euvolemic but is on pressors. When should you transfuse her?
        A. When the Hgb is <9, per the GDT trial
        B. When the Hgb is <7, per the TRICC trial
        C. Now
        D. 2 days ago

2. A trauma patient just rolled in with a sword stuck in his RUQ. He has an Hgb of 12 but is lethargic, cold, clammy, and tachycardic. When should you transfuse him?
        A. When the Hgb is <9, per the GDT trial
        B. When the Hgb is <7, per the TRICC trial
        C. Now
        D. 10 minutes ago

3. What is the most appropriate order for a patient who is scheduled to undergo a coronary artery bypass graft in 10 days?
>   A. Type and screen only
>   B. Type and cross 2 U
>   C. Type and cross 10 U
>   D. None of the above

Answers

1. **B**. This is a euvolemic patient in the ICU with no evidence of bleeding. The TRICC trial applies. Hold off on transfusion.

2. **D**. You are already behind because the patient is in shock. The patient has probably already lost at least 30% of the blood volume, regardless of the Hgb.

3. **D**. This patient will need to be typed and crossed for blood given the high likelihood of bleeding, but not until closer to the operation. The blood bank will not reserve the blood for this patient for 10 days.

SUGGESTED READINGS

Hébert PC, Wells G, Blajchman MA, et al. A multicenter, randomized, controlled clinical trial of transfusion requirements in critical care. *N Engl J Med*. 1999;340(6):409–417.
Rivers E, Nguyen B, Havstad S, et al. Early goal-directed therapy in the treatment of severe sepsis and septic shock. *N Engl J Med*. 2001;345(19):1368–1377.

A 70-year-old Man With "Bad Blood"

Emily Miraflor, MD, Louise Y. Yeung, MD, Brian C. George, MD, and Alden H. Harken, MD

Ephraim Hatfield IV is a 70-year-old male from Tug Fork, West Virginia, whose chief complaint is "bad blood." One week ago the patient recounts an attempt on his life where "I left a bunch of blood on the pavement." At your hospital, he received multiple blood transfusions. Following discharge, the patient noted that "my eyes turned yellow and my urine turned brown." The patient believes that he received "bad blood"—perhaps even from a McCoy donor.

1. **Explain the primary reason to transfuse blood.**

2. **Name an alloantigen that, when present in donor blood, can precipitate a transfusion reaction.**

3. **Did the patient in the vignette above have an acute or delayed reaction?**

TRANSFUSION REACTIONS

Answers

1. The only reason to transfuse blood is to increase oxygen-carrying capacity via hemoglobin. So, what we'd really like to do is transfuse pure hemoglobin. That has been tried. The 64,000 molecular weight hemoglobin tetramer breaks up to provoke an osmotic diuresis that rapidly abbreviates the therapeutic effect. So, we transfuse hemoglobin encapsulated in red cells.

   One unit of packed red blood cells can be expected to increase a patient's hemoglobin by approximately 1 g/dL, or the hematocrit by approximately 3%.

2. Unfortunately, 1 U of transfused blood contains a whole lot more than hemoglobin—and most of this stuff, you don't want. The stuff you don't want comes in 2 categories:

   A. The stuff the donor was born with
   B. The stuff the donor acquired

   A. **Born with**: Red blood cells come in multiple flavors. We focus on the A and B red cell antigens, but a short list of additional proteins includes C, D, E, c, e, K, k, JK^a, JK^b, s, Fy^a, Fy^b, and M. Therefore, every unit of transfused blood is at least a little mismatched.

   B. **Acquired**: What you do not want to do, when you receive a blood transfusion, is to dwell on the possible escapades of donors during the weeks before they offered up their blood. Perhaps the donor was a Mr. Rogers or a Mother Teresa who spent his or her life in church or school, but more likely, the donor enjoyed a more stimulating life. Now, in the absence of a Facebook page on the social antics of your blood donor, you—the blood recipient—are at the mercy of the blood bank laboratory technicians. Fortunately, the people who work in transfusion laboratories do not go to wild parties; their idea of excitement is to identify an arcane antibody in a crossmatch. These protectors of the faith can recite alloantibodies as effortlessly as their church catechisms.

The usual suspects are:

1. Pathogens:

    A. Bacteria—most bacteria survive happily in blood.

    B. Viruses—CMV, Epstein-Barr, hepatitis A, B, and C, HIV-1 and HIV-2, and human T-cell lymphotropic virus (HTLV)-1 and HTLV-2.

    C. Parasites—Chagas and malaria.

    D. Others: Creutzfeldt-Jakob disease has been associated with lots of things, including blood transfusions.

2. Non–red blood cell culprits:

    A. Leukocytes

    B. Platelets

    C. Immunoglobulins

    D. Cytokines

3. Transfusion reactions can be categorized as acute or delayed. Some, like hemolytic transfusion reactions, can be both. This patient had a delayed reaction with likely hemolysis.

Acute Transfusion Reactions

The Centers for Disease Control and Prevention (CDC) have characteristically catalogued these reactions into a sociobiological spectrum:

Level I: No big deal

Presentation: Maculopapular rash, flushing, pruritus, and urticaria.
Response: Give antihistamine and proceed.

Level II: Start to worry

Presentation: Bronchospasm, laryngeal tightness, hoarseness, and stridor.
Response: If possible, abort the transfusion and give β- and α-adrenergic agonists.

Level III: Drama

Presentation: Hypotension, disseminated intravascular coagulation (DIC), and hemoglobinuria.
Response: Stop the transfusion immediately! Give calcium gluconate or calcium chloride (it doesn't matter which), warm the patient, and give an α- or β-adrenergic agonist.

Delayed Transfusion Reactions

Like people, formed blood elements (leukocytes and platelets) can be happy, irritated, or overtly hostile. Much like a hibernating polar bear, most marginating neutrophils are tough to arouse. But, when you irritate them, they are capable of stirring up a lot of trouble—especially at home. Not surprisingly, self-satisfied quiescent white cells become aggrieved when they are drawn unceremoniously into a plastic, calcium-depleted bag. They get testy. And the longer they hang out in this foreign environment, the less neighborly they get. Your typical blood bank director will therefore not keep blood longer than a 42-day stay.

A transfused activated neutrophil expresses a sticky Velcro of adhesion molecules that facilitates lodging in the pulmonary endovasculature, where they blow big holes and promote interstitial fluid loss. This is the pathogenesis of transfusion-related acute lung injury (TRALI). These same neutrophils can also result in graft-versus-host disease, another type of delayed transfusion reaction that can be seen several weeks after a transfusion. A third type of delayed transfusion reaction is termed "posttransfusion purpura," which is simply a delayed thrombocytopenia (usually 1 or 2 weeks later). There is no reason to inflict this kind of damage on any patient, so all blood transfusions should be leukodepleted with a filter.

Hemolytic Transfusion Reactions

When an unfortunate patient already has (acute) or develops (delayed) antibodies to ABO-incompatible or other allotypic red cell antigens, rapid red blood cell destruction will ensue. The clinical manifestations of this hemolysis include chills, fever, hypotension, hemoglobinuria, and DIC, which can be most easily recognized by oozing at the IV site.

DON'T BE INTIMIDATED TO GIVE BLOOD

Blood bank directors thrive on detailed complexity. Surgeons like things simple. When your patient requires additional oxygen-carrying capacity, give blood. If you perseverate yourself into paralysis by conjuring all of the catastrophic and cataclysmic components of the contagious colostrum we, with inspirational innocence, term a "blood transfusion," your patient will succumb to deficient oxygen delivery—while you watch!

TIPS TO REMEMBER

- The sole reason to transfuse blood is to increase oxygen-carrying capacity.
- All blood transfusions are at least a little mismatched.
- Treat minor transfusion reactions with an antihistamine.
- Treat major transfusion reactions with α- and β-adrenergic agonists.

- With a suspected transfusion reaction, send blood specimens from both the patient and the transfused blood specimens to the lab.
- Acute DIC is most easily recognized as oozing at the IV site.

COMPREHENSION QUESTIONS

1. A 55-year-old male is still on the ventilator 3 days following an open aortobi-femoral graft. His Hbg is 7 g/dL. You decide to give him 2 U of packed red blood cells. The most likely benefit will be an increase in which of the following?

    A. Po_2 95 → 110 mm Hg
    B. O_2 saturation 95% → 98%
    C. CaO_2 by 25%
    D. Hbg 7 → 14 g/dL
    E. Hct 20% → 35%

2. DIC can be most easily recognized by which of the following?

    A. Low platelet counts
    B. Bleeding around a peripheral IV site
    C. Low hematocrit
    D. Elevated D-dimers

3. You should stop a transfusion if the patient develops which of the following?

    A. A rash
    B. Pruritus
    C. Hoarseness

4. Pharmacologic treatment of an acute transfusion reaction could include any of the following *except* which of the following?

    A. Acetaminophen
    B. Epinephrine
    C. Phenylephrine
    D. Diphenhydramine

Answers

1. **C.** More red blood cells increase the content of oxygen being carried in the blood. The oxygen saturation of that blood remains the same, as does the partial pressure of oxygen. The Hgb should rise by 1 g/dL for each unit, while the Hct will rise just 3% for each unit.

2. **B.** While these other elements can also be present, they are nonspecific and require a lab test. It is worth first checking the peripheral IV site.

3. **C.** A rash and pruritus are CDC level I–type reactions. You should give an antihistamine and then monitor the patient while you continue the transfusion.

4. **A.** Antihistamines such as diphenhydramine are first-line pharmacologic agents for all levels of transfusion reactions. For more severe reactions, α- and β-agonists are also indicated.

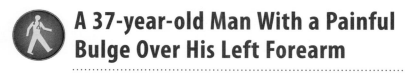

A 37-year-old Man With a Painful Bulge Over His Left Forearm

Eric N. Feins, MD

A 37-year-old man presents to the emergency department complaining of a painful bulge over his left forearm. He states that he noticed some redness around the area 1 week ago, and then over the past few days it has become more swollen and painful, but it has not drained anything. He denies fevers, but thinks he's had some occasional chills. He has no other medical problems and denies injecting drugs.

On physical exam, he is afebrile, HR 95, and BP 115/75. He has overall good hygiene and is well kempt. Over the dorsolateral aspect of his left forearm there is a 3-cm erythematous, fluctuant mass. It is extremely tender to light palpation and is mobile. Nothing can be expressed from the mass on palpation. There is also a 4- to 5-cm margin of erythema surrounding the mass without any evidence of streaking up the arm.

1. What, if any, additional imaging would you obtain?

2. Can you drain this abscess in the ED, or should it be done in the OR?

3. Is antibiotic therapy warranted for this patient?

SUPERFICIAL ABSCESS

Not all superficial abscesses are created equal and host factors often explain their etiology and severity. Superficial abscesses can arise in otherwise healthy individuals who develop skin breakdown (ie, abrasion, cut, surgical incision) that allows the entry of pathogenic bacteria. These are typically simpler to manage because the patient lacks risk factors and is immunocompetent. In contrast, patients with a history of injection drug use are at risk for recurrent superficial infections and abscesses. Immunocompromised patients (ie, diabetics) are also at risk for developing more severe infections due to their impaired host defenses.

Host factors influence the microbiology of superficial abscesses. Simple abscesses in immunocompetent patients are typically due to skin flora: *Staphylococcus* and *Streptococcus*, although gram-negative and anaerobic bacteria, can be involved. Methicillin-resistant *Staphylococcus aureus* (MRSA) is becoming increasingly common in some regions and is particularly prevalent in recently hospitalized patients, injection drug users, and diabetics. *Pseudomonas aeruginosa* is common in diabetics with abscesses (often on the feet), and is quite virulent if not treated. This is important to consider if antibiotics will be prescribed (see below).

Answers

1. A bedside ultrasound can be a useful adjunctive test. Ultrasound will give you 3 important pieces of information:

   A. *Whether there really is a drainable collection*: It can sometimes be difficult to determine on physical exam if an abscess is actually present, or if you are just feeling inflamed tissue from a cellulitis (ie, induration). Both cellulitis and abscesses will have warmth, redness, and tenderness (general markers of inflammation), and some abscesses will not have obvious fluctuance. In these cases of uncertainty ultrasound can confirm/rule out the presence of an abscess that needs drainage.

   B. *Size and depth*: If there is concern about how big and/or deep the abscess is, an ultrasound will help. This is important if you are concerned the abscess is so big or deep that it requires incision and drainage (I&D) in the OR.

   C. *Surrounding structures*: Sometimes abscesses are located near important structures (ie, blood vessels). In these cases, ultrasound can help you avoid such structures during a drainage procedure.

   For this particular patient with these physical findings ultrasound would not be necessary because it is clear that there is an undrained abscess, and it is not big enough or deep enough to require I&D in the OR.

2. This patient requires formal I&D of his undrained abscess under local anesthesia in the ER. This represents "source control," which is an important principle for the treatment of infections.

   In some cases it is more appropriate to drain a superficial abscess in the OR. The following are relative contraindications to a bedside I&D of a superficial abscess:

   A. *Size/depth*: There is no fixed size cutoff, but generally, abscesses that are too large or too deep to anesthetize with local anesthesia and/or require an extensive debridement should be done in the OR.

   B. *Location*: Abscesses in sensitive locations may require I&D in the OR due to the need for sedation or general anesthesia. In particular, this includes perirectal abscesses. While some are superficial enough to drain under local anesthesia, many are deeper and close to critical structures (ie, anal sphincter). These often require general anesthesia for patient comfort, to attain adequate exposure, and to evaluate for fistulae.

   C. *Patient anxiety or pain tolerance*: Some patients cannot tolerate bedside drainage, due to either their expected intolerance of pain or their baseline anxiety about the procedure. The operating room is the appropriate place for these patients as it allows for improved analgesia and optimal conditions to minimize procedure length.

Adequate drainage of an abscess requires several important components:

A. *Incision*: Your incision must be large enough to ensure adequate drainage. The incision need not extend over the entire length/diameter of the abscess, although if in doubt, you should err on the side of larger. There is no hard rule for incision size, but as an example, a 3-cm abscess might be adequately drained with a 2- or 3-cm incision.

B. *Deloculation*: After opening the cavity, gentle exploration with a cotton-tipped probe and curved hemostat (clamp) is necessary to break up any loculations within the cavity. The patient may require additional deep injection of local anesthetic.

C. *Packing*: After initial drainage the cavity must be kept open to allow for further drainage of leftover fluid/debris. This involves loosely packing the cavity with 0.25- or 0.5-in wide packing ribbon. Insert enough to keep the cavity open, and leave the ribbon extending out of the skin to prevent the skin edges from closing. Premature skin closure can lead to abscess recurrence. The abscess will heal by secondary intention.

Sending a wound culture is always a good idea. If the patient has a soft tissue infection (ie, cellulitis) in addition to an abscess, the culture data can help you narrow the initial empiric treatment. While patients without soft tissue infection will usually improve with drainage alone, if the patient later develops worsening soft tissue infection, then antibiotic therapy could be started and directed toward the culture data.

3. The 2 main determinants of whether antibiotic therapy is warranted are: *(A) presence of surrounding soft tissue infection and (B) host-related factors.*

A. *Presence of soft tissue infection*: Cellulitis, the most common form of soft tissue infections associated with superficial abscesses, requires treatment with antibiotics. In the patient presented here, there is a significant degree of surrounding erythema/tenderness consistent with cellulitis. Therefore, he will require antibiotic therapy. In many cases, abscesses do not have significant surrounding erythema, warmth, or redness, suggesting absence of cellulitis. In these cases, antibiotics are not warranted.

B. *Host-related factors*: In immunocompetent patients there is no need for antibiotics after abscess drainage, assuming there is no surrounding cellulitis. For them, we rely on their immune defenses to completely eradicate the infection after drainage. However, in immunocompromised patients (ie, diabetics) it is reasonable to consider a short course of antibiotics, and this can be discussed with a senior resident.

Antibiotic choice: For the immunocompetent host with a simple, drained abscess and surrounding cellulitis, empiric coverage with an oral β-lactam antibiotic is appropriate to cover staphylococcal and streptococcal organisms: dicloxacillin or cephalexin (even if penicillin-allergic but without any immediate hypersensitivity reaction). If there is concern for MRSA (see above) or the patient has an allergy to penicillin, alternative oral antibiotic option is clindamycin or TMP-SMZ.

Patients with extensive, severe cellulitis and signs of systemic toxicity (ie, fevers, abnormal vital signs, etc) should receive parenteral antibiotics that cover MRSA as well as gram-negative and anaerobic bacteria. Two typical antibiotic regimens are:

- Vancomycin (MRSA coverage), *and*
- Piperacillin–tazobactam *or* ticarcillin–clavulanate (gram-negative + anaerobic coverage)

Or

- Vancomycin (MRSA coverage), *and*
- Ceftriaxone *or* ciprofloxacin (gram-negative coverage), *and*
- Metronidazole (anaerobic coverage)

Diabetics often have more severe soft tissue infections involving *Pseudomonas*. These typically require treatment with an antipseudomonal antibiotic, such as piperacillin–tazobactam or cefepime.

The patient presented here has significant surrounding cellulitis that is concerning, although he has no systemic signs of infection. A reasonable treatment plan after I&D is to start an oral antibiotic (dicloxacillin or cephalexin) and admit the patient for 12 to 24 hours to ensure improvement of the cellulitis after a day of antibiotic treatment.

TIPS TO REMEMBER

- Bedside ultrasound is a useful modality for both diagnosis and procedural planning.
- The length of the incision for an abscess can vary but should be large enough to ensure adequate drainage.
- After incision, adequate drainage requires you to break up the loculations and loosely pack the cavity with gauze or other packing material.
- Assuming an abscess is adequately drained, the main indications for antibiotic therapy are: (1) presence of surrounding cellulitis, (2) severe infection with systemic signs of illness, or (3) patient immunocompromise (eg, from diabetes).

COMPREHENSION QUESTIONS

1. To ensure adequate drainage of a superficial abscess, which of the following is/are important component(s)? (Choose all that apply.)
    A. Skin incision large enough to ensure adequate drainage
    B. Deloculation of abscess cavity
    C. Antibiotic treatment
    D. Loose packing

2. Which of the following are contraindications to I&D of a superficial abscess under local anesthesia? (Choose all that apply.)
    A. Immunocompromised patient
    B. History of injection drug use
    C. Large size
    D. Sensitive location
    E. Location requiring extensive exposure

Answers

1. **A, B, D**. Antibiotic treatment is most important for treatment of surrounding cellulitis, not for drainage of an abscess.

2. **C, D, E**. Immunocompetency and history of drug use are risk factors for more severe infection, but do not preclude drainage of the abscess under local anesthesia.

Three Patients All Present With Issues Related to Laboratory Tests

Abigail K. Tarbox, MD and Mamta Swaroop, MD, FACS

Case 1: Mr. Jones is a 51-year-old male who comes to your office for a screening colonoscopy. He tells you that he had a friend who had a colon perforation from a colonoscopy and he is reluctant to undergo one himself. He has heard that there is a new blood test for colon cancer and asks you why he can't have this instead. You do a quick search for this test and learn that it has low sensitivity but high specificity.

Case 2: Mrs. Smith has been on a therapeutic heparin drip with a goal partial thromboplastin time (PTT) of 60 to 80. For the last 3 lab draws, her values have been 70, 73, and 69. Because her PTT has been at goal, you have not changed the rate of her drip. On her next set of labs her PTT suddenly becomes 133.

Case 3: Jane Doe has a urine specimen with the following results:

2 to 3 white blood cells

50,000 bacteria per high-power field

Negative nitrite

Negative leukocyte esterase

Multiple squamous epithelial cells

1. Should you order this new blood test for Mr. Jones?

2. What is the next step in evaluating Mrs. Smith's newly elevated PTT?

3. Does Jane Doe have a urinary tract infection?

LABS 101

Doctors spend a significant portion of their time ordering and interpreting various lab tests, but knowing when and which test to order is not always easy. As a general rule with any diagnostic testing, it is important to ask the following questions: "What am I looking for?" and "How will the results change the management of this patient?" The sensitivity, specificity, positive predictive value, and negative predictive values are all critical statistics that help you determine the answers to those questions (Table 18-1).

It should be noted that the positive predictive value and negative predictive values will be affected by the prevalence of the condition. Hence, when ordering tests for something very rare, the likelihood of a false test goes up. This is demonstrated in Table 18-2, where for the same specificity and sensitivity the positive predictive value increases dramatically as the disease prevalence goes from 2% in

Table 18-1. Calculations of Predictive Value, Sensitivity, and Specificity

Test Result	Disease	No Disease	
Positive	A (true-positive)	B (false-positive)	Positive predictive value (PPV) = A/A + B
Negative	C (false-negative)	D (true-negative)	Negative predictive value (NPV) = D/C + D
	Sensitivity = A/A + C	Specificity = D/B + D	

Table 18-2A to 20% in Table 18-2B. Awareness of such principles will maximize your likelihood of testing your patients appropriately.

It is also important to note that laboratory tests that measure a continuous variable (eg, CBC, chemistries, LFTs) are subject to unavoidable systematic error intrinsic to the method by which the reference range is determined. For these types of tests the thresholds used to distinguish a "normal" result from an "abnormal" result are determined based on large samples of data from healthy

Table 18-2. Effect of Disease Prevalence on Positive and Negative Predictive Values

Test Result	Disease	No Disease	Total
A			
+	99	49	Positive predictive value (PPV) = 99/148 = **0.66**
−	1	4851	Negative predictive value (NPV) = 4851/4852 = 0.99
	Sensitivity = (99/100) × 100 = 99%	Specificity = (4851/4900) × 100 = 99%	
B			
+	990	40	PPV = 990/1030 = **0.96**
−	10	3960	NPV = 3960/3970 = 0.99
	Sensitivity = (990/1000) × 100 = 99%	Specificity = (3960/4000) × 100 = 99%	

The bolded results show the effect of disease prevalence on PPV.

individuals, with the middle 95% of the values simply defined as normal. In other words, the reference range is calibrated for a specificity of 95%, which means that 5% of healthy individuals would be expected to have a falsely positive test result (ie, the result is outside the reference range even though they don't have the disease). This has important clinical implications. If you order 20 tests (the labs included with a CBC with differential and a basic metabolic panel will generally cross this threshold), you should expect on average 1 value to be outside the reference range. Since "abnormal" values often lead to further testing, some of which are invasive, a false-positive lab test can be associated with substantial risk. While it may seem you are being more thorough when you reflexively order every lab available, taking the time to order only a limited number of labs is actually protective and is therefore better patient care.

Answers

1. Before you order any test you should ask yourself:

   A. "What am I looking for?"

   B. "How will the results change the management of this patient?"

   In trying to answer these questions, we should first examine the test characteristics. This test has a low sensitivity, which means that it is less likely to be positive in disease. But the test is specific, which means that a positive result is most likely a true-positive. Furthermore, colon cancer has a relatively high prevalence, increasing the positive predictive value.

   Based on these statistics it may at first glance appear that a positive test result might be useful—after all, it is highly specific and a positive result therefore most likely reflects the presence of disease. With this information we can answer question A: You could use this test to find what you are looking for. But in examining the second question regarding the impact the test result might have on patient management, things get a little more complicated. Indeed, on further examination it becomes clear that a positive result would not change management because it would require a colonoscopy to localize the tumor. If we examine the opposite outcome where this poorly sensitive test is negative, we cannot make any conclusions about the presence or absence of disease and—you guessed it—a colonoscopy would be needed. So, while this test might be able to help find colon cancer, it would not change the management of the patient. You should therefore explain this to the patient, decline to use the new test, and encourage the patient to undergo a colonoscopy.

2. You have measured 3 consecutive PTT values in the therapeutic range and now there is suddenly a value way above your goal. It is important to first confirm that the drip rate did not change, as a result of either a miscommunication or a nursing error. If the rate has remained the same, then it is likely that some type

of lab error has occurred. A very common instance in the case of PTT testing is that the sample sent to the lab was drawn off of a line through which heparin was infusing. A repeat sample should be sent.

Similar situations can occur with almost any medication or infusion going through an intravenous line. For example, one may see falsely elevated glucose levels in patients receiving TPN when the blood sample was drawn off of the line. In such a case, correlation with finger-stick glucose levels is advised.

Other lab abnormalities that can occur are hemolysis in the sample tube, resulting in falsely elevated potassium levels, falsely elevated lactic acid levels from the sample being drawn from a vein in an arm with a tourniquet on it for an extended time, or pseudohyponatremia in the presence of extremely high glucose levels.

3. First, let us review urine testing. There are 2 common urine tests—urinalysis and urine culture. A urinalysis looks at the following: appearance, pH, specific gravity, protein, glucose, ketones, red blood cells, leukocyte esterase, nitrites, bile, and urobilinogen. Additional elements of a urinalysis analyzed at the microscopic level are white blood cells, urinary casts, yeast, and epithelial cells.

The interpretation of urinalysis is not as easily defined as for some other tests. Each element of the urinalysis should be integrated into a whole, balancing those elements that suggest infection against those that argue against. Ms. Doe has some elements of her urinalysis that might suggest a urinary tract infection, such as the presence of bacteria and the presence of leukocytes. This is counterbalanced by the presence of squamous epithelial cells, negative leukocyte esterase, and negative nitrate. But how do we integrate these conflicting data?

Bacteria often appear in urine specimens. Normal microbial flora of the vagina in the female and the external urethral meatus in both sexes can rapidly multiply in urine standing at room temperature. Bacteriuria alone is therefore not diagnostic and, in a case of suspected urinary tract infection, requires culture to determine if it represents a pathogen or contamination. A bacterial count of more than 100,000/mL of 1 organism reflects significant bacteriuria and, in the setting of other positive findings on the urinalysis, a likely urinary tract infection. The presence of multiple organisms is usually indicative of contamination.

Leukocytes (white cells) may appear with infection in either the upper or lower urinary tract or with acute glomerulonephritis. White cells may also be contaminants from other, non-urinary tract sources. For example, samples may be contaminated with white cells from the vagina (often present in vaginal and cervical infections), or white cells from the external urethral meatus (in both men and women). Yet the presence of squamous epithelial cells indicates likely contamination from the skin surface or from the outer urethra. In general, 2 or more leukocytes per high-power field in urine that does not include any other markers of contamination suggest that the specimen is abnormal. Higher numbers of leukocytes are even more convincing in this regard.

Nitrates and leukocyte esterase are more specific tests of urinary tract infection. Nitrates are the by-product of some bacteria, especially gram-negative rods such as *E coli*. Leukocyte esterase is normally contained within white blood cells and its presence indicates likely pyuria. Its absence, in contrast to nitrates, strongly argues against a urinary tract infection, especially in the absence of other compelling markers. As with all urinalysis data both leukocyte esterase and nitrate results should be integrated with other available data prior to drawing a final conclusion.

Lastly, a urinalysis should also be interpreted in the context of a patient's clinical picture, including whether the patient is having symptoms of a UTI such as fevers, dysuria, or increased urinary frequency, urgency, or hesitancy. If the patient is symptomatic, then a urinalysis may not even be needed, and if performed, may require less criteria to be considered positive.

In our example, Ms. Doe's urinalysis likely reflects a contaminated specimen. The squamous cells indicate contamination, she has relatively few white cells, leukocyte esterase and nitrate are negative, and the bacterial count is below the standard cutoff for urinary tract infections. Although she has 3 to 5 white cells, this is difficult to interpret in the context of contamination. Lastly, both negative leukocyte esterase and nitrate support the negative laboratory diagnosis.

TIPS TO REMEMBER

- Judicious use of laboratory testing is essential to providing safe and cost-effective care to patients.
- In the case of unexpected lab value results that are inconsistent with the clinical picture, remember that sampling errors can occur and that the context of the patient's condition should help guide you in interpreting that result.

COMPREHENSION QUESTIONS

1. A D-dimer test is highly sensitive for recent clotting, but it is not very specific (eg, it can be due to sepsis). Given this information, for which patient would it be reasonable to order a D-dimer test to screen for a DVT? Why?

    A. A 55-year-old male patient with a history of peripheral vascular disease who is postoperative day 7 from an aortic aneurysm repair

    B. A 65-year-old woman with an IVC filter and on chronic anticoagulation for a history of DVT who complains of R calf pain

    C. A 43-year-old patient who was diagnosed yesterday with a subsegmental pulmonary embolus

    D. A 23-year-old healthy woman with no known risk factors for DVT who presents to the ER with unilateral leg swelling

2. A patient is postoperative day 1 from a pulmonary wedge resection. You stop to check on your patient and find that he is pale, tachycardic, and confused. Among other orders you ask the nurse to draw a stat CBC, chem 10, coagulation studies, and LFTs. When the labs come back, you see that he has an elevated total bilirubin of 2.5. This is an example of which of the following?
>   A. The limitations of the test characteristics for total bilirubin
>   B. A finding that is difficult to interpret
>   C. A normal result
>   D. A false-positive
>   E. A true-positive

Answers

1. **D**. Before ordering a test you must determine if the test actually measures what you are looking for. A d-dimer will always be elevated in a postoperative patient due to both stress and clot. It will also be elevated in a patient with a known PE. In both A and C the test doesn't measure anything that isn't already known. It is also imperative to determine how the result will change management. While B might have a new DVT, she is already being maximally treated for it and a positive result would not prompt any changes in management. While your pretest probability for a DVT might be low in D, a positive result might prompt additional diagnostic workup.

2. **B**. When ordering these many tests, there is a very high (>90%) chance of false-positives. While the measured total bilirubin is outside the "normal" reference range, we cannot know without further testing whether this value represents clinically significant pathology, if it is this patient's normal baseline, or if it is simply lab error. Unfortunately, once an abnormal value is detected, there is an increased chance that the team will feel that the patient requires additional workup (in this case possibly an ultrasound).

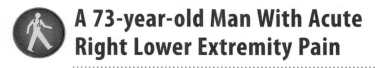

A 73-year-old Man With Acute Right Lower Extremity Pain

Joel T. Adler, MD and
Virendra I. Patel, MD, MPH

A 73-year-old male presents to the emergency department with 5 hours of acute right lower extremity pain. Mr. P tells you that the pain came "out of nowhere" while he was reading the morning newspaper. His past medical history is notable for atrial fibrillation, coronary artery disease, and diabetes. He takes warfarin, a baby aspirin, and a statin, and he has an 80-pack-year smoking history.

1. **What other parts of the history are relevant?**
2. **What is the blood supply to the lower extremities?**
3. **What findings on physical examination differentiate acute from chronic limb ischemia?**
4. **What further testing would you want in this patient?**
5. **What are the most common causes of acute limb ischemia?**
6. **What can be done to treat this patient?**
7. **What is compartment syndrome?**

ACUTE LIMB ISCHEMIA

Answers

1. You first need to understand the pain: the quality, timing, location, onset, and severity. Has he had the pain before? Does he have associated numbness, tingling, or swelling? Does he have pain at rest? Has he ever had pain in the back of his calves, thighs, or buttocks associated with walking? Did it come on suddenly, or has it been worsening over the past few days? Is there any recent trauma to the area?

   In terms of past medical history, a history of cardiac or vascular disease is key information: atrial fibrillation, angina/MI, claudication/ulceration, and transient ischemic attacks/strokes. Also notable is a history of cardiac or peripheral revascularization. Current medications are important, as is a personal or family history of cardiac disease, vascular disease, or a hypercoagulable state. Much of the past history gives you an idea as to the cause of ischemia, potential intraoperative challenges, and the perioperative risk associated with intervention.

   This is also an appropriate time to gather a quick vascular-oriented review of symptoms. Questions should cover the carotids (visual changes, word-finding difficulties, transient ischemic attacks, or strokes with paralysis or paresthesias), aorta (abdominal or back pain, family or personal history of abdominal aortic aneurysm [AAA]), and peripheral vasculature (claudication, rest pain, ulceration). This is by no means comprehensive, but remember that vascular disease involves numerous territories simultaneously.

On further questioning, Mr. P reveals that the pain behind his right calf started abruptly 5 hours ago. He has been able to walk around, but he notes that the leg is feeling weaker. His activity is so limited at baseline that he normally walks only a few blocks before becoming quite dyspneic. He notes no claudication otherwise, and his vascular review of symptoms is otherwise negative.

He has an 80-pack-year history of smoking, and he also has a history of atrial fibrillation. His warfarin dosing is managed by his PCP, but he takes it regularly with his last INR "above 2."

2. The lower extremity circulation begins with the common iliac artery. After the internal iliac branches, the external iliac comes forward and laterally within the pelvis and eventually crosses under the inguinal ligament. After the inferior epigastric and circumflex iliac arteries branch, it is called the common femoral artery (immediately proximal to the inguinal ligament). The next important branch point is the profunda femoris artery, which takes off posterolaterally from the common femoral artery to supply the thigh and deep muscles of the upper leg.

The superficial femoral artery continues and passes through the adductor (Hunter's) canal. At the level of the adductor hiatus, it wraps behind the knee to become the popliteal artery, which is often referenced in relation to the knee joint, that is, above versus below the knee popliteal. Below the knee, the popliteal artery splits into 3 arteries (the "trifurcation"). The most common pattern begins with a 2-way split into the anterior tibial artery and the tibioperoneal (TP) trunk. The TP trunk then becomes the peroneal artery and the posterior tibial artery. All 3 of these arteries reach the foot: the anterior tibial artery runs laterally and eventually becomes the dorsalis pedis artery, the posterior tibial artery runs medially and can be felt behind the ankle (still called the posterior tibial artery), and the peroneal artery follows the fibula down to the ankle and bifurcates into medial and lateral branches, which provide collaterals to the foot.

The basic anatomy is fairly consistent (see Figure 19-1). Collateralization is crucial for patients with atherosclerotic disease, as it provides continued blood supply and also serves as a "detour" during acute occlusion. It is most commonly seen around major branch points: the external iliac filling through the pelvis (from the internal iliac artery), the superficial femoral artery reconstituting via the profunda femoris artery, and the foot filling through patent tibial vessels.

3. A pulse examination is essential. There are various scoring systems for pulses (0-2, 0-4, etc). If your scale may be unclear, document in words the pulse examination (easily palpable, barely palpable, dopplerable, etc). If unable to find a

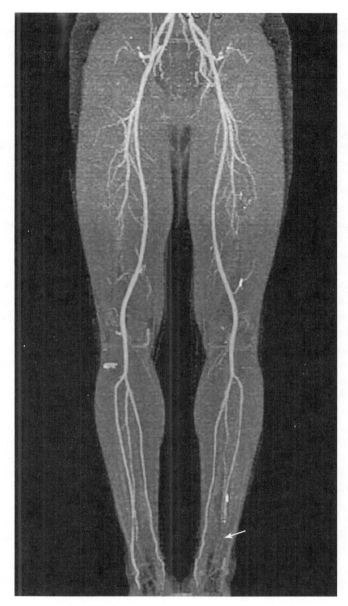

Figure 19-1. Arterial circulation of the lower extremities. The left anterior tibial artery (arrow) is noted to be diseased. (Reproduced with permission from Brunicardi FC, Andersen DK, Billiar TR, et al. *Schwartz's Principles of Surgery*. 9th ed. New York: McGraw-Hill; 2010 [Figure 23-59].)

Table 19-1. Mr. P's Pulse Examination

	Femoral	Popliteal	DP	PT
R	2+	Absent	Absent	Absent
L	2+	1+	Dopplerable	Dopplerable

pulse by palpation, use a Doppler probe and note the characteristic of the sound. It is rare to have acute limb-threatening ischemia without a major pulse deficit.

If a patient has acute peripheral ischemia, the "6 P's" are common examination findings: pain, pallor, poikilothermia (coolness), pulselessness, paresthesia, and paralysis. Paralysis is a late sign that warrants emergent intervention. Chronic ischemia is evidenced by hairless legs, symmetrically cool feet, dependent rubor, diminished pulses, and nonhealing distal ulcers or gangrene.

A commonly used measure of peripheral vascular disease is the ankle-brachial index (ABI). It is the ratio of the systolic blood pressure of the brachial artery to that of either the posterior tibial or dorsalis pedis artery. An ABI of 0.9 to 1.2 is considered normal. ABIs from 0.7 to 0.9 suggest mild disease, 0.7 to 0.4 imply moderate disease (usually associated with claudication), and less than 0.4 denote critical limb ischemia (rest pain). Of note, an ABI of greater than 1.2 signifies arterial calcification; in such instances, ABIs are not helpful. This is especially common in patients with diabetes and end-stage renal disease. Don't let this fool you into thinking the patient has healthy arteries.

Back to our patient. On examination, you note the following pulses (see Table 19-1).

Mr. P's right leg is notably cooler than the left, starting immediately above the knee. He has some small ulcerations on the first 3 toes of the left foot without evidence of infection, and there is a lack of leg hair starting halfway down the tibia bilaterally. He has weakness on movement of his right ankle, and his sensation is intact except for the web space between the first and second toes. His calves feel soft bilaterally. ABIs are >1.3 bilaterally.

From the examination you deduce that he has an acute arterial occlusion, likely at the level of Hunter's canal. Your patient clearly has chronic peripheral vascular disease as well, indicated by weakened peripheral pulses, a history of claudication, lack of leg hair, and the ulcerations of the toes on the asymptomatic leg. He requires urgent revascularization of the right leg because of the acute ischemia.

4. Basic laboratory workup is important, especially renal function tests, coagulation studies, creatinine kinase, and a urinalysis. Knowing the general function of a patient's kidneys allows decisions about further imaging (CT angiogram, intraoperative angiogram, or duplex ultrasound). Creatinine kinase and a urinalysis are helpful when you suspect rhabdomyolysis associated with prolonged ischemia or compartment syndrome.

A complete blood count, coagulation studies, basic metabolic panel, and urinalysis are within normal limits except for the following:

INR 1.8

PTT 32.7

Cr 1.3

CK 10451

EKG atrial fibrillation with rate in the high 80s

Unfortunately, you have no other lab values for comparison purposes. The INR indicates that he is not therapeutically anticoagulated at this time. The elevated creatinine is indicative of underlying renal insufficiency and should be addressed by pretreatment with acetylcysteine (Mucomyst) and sodium bicarbonate. The elevated CK indicates ongoing muscle death from ischemia. His urinalysis is presently normal, but it will be important to closely monitor his urine for renal injury.

5. These are commonly divided into 4 categories: embolus, thrombosis, trauma, and dissection (see Table 19-2).

6. After acute arterial occlusion is diagnosed, there are 2 priorities: systemic anticoagulation to prevent further propagation and urgent revascularization to reestablish blood flow to the extremities.

Anticoagulation is usually achieved with intravenous heparin (rather than low-molecular-weight heparin). Revascularization is simple in principle, but

Table 19-2. Common Causes of Acute Limb Ischemia

Embolus	Thrombosis	Trauma	Dissection
Atrial fibrillation	Atherosclerosis	Blunt	Proximal dissection
Endocarditis	Hypercoagulable states (antiphospholipid antibodies, hyperhomocysteinemia, and heparin-induced thrombocytopenia)	Penetrating	
Valves (either diseased or prosthetic)		Iatrogenic	Postintervention dissection (arterial catheterization)
Myocardial infarction			
Aneurysm (atherosclerotic debris or blood clot)	Low-flow state		
	Aneurysm thrombosis (popliteal aneurysm)		
Paradoxical embolus (patent foramen ovale)			

quite complicated in practice due to the myriad of options available. If clinically stable and appropriate from the standpoint of renal function, CT angiography is used to establish the level of the occlusion; simultaneously, the proximal and distal vasculature are assessed for other occlusions and possible bypass targets.

Thromboembolectomy is traditionally achieved by direct cutdown and embolectomy with Fogarty catheters. A lysis catheter with infusion of lysis agent (tissue plasminogen activator [tPA], urokinase, streptokinase, etc) can also be used in patients who have intact sensation and motor function, especially for patients in whom the risk of general anesthesia is felt to be high. Fogarty catheters can be used for embolectomy under local anesthesia as well.

All management decisions should be based on consultation with a vascular surgeon, and this depends on the acuity of presentation and anatomy.

Back to our patient. A CT angiography demonstrates an acute occlusion in Hunter's canal. The length of the occlusion is relatively short, and there appears to be some reconstitution of flow below the level of the occlusion. Mr. P has single-vessel runoff to his foot via the posterior tibial artery. Because he is in atrial fibrillation and is subtherapeutic on warfarin, he is brought to the operating room for a direct cutdown and thromboembolectomy with Fogarty catheters. A lysis catheter is not entertained because he is having leg weakness with an elevated CK. The operation is successful in restoring flow to the foot, and completion angiography demonstrates good flow in the posterior tibial artery. On leaving, the posterior tibial pulse is now dopplerable.

7. Compartment syndrome results from an ischemia–reperfusion injury after revascularization. This results in tissue swelling and entrapment by the fascia. This in turn can cause *more* ischemia by causing occlusion in extreme circumstances as the blood vessels are externally compressed. This results in more muscle death, release of myoglobin, and potential for renal injury and loss of the limb.

There are 4 compartments of the leg: anterior, lateral, deep posterior, and superficial posterior. The anterior compartment is the most commonly affected (anterior tibial artery, deep peroneal nerve, and the 4 extensor muscles of the foot) (see Figure 19-2).

Traditionally, compartment pressures greater than 30 mm Hg have been considered an indication for intervention. However, there are increasing data to suggest that the delta pressure (difference between diastolic pressure and compartment pressure) is a more accurate predictor of compartment syndrome. A difference of 20 mm Hg is the generally accepted value.

A 4-compartment fasciotomy can be performed by making an incision 2 fingerbreadths (4–5 cm) medial (deep and superficial posterior compartments) and lateral (anterior and lateral compartments) to the tibia. Once down to muscle, a long scissors can be used to split the fascia and assess the quality of the underlying muscle.

Back to the patient. Postoperatively, our patient's pain is well controlled. At 4:00 the following morning, you are asked to evaluate him for worsening pain and

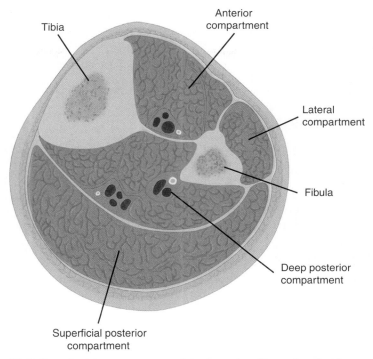

Figure 19-2. Four fascial compartments of the lower leg. (Reproduced with permission from Brunicardi FC, Andersen DK, Billiar TR, et al. *Schwartz's Principles of Surgery.* 9th ed. New York: McGraw-Hill; 2010 [Figure 23-62].)

an inability to move his right foot again. On examination, the arterial pulses are still dopplerable, but Mr. P notes weakness and numbness of the right foot. The calf feels "rock hard" and is tender to palpation, and you suspect compartment syndrome. Compartment pressures are measured at greater than 30 mm Hg. He is brought emergently to the operating room for 4-compartment fasciotomies.

Measuring the CK may or may not have been useful because of the recent operation. However, fasciotomies can be limb-saving and are indicated in this situation. Trending CK postoperatively after fasciotomies is common practice to ensure that there is no ongoing ischemia. Second-look operations are also common.

TIPS TO REMEMBER

● Acute peripheral ischemia is a surgical emergency that can result in limb loss if not treated expeditiously.

- Once the diagnosis is made, therapeutic anticoagulation is indicated. Further workup and planning is dictated by the clinical presentation, past medical history, health of the patient, and further imaging.
- Compartment syndrome is also a surgical emergency managed by fasciotomies and conscientious wound care.

COMPREHENSION QUESTIONS

1. Of the signs and symptoms of acute leg ischemia, which is typically the last one to occur?
   - A. Pain
   - B. Pallor
   - C. Poikilothermia
   - D. Pulselessness
   - E. Paresthesia
   - F. Paralysis

2. What is the cutoff on ABI for critical leg ischemia?

3. True/false: acute limb ischemia is associated with ulcerations.

4. Which is *not* a fascial compartment of the leg?
   - A. Anterior
   - B. Lateral
   - C. Medial
   - D. Deep posterior
   - E. Superficial posterior

Answers

1. **F.** Paralysis is a late finding suggesting muscle necrosis and nerve injury, both of which take a substantial period of time. The other signs and symptoms tend to evolve much sooner.

2. **0.4** is the usual cutoff for critical limb ischemia, and it usually causes rest pain. This is time for either endovascular or open intervention to improve flow to the distal extremities to improve rest pain and/or prevent gangrene.

3. **False.** *Acute* limb ischemia is not associated with ulcerations unless superimposed on ischemia that is also chronically present. The chronicity of peripheral ischemia matters, especially when considering the appropriate intervention in the acutely cold extremity.

4. **C.** The medial compartment does not exist in the leg.

A 36-year-old Woman Status Post Motor Vehicle Accident While Intoxicated

Shamim H. Nejad, MD and
Nadia Quijije, MD

A trauma alert is called for a 36-year-old woman brought in by ambulance after intentionally crashing her car into a tree while intoxicated. On physical examination, her vitals are: T 98.6, BP 165/80, HR 115, RR 16, O_2 88% on RA, and 96% with 3 L NC. She is slightly lethargic and disoriented to time, but able to answer simple questions. She complains of acute pain in her chest along with a mild headache. She displays no evidence of diaphoresis or tremor and denies feeling anxious or nauseated. Pupils are reactive, without any evidence of nystagmus. The remainder of the neurological and general examination is normal.

The patient gives a history of binge-type drinking, in which she consumes "a lot" of vodka every weekend. She denies daily drinking, however also reports that alcohol helps her sleep at night. She reports 1 previous detox approximately 1.5 years ago. She also notes losing 1 job in the past due to her alcohol use, along with it affecting past relationships, and legal complications due to assaulting others while intoxicated. She denies a history of past delirium tremens or alcohol withdrawal seizures. She denies any history of benzodiazepine, cannabis, cocaine, heroin, or other drug use.

Her injuries include multiple left-sided rib fractures and a subarachnoid hemorrhage for which she is started on levetiracetam (Keppra) for seizure prophylaxis. She is found to have a blood alcohol level (BAL) of 3600 mg/L in the emergency department, along with an AST of 235 U/L, an ALT of 120 U/L, and a normal mean corpuscular volume (MCV) of 95.

1. Name 4 symptoms or signs of alcohol withdrawal.

2. Is she at high risk of developing alcohol withdrawal syndrome (AWS)? How can you tell?

3. What is the treatment of symptoms due to alcohol withdrawal?

4. For a patient with AWS, when should psychiatry be consulted?

ALCOHOL WITHDRAWAL

Answers

1. Long-term exposure to ethanol results in adaptive changes in several neurotransmitter systems. Abrupt withdrawal of ethanol results in nonphysiologic levels of these neurotransmitters, which in turn cause the signs and symptoms

Table 20-1. Alcohol Withdrawal Symptom Clusters

Symptom Cluster	Symptoms	Pathophysiology	Treatment
Type A	**Anxiety,** restlessness, nausea, general malaise, *minor* tremor	Decreased GABA	**GABA agonist administration** (ie, benzodiazepines, phenobarbital, etc)
Type B	**Tremor, tachycardia, hypertension,** diaphoresis, fever	Excess noradrenaline	**β-Blockers, α-agonists,** antihypertensives
Type C	**Confusion,** paranoia, hallucinations, agitation	Excess dopamine	**Dopamine antagonist** (ie, intravenous haloperidol, atypical agents)

The bold words represent the most prevalent symptoms and the primary form of treatment respectively.

of alcohol withdrawal. Understanding the basics of these changes not only can help guide your choice of therapy but also can help you appreciate alarming versus less concerning signs.

The changes in neurotransmitter systems can be clustered as shown in Table 20-1.

Chronic exposure to alcohol results in an increase in glutamatergic reaction and decrease in GABA activity. When alcohol is abruptly removed, decreased GABA activity leads to symptoms of anxiety and restlessness, referred to as *uncomplicated* AWS. Concomitantly, excess glutamate stimulates an increase in

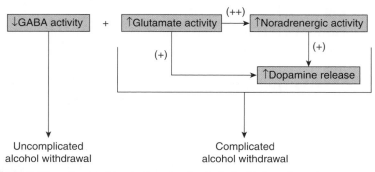

Figure 20-1. Neurotransmitter dysfunction in alcohol withdrawal syndromes.

Table 20-2. Alcohol Withdrawal Syndromes

Stages	Clinical Findings	Onset (h)
Uncomplicated (early)	Tremulousness, mild anxiety, headache, diaphoresis, palpitations, anorexia, GI upset	1–36
Complicated		
Alcohol withdrawal seizure	Generalized tonic–clonic seizures, status epilepticus (rare)	1–48
Alcoholic hallucinosis	Visual, auditory, and/or tactile hallucinations; paranoia; delusions	1–48
Delirium tremens	Delirium, tachycardia, hypertension, agitation, fever, diaphoresis	24–96

noradrenaline and dopamine, as shown in Figure 20-1. Increased noradrenaline results in Type B symptoms resulting in increased sympathetic activity (see Table 20-1). Increased dopaminergic activity leads to Type C symptoms, a contributor to alcohol hallucinosis and, in conjunction with severe Type B symptoms, delirium tremens (alcohol withdrawal delirium). Seizures, alcoholic hallucinosis, and delirium tremens are AWSs referred to as *complicated* AWS (see Table 20-2).

2. Knowing the risk factors for complicated alcohol withdrawal symptoms can help you obtain an appropriate history, decide when and how to initiate alcohol withdrawal prophylaxis, and guide your therapy of early symptoms.

   Major risk factors:

   - A history of past alcohol withdrawal seizures and/or delirium tremens
   - Heavier and longer alcohol consumption history
   - Elevated MCV
   - Elevated AST:ALT ratio

   Context-dependent risk factors:
   - More days since the last drink (2 or more days of cessation)
   - Elevated blood alcohol on admission
   - Decreased platelets
   - Decreased albumin
   - History of falls, particularly presentations with long bone fractures
   - Patients with burn-related injuries
   - Age >35 years

   The last item bears some additional explanation. While patients below the age of 35 years may experience symptoms of uncomplicated alcohol withdrawal, the development of any type of meaningful complicated alcohol withdrawal symptoms tends to be rare. The exception to this general rule is when patients have a history of traumatic brain injury (lowers the seizure threshold), or when chronic heavy use was initiated in teenage years, which generally results in abnormal CNS development.

It is imperative that alcohol dependence be identified early in order to perform adequate prophylaxis and prevent AWS (particularly complicated alcohol withdrawal symptoms). Data regarding the use of alcohol should be elicited during the intake history of all patients. If the patient is alert and able to clearly communicate, the fastest option is to start with a single alcohol use screening question: "How many times in the last 2 weeks have you had 'X' or more drinks in a day?" (X is 5 for men and 4 for women). If the patient has had these many drinks at any point in the last 2 weeks, then additional questioning should be performed. The CAGE or T-ACE questionnaires are particularly useful, simple, and efficient screening tools (Table 20-3). If these more detailed screening tests are positive for chronic alcohol use, then you need to assess the patient's risk for alcohol withdrawal. Relevant data include quantity of alcohol consumed, duration of use, the longest period of sobriety in the last 6 months, past history of withdrawal symptoms during periods of sobriety, past detox, and last detox complications.

Table 20-3. The CAGE and T-ACE Screening Tools

CAGE		T-ACE	
C	Have you ever felt you should **cut down** on your drinking?	T	**Tolerance**: How many drinks does it take to make you feel high?
A	Have people **annoyed** you by criticizing your drinking?	A	Have people **annoyed** you by criticizing your drinking?
G	Have you ever felt bad or **guilty** about your drinking?	C	Have you ever felt you ought to **cut down** on your drinking?
E	**Eye-opener**: Have you ever had a drink first thing in the morning to steady your nerves or to get rid of a hangover?	E	**Eye-opener**: Have you ever had a drink first thing in the morning to steady your nerves or get rid of a hangover?

The CAGE can identify alcohol problems over the lifetime. Two positive responses are considered a positive test and indicate further assessment is warranted.

The T-ACE, which is based on the CAGE, is helpful in identifying range of use, including lifetime use and prenatal use. A score of 2 or more is considered positive. Affirmative answers to questions A, C, or E = 1 point each. Reporting tolerance to more than 2 drinks (the T question) = 2 points.

Many patients feel that their care may be compromised if they notify their surgical team of their actual alcohol consumption. A nonconfrontational approach, with clear communication to the patient that this information is needed for optimal medical care (and to prevent morbidity and mortality) and will not be used to judge him/her, is advised. In all cases, collateral history from friends and family should be obtained if possible; however, the accuracy of this information should also be weighed.

While history from the patient or the patient's family can be helpful, objective data can also provide additional information regarding the risk of AWS. These objective data are particularly important if the patient is unable to provide any history due to a compromised mental status or the severity of illness. Physical examination can reveal tremors, diaphoresis, nystagmus, or autonomic hyperactivity. Laboratory results can be particularly helpful in the evaluation of the risk for development of alcohol withdrawal delirium (DTs). Relevant labs include admission BAL, urine toxicology screen, AST:ALT ratio, MCV, Hct, platelet count, albumin, and B_{12}. All of these labs are imperative for the evaluation of the risk for development of alcohol withdrawal delirium (DTs).

3. As in all medical patients, treatment should be individualized to symptoms and severity. Clinical examination can be centered on evaluating symptom clusters (see Table 20-1). Type A symptoms are those of CNS excitation and are most commonly treated with benzodiazepines. Type B symptoms are those of noradrenergic excess (diaphoresis, tremor, tachycardia, hypertension, fever). They are best controlled with the use of β-blockers in patients with concern for demand ischemia, and with α-agonists (dexmedetomidine, clonidine) or other antihypertensive medications for symptoms of significant hypertension. Type C symptoms are those due to a hyperdopaminergic state (confusion, paranoia, hallucinations, and agitation) and are treated with the use of dopamine antagonists.

When treating a patient with alcohol withdrawal, you must first treat any Type B emergencies (severe tachycardia, hypertensive crisis) or Type C emergencies (agitation, hallucinations), and then review clinically to ensure that Type A symptoms are also well controlled. In the absence of emergent signs, Type A symptoms are primarily evaluated and treated as described below.

In early uncomplicated AWS, benzodiazepines are helpful in controlling signs and symptoms. Long-acting benzodiazepines (such as chlordiazepoxide and diazepam) are helpful secondary to their slower elimination half-life and self-tapering properties, possibly providing for a smoother course of alcohol withdrawal symptoms. Patients with impaired liver function may benefit from shorter-acting agents (such as lorazepam and oxazepam) that only undergo glucuronidation and not hepatic oxidation (see Table 20-4).

Benzodiazepine dosing is nonstandardized due to significant individual variability in dosages required for symptom control, along with differences in underlying medical and surgical illness that may predispose the patient to

Table 20-4. Commonly Utilized Benzodiazepines for Type A Symptoms of Alcohol Withdrawal

Agent	Usual Starting Dose	Elimination Half-life (Including Active Metabolites)
Lorazepam	0.5–2 mg IV/PO q 4 h PRN or standing	10–20 h
Diazepam	5–10 mg IV/PO q 4 h PRN or standing	Diazepam: 20–75 h Nordiazepam: 36–100 h
Chlordiazepoxide	25–100 mg PO q 2 h PRN or 25–50 mg PO q 6 h standing (maximum: 100–300 mg/day depending on alcohol use severity and underlying medical/surgical illness)	Chlordiazepoxide: 5–30 h Diazepam: 20–75 h Nordiazepam: 36–100 h Temazepam: 8–20 h Oxazepam: 5–15 h

increased risk of using sedating medications. The clinician's goal is to lightly sedate the patient to control symptoms of hyperarousal.

Benzodiazepines should never be dosed for nonspecific signs of tachycardia and hypertension. These 2 signs may be secondary to a variety of other medical etiologies besides alcohol withdrawal. Furthermore, benzodiazepines do not actually affect the noradrenergic system and so are not effective agents for these abnormalities.

Once symptoms and signs are well controlled, the dosage is tapered. For shorter-acting benzodiazepines, doses should be reduced by 25% per day. For longer-acting agents, doses can be reduced by as much as 30% to 50% per day to allow for auto-tapering and the prevention of a buildup of active metabolites. Some institutions utilize symptom-triggered protocols for the administration of benzodiazepines; however, there have been no trials to date validating this method in the acute medically and surgically ill patient. In certain instances, these protocol-based methods have even been shown to lead to complications in the general hospital setting.

In addition to the medications described above, patients who chronically use alcohol should be treated with the use of intravenous (or intramuscular) thiamine. Administration of at least 200 mg daily is indicated for the prevention of Wernicke encephalopathy and Korsakoff psychosis. Dosages below this, or administered via the enteral route, are ineffective.

4. Consultation should be provided at any time when the primary surgical team would like assistance for symptoms of alcohol withdrawal. In addition, other

times in which consultation with the psychiatry consultation service may be helpful include:

- In the preoperative period, including for anticipated elective operations
- In the perioperative period when there is concern that autonomic hyperactivity may lead to demand ischemia, MI, respiratory compromise
- In the postoperative period when it is felt that AWS is compromising the safety and stability of a patient
- When alcohol withdrawal may lead to worsening mental status and agitation

TIPS TO REMEMBER

- Assessment of alcohol use should be obtained at the earliest possible time.
- Seizures, hallucinations, and delirium tremens differentiate complicated alcohol withdrawal from uncomplicated alcohol withdrawal.
- Untreated and severe Type B and C symptoms may lead to complicated withdrawal. It may be difficult to separate these symptom clusters entirely as they represent dynamic neurotransmitter systems that are interrelated and, importantly, may become dysfunctional from other medical/surgical etiologies.
- Benzodiazepines are used as prophylaxis and/or treatment of uncomplicated AWS. Type A symptoms are most effectively treated with benzodiazepines.
- Patients with a previous history of seizures and/or DTs are at especially high risk for alcohol withdrawal delirium and these patients should be covered via prophylaxis if possible, with adequate coverage of Type B and C symptoms, should they develop.
- Complicated AWS requires urgent psychiatric consultation.

COMPREHENSION QUESTIONS

1. Which of the following describes symptoms of complicated alcohol withdrawal?
   A. Slurred speech, ataxia, and nystagmus
   B. Agitation, diaphoresis, and presence of visual hallucinations
   C. Anxiety, restlessness, mild tremor, and nausea
   D. Lacrimation, diarrhea, diaphoresis, and myalgia

2. Which of the following describes symptoms of early alcohol withdrawal?
   A. Breath smelling of alcohol, slurred speech, and ataxia
   B. Agitation, hypertension, and tactile hallucinations
   C. Tremors, mild anxiety, and diaphoresis
   D. Lacrimation, diarrhea, diaphoresis, and myalgias

3. Of the following, which is the highest-risk patient for alcohol withdrawal delirium?
> A. A 20-year-old man, (+) BAL, elevated AST:ALT ratio, normal MCV, consumes 6 beers/day for the last month
> B. A 40-year-old woman, (−) BAL, drinks 1 to 2 drinks/week, no history of DUIs
> C. A 50-year-old man, (+) BAL, elevated AST:ALT ratio, elevated MCV, consumes 6 beers/day for the last month
> D. A 55-year-old man, (+) BAL, normal MCV, normal liver function tests

4. Which of the following is a long-acting benzodiazepine?
> A. Chlordiazepoxide
> B. Oxazepam
> C. Lorazepam
> D. Midazolam

Answers

1. **B**. Seizures and hallucinations, along with autonomic dysfunction and the presence of delirium, are signs and symptoms of complicated alcohol withdrawal. Choice A describes benzodiazepine intoxication. Choice C describes uncomplicated alcohol withdrawal. Choice D represents symptoms of opioid withdrawal.

2. **C**. Tremulousness, anxiety, headache, palpitations, anorexia, nausea, and GI upset are all signs and symptoms of uncomplicated alcohol withdrawal.

3. **C**. While both A and C carry the highest risk of the scenarios presented, the patient in answer C is greater than 35 years old (increased risk factor) versus the patient in A, in which his younger age should provide some protection. In addition, the patient in C has an elevated MCV in the presence of an elevated AST:ALT ratio, likely corresponding to a longer and heavier drinking history.

4. **A**. Chlordiazepoxide has a half-life of 30 to 100 hours. Choices B and C are all intermediate-acting benzodiazepines, and D is a short-acting benzodiazepine.

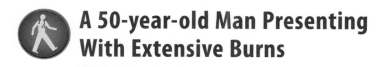

A 50-year-old Man Presenting With Extensive Burns

Jeremy Goverman, MD, FACS and Shawn P. Fagan, MD, FACS

A 50-year-old, 75-kg, male is brought into the emergency department by EMS. He was found ambulating at the scene of a house fire approximately 2 hours prior. He is noted to have circumferential third-degree burns to his entire right and left upper extremities as well as his entire head and neck. In the emergency department he is alert and oriented, and complains of a dry mouth.

1. **What is the first step in assessing this patient?**

2. **How large is this patient's burn?**

3. **According to the Parkland formula, how much fluid will this patient need during the first 8 hours? Next 16 hours? What is the initial intravenous fluid rate?**

4. **Should this patient be transferred to an American Burn Association–verified Burn Center?**

5. **Why is it important to know if a burn is circumferential? What procedure would you perform?**

BURNS

Answers

1. As with every trauma, begin with ATLS protocol and assessment of ABCs. In this case the patient will require intubation for airway protection. Given the size (>20%) and location of the burn, the patient will require large-volume resuscitation and will likely develop significant facial and airway edema. Elective intubation prior to the development of airway edema is common practice for larger burns.

2. The rule of 9's allows for a simplified approach to calculate total body surface area (TBSA) for a burn (Figure 21-1). The Lund and Browder method (which utilizes a chart) is commonly used for estimation of burn size in children.

    In the case above, each upper extremity is 9, head is 9, neck is 1 = 28% TBSA.

3. The Parkland formula is a formula used for the initial fluid resuscitation of a burn patient with >20% TBSA. It estimates the overall fluid total as 4 mL × % TBSA × weight (kg). Half of this volume is to be administered in the first 8 hours post burn, while the second half of this volume is to be administered over the next 16 hours.

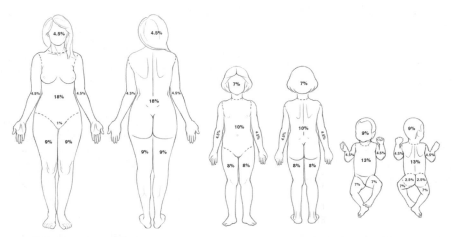

Figure 21-1. The rule of 9's. (Reproduced with permission from Kaufman MS, Stead LG, Stead SM, et al. *First Aid for the Surgery Clerkship*. 2nd ed. New York: McGraw-Hill; 2009:299 [Figure 18-1].)

The Parkland formula should only serve as a guide to resuscitation. Global (ie, lactate, base deficit, pH) and regional (ie, urine output, mental status) parameters of perfusion should be followed and trended in order to fine-tune the resuscitation volumes. Typically crystalloid is used for the first 8 hours and varying quantities of colloid (ie, albumin) are added in according to patient needs and surgeon preference. As resuscitation volumes approach and exceed 6 cm³/% TBSA/kg, the incidence of compartment syndromes and intra-abdominal hypertension increases. In such cases, the addition of colloid may allow for slightly less overall fluid administration.

In this case 4 mL × 28% third-degree burn × 75 kg = 8400 cm³. This is the total fluid to be given over 24 hours (4200 cm³/first 8 hours, 4200 cm³/next 16 hours). Since the patient presented 2 hours post injury, the first 4200 cm³ should be given over 6 hours. IVF rates would be 700 cm³/h (first 6 hours), and 262.5 cm³/h (second 16 hours).

4. Yes; because this second-degree burn involves the face, this patient should be transferred to a burn center. According to the American Burn Association the following 10 items require transfer to a burn center:

   1. Partial thickness burns greater than 10% TBSA.

   2. Burns that involve the face, hands, feet, genitalia, perineum, or major joints.

   3. Third-degree burns in any age group.

4. Electrical burns, including lightning injury.

5. Chemical burns.

6. Inhalation injury.

7. Burn injury in patients with preexisting medical disorders that could complicate management, prolong recovery, or affect mortality.

8. Any patient with burns and concomitant trauma (such as fractures) in which the burn injury poses the greatest risk of morbidity or mortality. In such cases, if the trauma poses the greater immediate risk, the patient may be initially stabilized in a trauma center before being transferred to a burn unit. Physician judgment will be necessary in such situations and should be in concert with the regional medical control plan and triage protocols.

9. Burned children in hospitals without qualified personnel or equipment for the care of children.

10. Burn injury in patients who will require special social, emotional, or rehabilitative intervention.

5. Escharotomy: A circumferential second- or third-degree burn, on extremities or digits, has the potential to compromise circulation. A significant burn on the anterior torso has the potential to compromise ventilation. Prompt attention to such burns can prevent serious complications. The appropriate anatomic sites for escharotomies vary; however, a proper escharotomy should extend into normal skin on either end of the incision and penetrate through the dermis up to the subcutaneous tissue. The ultimate goal is decompression, while at the same time minimizing exposure of, or damage to, neurovascular structures. When possible, escharotomies should be located at the sites of standard fasciotomy incisions. This facilitates evaluation and treatment of compartment syndrome, which may accompany a massive fluid resuscitation.

TIPS TO REMEMBER

- Rule of 9's: head 9%, each upper extremity 9%, each lower extremity 18%, anterior chest + abdomen 18%, and back 18%.

- First-degree burns are not included in TBSA calculations.

- <20% TBSA does not require large-volume resuscitation (ie, Parkland formula).

- Parkland formula = 4 mL × % TBSA × weight/kg; give one half in the first 8 hours post injury.

- Burn depth often progresses over the first 24 hours post burn.

- Massive fluid resuscitation has the potential to cause secondary compartment syndrome, that is, orbital, abdominal, extremity. Treatments include increasing colloid as fluid, lateral canthotomy, paralysis, abdominal decompression, and escharotomy/fasciotomy.

COMPREHENSION QUESTIONS

1. A 33-year-old man is noted to have first-degree burns to his entire left leg, third-degree burns to his entire right leg, as well as second- and third-degree burns to his entire anterior chest and abdomen. Which of the following statements is *false*?
    A. He may require escharotomies to his chest.
    B. He will require large-volume resuscitation (ie, Parkland formula).
    C. He has a 54% TBSA burn.
    D. He fulfills the ABA criteria for transfer to a burn center.

2. A 20-year-old female is seen in the emergency department after scalding herself with hot soup. She is noted to have blistering of her anterior thigh with involvement of her genitals. Which of the following is most likely true?
    A. She has an 18% TBSA burn.
    B. She may require large-volume resuscitation (ie, Parkland formula).
    C. She fulfills the ABA criteria for transfer to a burn center.
    D. She should be resuscitated with albumin.

3. A 50-year-old male electrical worker was involved in a high-voltage electrical injury at approximately 8 AM. He was intubated in the field by EMS and transferred to the local emergency department where he was given 4 L of lactated Ringer's solution and quickly transferred to a regional verified burn center. The patient arrived to the burn center at 1 PM and is noted to have a 40% TBSA burn. He is 100 kg. What should his initial fluid rate on arrival to the burn center be?
    A. 1000 cm³/h
    B. 1333 cm³/h
    C. 800 cm³/h
    D. 500 cm³/h

Answers

1. **C.** Only second- and third-degree burns are included in calculations of TBSA. Leg (18%) + anterior chest (9%) + anterior abdomen (9%) = 36% TBSA.

2. **C.** Burns that involve the genitalia, perineum, face, hands, or feet fulfill criteria for burn center transfer.

3. **B.** Total fluid requirement first 24 hours = 4 (40 × 100) = 16,000 cm³. Therefore, 8 L (one half the total resuscitation volume) must be given in the first 8 hours. The patient has already received 4 L in the first 5 hours; therefore, he requires an additional 4 L over the next 3 hours: 1.33 L/h.

SUGGESTED READING

Herndon D. *Total Burn Care*. 4th ed. Philadelphia, PA: Elsevier, Inc; 2012.

A 56-year-old Man 6 Days Status Post Colectomy With New Pelvic Discomfort

Michael F. McGee, MD and
Brian C. George, MD

You evaluate an otherwise healthy 56-year-old man in the emergency department with a 4-day history of worsening left lower quadrant abdominal pain and fever. He has no evidence of peritonitis or sepsis. Computed tomography (CT) imaging of the abdomen and pelvis reveals sigmoid diverticulitis without abscess. The patient is admitted for a trial of bowel rest and broad-spectrum intravenous antibiotics. After 48 hours, the patient worsens clinically and undergoes sigmoid colectomy, end colostomy, and oversewing of the distal rectal stump (Hartmann procedure).

Six days later, while on call for the general surgery service, you are asked to evaluate the same patient who has been recovering uneventfully until now. He complains of new mild pelvic discomfort, anorexia, and difficulty voiding. His bowel function has not yet returned. He has a low-grade fever, mild tachycardia, and moderate right lower quadrant tenderness to deep palpation. A CBC with differential reveals leukocytosis with neutrophil predominance. CT of his abdomen and pelvis with oral and intravenous contrast reveals a 6-cm rim-enhancing pelvic fluid collection surrounding the rectal stump (see Figure 22-1).

1. Does this patient have an abscess or does he have a phlegmon?

2. Would this fluid collection be classified as primary, secondary, or tertiary?

3. Why does this patient have an ileus?

4. Is it reasonable to treat this patient with antibiotics alone?

5. What class of microbes should you cover with antibiotics?

6. Would you order this patient's CT with oral, IV, or both types of contrast?

7. Based on the available CT imaging, do you think your interventional radiology (IR) colleagues would agree to drain this abscess percutaneously?

INTRA-ABDOMINAL ABSCESS

Answers

1. An intra-abdominal abscess (IAA) is a contained collection of infected fluid within the confines of the peritoneal cavity, with or without associated pockets

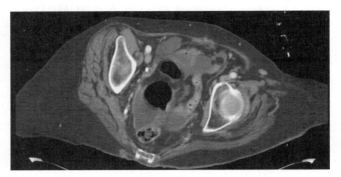

Figure 22-1. Axial CT of a postoperative pelvic fluid collection.

of gas. A phlegmon, in contrast, is an inflammatory mass without identifiable fluid. The patient in the case vignette has IAA.

2. There are several ways to classify IAA, although the etiologic classification is the most common:

- Primary IAAs are monomicrobial infections that arise spontaneously without any identifiable breach of the gastrointestinal tract. Spontaneous bacterial peritonitis is an example of a primary IAA.

- Secondary IAAs result from spontaneous, surgical, or iatrogenic violation of the gastrointestinal tract and account for the overwhelming majority of abscesses encountered by the surgeon. Diverticular abscesses are a common example of secondary IAA.

- Tertiary IAAs are recurrent infections following treatment of primary or secondary abscesses. These recalcitrant IAAs typically contain antibiotic-resistant nosocomial infections.

Given the relative infrequency of primary and tertiary abscesses, this chapter will focus on secondary IAA, and more specifically on intraperitoneal secondary IAA, which is present in the patient in the case vignette.

3. IAA may present with a wide range of clinical manifestations. Classic findings for spontaneous IAA include fever, lethargy, leukocytosis, and abdominal pain or fullness. Rarely, IAA may present with overt peritonitis or sepsis. The local inflammation can cause changes in bowel habits, including nausea, vomiting, diarrhea, or constipation. Similarly, a prolonged postoperative ileus can often be the initial manifestation of postoperative IAA, as is the case in this vignette. Subphrenic abscesses can cause hiccups and a sympathetic pleural effusion, while pelvic abscesses can cause tenesmus, lower back pain, and urinary retention. Physical exam may reveal focal tenderness or occasionally a palpable abdominal mass, while low pelvic abscesses may be palpated on digital rectal exam.

4. Generally no. Systemic antibiotic therapy is thought to have poor penetration into an abscess cavity for several reasons. First, host neutrophils form an inflammatory rind of fibrin that encases and entraps the collection, walling the cavity off from host circulation and preventing penetration of circulating antibiotic. It also markedly reduces the oxygen available in the cavity, and as a consequence of these anaerobic conditions, the abscess cavity contents are usually acidic. This acid further reduces the efficacy of any antibiotic that does manage to penetrate the cavity.

For these reasons, classical surgical dogma states that antibiotics alone are not helpful and recommend source control via abscess drainage. Antibiotics should still be used, but only as adjunctive treatment for IAA in order to prevent extension of infection into the surrounding soft tissue. There are a few narrow circumstances, however, where it may be appropriate to violate the classical dogma and treat with antibiotics alone. For example, immunocompetent patients who only have small abscesses and do not have any other concerning signs (eg, peritonitis, sepsis) may not require drainage for full recovery. It bears emphasizing, however, that any patient with sepsis, peritonitis, or evidence of end-organ dysfunction requires emergent (likely surgical) drainage—in those cases, antibiotic therapy alone is typically not helpful.

5. Virtually all secondary IAAs contain gut flora. Common aerobes include *Escherichia coli*, *Enterococcus*, and *Klebsiella* species while common anaerobes include *Bacteroides fragilis* and *Peptostreptococcus* species. Suitable first-line antimicrobials include piperacillin–tazobactam, ticarcillin–clavulanate, ertapenem, or tigecycline as single-agent therapy, or combinations of metronidazole with cefazolin, cefuroxime, levofloxacin, or ciprofloxacin.

6. Both types of contrast should be used. Contemporary CT imaging can accurately diagnose IAA with a sensitivity and specificity that exceeds 90%. In the stable patient without indication for immediate surgical exploration, cross-sectional imaging presents important data to the surgeon regarding underlying abscess etiology and may provide nonoperative treatment alternatives that may obviate or temporize surgery until conditions are ideal. In special circumstances, ultrasound may play an ancillary role in diagnosing IAA with slightly lower accuracy rates compared with CT or MRI.

IAAs are defined on CT as a fluid collection with or without associated pockets of gas. An abscess is in contradistinction to a phlegmon, which is an inflammatory mass without identifiable fluid. Enteral contrast (either oral or rectal) can be a helpful adjunct that distinguishes loops of bowel from the abscess cavity and may provocatively assess anastomoses for leaks or fistulae. Intravenous contrast provides a pathognomonic "rim enhancement" that is seen along the outer rind of the abscess cavity. Abscess architecture can be classified as simple or loculated, referring to the degree of internal pockets or presence of septae. The location of the abscess, both absolute and relative to other organs, can be assessed and may diagnose the pathology responsible for the abscess (see Figure 22-2).

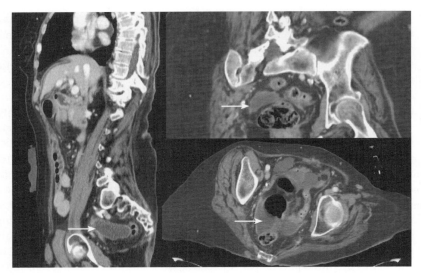

Figure 22-2. Axial, coronal, and sagittal CT reconstructions of a postoperative pelvic abscess.

7. The development of percutaneous image-guided drainage techniques in the early 1980s has markedly impacted the management of IAA. Prior to the advent of cross-sectional imaging, the diagnosis and management of IAA often required surgical reexploration that conveyed mortality rates as high as 40%.

   IAA with favorable characteristics can often be managed with image-guided drain placement. Ideally, the target fluid collection must be well circumscribed and have radiographic characteristics of an abscess, rather than free ascites. There must be a radiographic window that permits a safe percutaneous trajectory for real-time image-guided needle passage without causing injury to other structures. Abscesses typically must be larger than 4 cm for consideration of drain placement, although smaller abscesses can be aspirated without placement of a drain or treated with antibiotics alone. Solitary, noncomplex, nonloculated abscesses are ideal candidates for successful image-guided drainage procedures with success rates of approximately 80%.

TIPS TO REMEMBER

- IAAs with sepsis, peritonitis, or failing nonoperative management typically require prompt resuscitation and surgical exploration.
- Image-guided drain placement is suitable for stable patients with confirmed abscess >4 cm. Smaller fluid collections can be aspirated under image guidance or treated with antibiotics alone.

- Antibiotic therapy alone is only helpful for small abscesses or phlegmons. Larger abscesses require drainage via percutaneous or surgical approaches with antibiotics relegated to an adjunctive role.
- Some abscess locations will not permit a safe radiographic window or trajectory for image-guided drainage and may require surgical drainage.

COMPREHENSION QUESTIONS

1. A 16-year-old male with a 3-week history of right lower quadrant pain presents to the emergency department. An abdominopelvic CT shows a 6-cm phlegmon adjacent to an inflamed appendix with small pockets of free air. He is febrile, mildly tachycardic, and normotensive without peritoneal signs. The next step of management should be which of the following?
    A. Begin intravenous piperacillin–tazobactam.
    B. Appendectomy.
    C. Arrange for image-guided percutaneous drain placement.
    D. Colonoscopy.

2. A 32-year-old woman with Crohn disease has been receiving inpatient intravenous steroids and antibiotics for 2 weeks. She suddenly develops fever and worsening abdominal pain. CT reveals a 6-cm rim-enhancing fluid collection adjacent to a thickened, inflamed terminal ileum. The next step of management should be which of the following?
    A. Continue antibiotics and observe.
    B. Terminal ileal resection and operative abscess drainage.
    C. Arrange for image-guided percutaneous drain placement.
    D. Start acetaminophen for fever and β-blocker for tachycardia.

3. A 55-year-old male presents to the emergency department with a 5-day history of worsening left lower quadrant pain. He is tachycardic and febrile with intense left lower quadrant tenderness. CT reveals a 7-cm left lower quadrant fluid and air collection adjacent to a segment of thickened sigmoid colon with multiple diverticula. After resuscitation and IV antibiotics his blood pressure is 85/60 mm Hg and he has left lower quadrant guarding. The next management step should be which of the following?
    A. Sigmoid colectomy.
    B. Broaden antibiotics to cover tertiary abscesses.
    C. Arrange for image-guided percutaneous drain placement.
    D. Repeat CT scan.

Answers

1. **A.** A chronic phlegmon without sepsis or peritonitis should be managed first with antibiotics and close observation. A chronic phlegmon may be hostile

(difficult and dangerous to operate on), and surgery is reserved for sepsis or failure of medical therapy. A phlegmon typically contains no drainable fluid and is not amenable to percutaneous drainage. Colonoscopy may eventually be necessary to evaluate for inflammatory bowel disease, but is not necessary acutely.

2. **C.** Image-guided drain placement would be ideal for the stable patient with a drainable abscess. This patient is worsening despite 2 weeks of antibiotics and continued antibiotic therapy alone will not help. In this high-risk patient, operation would be reserved for failure of percutaneous drainage, sepsis, or peritonitis. Acetaminophen and β-blockers may only mask symptoms and will not treat the patient's underlying pathology.

3. **A.** This patient requires abscess drainage. He is hypotensive, which determines the means by which you should drain the abscess. Hypotension makes image-guided drainage a risky procedure and is generally considered a contraindication. Instead, he should undergo prompt resuscitation and an emergent operation. Antibiotics play only an adjunctive role for a large drainable abscess. Short-interval re-imaging is wasteful, dangerous, and unhelpful in this hypotensive patient.

Section III.
Handling Inpatients

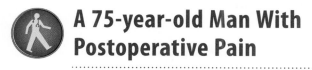

A 75-year-old Man With Postoperative Pain

Ezra N. Teitelbaum, MD

A 75-year-old, otherwise healthy man undergoes an elective right hemicolectomy for colon cancer. The case was converted from laparoscopic to open due to dense adhesions from a prior laparotomy. Six hours after the operation, you are paged by the patient's nurse because he is complaining of 8 out of 10 abdominal pain and his next dose of "prn" morphine is not available for another 2 hours.

When you arrive at the bedside, the patient is alert and answers all questions appropriately. He complains of a sharp pain along the length of his incision that was improved from 10 out of 10 to 6 out of 10 after receiving a dose of morphine 4 hours ago. In the past hour, however, the pain has been gradually increasing and is once again 10 out of 10. He is not nauseated and has not vomited.

His vital signs are: temperature 37.2°C, heart rate 85, blood pressure 150/90, and respiratory rate 12. His abdomen is soft with localized and appropriate tenderness along the length of the midline incision dressing. He is making 100 mL/h of clear yellow urine and, except for the pain, has been recovering well.

You review his medications and find he is ordered for "morphine 2 mg IV q6h prn pain." He has received a single dose since arriving to the surgical ward 4 hours ago.

1. **Why did you have to come see the patient and not simply provide a new order over the phone?**

2. **How would you change the order for his pain medications?**

3. **Name 3 common side effects of opioids.**

4. **Name 2 nonopiate medications that can be used in the immediate postoperative period (ie, when the patient is NPO).**

5. **When and how should this patient be transitioned to oral pain medications?**

POSTOPERATIVE PAIN MANAGEMENT

Answers

1. When evaluating a patient complaining of an unusual amount of pain, or pain that is persistent despite the administration of medication, your first thought should always be that the pain might be the result of a surgical complication. While the most common cause of pain in the immediate postoperative period is inadequate analgesia, this should always be considered a diagnosis of exclusion. Therefore, patients with refractory pain need to be evaluated *in person*, and orders to increase the dose of narcotics should never be given over the phone. On

your way to evaluate this patient you should be thinking of the possibility that bleeding, an anastomotic leak, or a missed bowel injury is responsible for his pain.

Your bedside history and physical exam should therefore focus on ruling out these serious complications. The fact that the patient's pain is localized to his incision, rather than the site of the anastomosis (likely the RUQ or RLQ) or diffusely over the entire abdomen, is reassuring, as is the fact that the pain is partially relieved by medication. The patient's vital signs are also within normal limits except for mild hypertension. Any fever, tachycardia, hypotension, or tachypnea in the immediate postoperative period is concerning and may be the result of hypovolemia (due to bleeding) or an inflammatory response (due to infection, anastomotic leak, or another complication). Hypertension in isolation is a common result of pain itself and is not immediately concerning (see Chapter 36 on postoperative hypertension for criteria for when you *should* be concerned).

The abdominal exam (or other surgery site–specific exam) is an essential component to differentiating between pain from inadequate analgesia and pain secondary to a complication. Patients with poorly controlled but uncomplicated pain should still have abdomens that are soft to palpation, especially away from the area of the incision. Your exam should thus start laterally (if you are examining a patient with a midline laparotomy) and proceed medially toward the incision. If the patient has an abdominal drain, then its output should be closely examined for bile, succus, stool, or frank blood.

If you are confronted with a patient with poorly controlled pain and any of these "warning signs," you should notify your senior resident or the attending immediately. While it's always good to come up with a plan for investigating potential complications (eg, checking a CBC to rule out bleeding) before making that call, such a workup should never be initiated on your own without keeping everyone "in the loop" about what is going on with a potentially sick patient.

2. After you have reassured yourself that this patient's pain is not due to a surgical complication, the next step is to look at the existing pain orders and the medication administration record (MAR) to see how you can best address the inadequate analgesia. In this case, the patient's morphine order has too low a dose and too long an interval between doses. For treating pain in an average patient after a laparotomy or other major surgery, an order of morphine 4 mg IV q3h or q4h is a good place to start. Keep in mind that younger adult patients and patients taking opioids chronically at home will typically require higher doses of narcotics. Conversely, elderly patients or those with renal insufficiency should be started on lower doses.

   In this patient, starting a patient-controlled analgesia (PCA) pump is an even better solution than simply increasing the dose and frequency of his morphine order. A PCA allows patients to control the administration of intravenous opioids themselves by pressing a button attached to the PCA pump. The physician indicates in the PCA order the dose that is given with each button press and a "lockout" interval that is required to elapse between presses before the pump will administer a second dose.

PCAs are ideal for pain management in the immediate postoperative period for several reasons. The patient is in control of his or her own medication administration, and thus the time between when the patient begins to experience pain and when he or she finally receives medication is greatly reduced. Second, by providing small, frequent doses, a PCA allows for better medication titration to the required level, helping to avoid the "peaks and valleys" of pain often caused when a q3h or q4h prn opioid schedule is used. Lastly, PCAs limit the risk of opioid overdose, as the patient must be alert enough to press the pump button in order to administer another dose. A good starting PCA dose for a standard patient is morphine 1 mg, with a lockout interval of 8 minutes. Hydromorphone (trade name Dilaudid) is the other most popular IV opioid and is approximately 7 times as potent as morphine. A standard PCA order would be Dilaudid 0.1 or 0.2 mg with the same lockout interval of 8 minutes.

So far we have only discussed the use of "prn" or "breakthrough" pain medication that is administered when requested by the patient (via either the patient's nurse or a PCA). The other, complementary, dosing option is a "standing" or "basal rate" in which patients receive the medication at a set time interval or continuously, regardless of whether they are in pain. In general, opioids should not usually be ordered in such a fashion due to the risk of narcotic overdose. Likewise, a basal administration rate on a PCA (by which patients get a set dose of narcotics every hour regardless of whether they press the pump button) should not be used except in special circumstances.

3. Opioids act on the central nervous system to depress consciousness and, ultimately, respiratory drive. Other than depressed mental status, the primary finding of opioid toxicity on physical exam is pinpoint and sluggishly reactive pupils. Opioid overdose is treated with IV naloxone; however, keep in mind that any narcotic overdose resulting in unresponsiveness or respiratory depression is a life-threatening emergency. Under no circumstance should you attempt to treat it on your own and if an inpatient is found in such a condition, a medical "code" should be called so that help arrives immediately.

Opioids can also cause delirium, especially in elderly patients. This can result in paradoxical agitation, confusion, and aggressive behavior. In older inpatients these side effects are often falsely attributed to dementia, even when the patient was not previously diagnosed with this condition. This is why it is extremely important to determine what the patient's baseline mental status was when evaluating abnormal behavior in the hospital.

Another opioid side effect of critical importance in general surgery is the slowing of bowel peristalsis, resulting in ileus and/or constipation. For this reason, the total amount of opioids used should be limited whenever possible, especially after a bowel resection. Additionally, patients who are receiving opioids and can take oral medications should be placed on a prophylactic stool softener (ie, "bowel regimen"), such as docusate (trade name Colace) 100 mg PO BID. Another option is the relatively new medication alvimopan (trade name Entereg), an opioid antagonist that acts selectively in the enteric nervous system and has been shown to reduce the length of ileus after colon resections.

4. In order to minimize the use (and consequently the risk) of opiates, adjunct analgesic medications are sometimes used. The 2 most common medications are NSAIDs and acetaminophen (Tylenol). These are most effective if written "around the clock," that is, they can serve as basal pain control while the opiates can be used for breakthrough pain. Numerous studies have demonstrated that this type of regimen results in lower total usage of opiates.

    Acetaminophen is most useful after the patient is eating, although there is a formulation that can be given per rectum (PR) if the patient tolerates this route of administration. An intravenous formulation of acetaminophen (trade name Ofirmev) was recently approved by the FDA for postoperative pain management. However, as this is a relatively new medication prevalence of usage varies between institutions, and you should check with your senior resident or attending before ordering it. Acetaminophen is usually well tolerated, although it does have the well-known risk of hepatotoxicity. Total acetaminophen dose should not exceed 4 g in 24 hours—remember that this total includes any acetaminophen given as part of a mixed formulation such as Percocet or Vicodin. Acetaminophen should also be minimized in those patients with existing hepatic disease or those who have just undergone a liver operation.

    Like acetaminophen, NSAIDs are also commonly added to a patient's medical regimen in order to minimize opiate usage. The only commonly used IV NSAID is ketorolac (trade name Toradol), which is dosed at 15 or 30 mg IV q6h. As discussed above, it is usually ordered in a scheduled (rather than prn) fashion. While effective, Toradol does, however, have several important side effects. Toradol (as well as the other NSAIDs) is a mild anticoagulant, and for this reason you should never initiate its use postoperatively without first discussing it with the senior resident or attending. Second, NSAIDs can reduce renal perfusion and should be avoided in patients with impaired renal function. Patients on Toradol should have a daily chemistry ordered to check for an increase in their creatinine levels. NSAIDs also inhibit bone growth and are generally avoided in patients with fractures.

5. Generally, patients should be transitioned to an oral pain regimen as soon as they are started on a diet. Some surgeons will start their patients on PO pain medication when they are advanced to liquids; however, others will wait until patients are taking a regular diet, so you should always check before making this change. The most commonly used postoperative oral pain medications are combinations of acetaminophen and an opioid. These include Percocet (acetaminophen and oxycodone), Vicodin (acetaminophen and hydrocodone), and Tylenol #3 (acetaminophen and codeine). Morphine and Dilaudid can also be prescribed in oral form, but these are generally reserved for patients with

Table 23-1. Standard Pain Medications and Their Relative Strengths

	Typical Dosing Range	Equianalgesic Dose
IV medications (brand name)		
Morphine	3-6 mg IV q4h prn pain	7 mg
	PCA: 1-2 mg with an 8 min lockout interval	
Hydromorphone (Dilaudid)	0.5-1 mg IV q4h prn pain	1 mg
	PCA: 0.1-0.2 mg with an 8 min lockout interval	
Ketorolac (Toradol)	15 or 30 mg IV q6h standing	N/A (not an opioid)
Fentanyl	10-50 μg IV q15min (used in the PACU b/c of its short half-life, should *never* be ordered on the surgical floor)	70 μg
PO medications (doses in each tablet)		
Percocet (5 mg oxycodone and 325 mg acetaminophen)	1 or 2 tablets PO q4h prn pain	3 tablets (or 15 mg oxycodone)
Vicodin (5 mg hydrocodone and 500 mg acetaminophen)	1 or 2 tablets PO q4h prn pain	3 tablets (or 15 mg hydrocodone)
Tylenol #3 (30 mg codeine and 300 mg acetaminophen)	1 or 2 tablets PO q4h prn pain	5 tablets (or 150 mg codeine)
Ibuprofen	400 mg tablet PO q6h standing	N/A (not an opioid)
Morphine (*oral formulation*)	Not typically used postoperatively	20 mg
Dilaudid (*oral formulation*)	Not typically used postoperatively	5 mg

chronic opioid usage (and thus tolerance) and are not used in standard postoperative situations. Oral NSAIDs, most commonly ibuprofen at 400 mg PO q6h, can be given in addition to the above medications, again in an effort to reduce the total opioid usage.

All opioids have different analgesic strengths per milligram and you should be generally familiar with the conversion factors between them. Table 23-1 shows a chart of standard pain medication doses and their relative strengths.

Although oral opioids have less severe side effects than those given IV, they still cause constipation. Patients should be placed on a bowel regimen when receiving them and be given a prescription for Colace (or another stool softener) on discharge.

TIPS TO REMEMBER

● Assume that patients with an unusually high level of pain after an operation have a surgical complication. Inadequate analgesia is a diagnosis of exclusion.

● PCAs are an effective delivery method for IV opioids in the immediate postoperative period. In general, PCAs should not be ordered with a basal rate (ie, a continuous infusion).

● All pain medications have side effects. Opioids can cause depression of consciousness and respiratory drive, and delirium in the elderly, and can cause or prolong ileus. NSAIDs can increase the risk of bleeding and can be nephrotoxic.

● When a patient's diet is advanced after surgery, he or she should be transitioned to oral pain medications as soon as possible.

● A prophylactic bowel regimen should be ordered for all patients receiving opioids and who are able to take PO medications.

COMPREHENSION QUESTIONS

1. In which of the following patient populations should ketorolac (brand name Toradol) *not* be used? (Choose all that apply.)
    A. Trauma patients with subdural hematomas
    B. Patients with type II diabetes
    C. Patients with chronic renal insufficiency
    D. Patients with dementia

2. Which of the following is an appropriate PCA order for a patient immediately after a laparotomy?
    A. Morphine 3 mg per dose, with a lockout interval of 2 minutes
    B. Dilaudid 1 mg per dose, with a lockout interval of 8 minutes
    C. Morphine 1 mg per dose, with a lockout interval of 8 minutes
    D. Dilaudid 0.2 mg per dose, with a lockout interval of 2 minutes

3. On postoperative day 1 after a laparoscopic gastric bypass, a patient is complaining of what you think is unusually intense epigastric pain. What other finding would make you most concerned for an anastomotic leak?
    A. Heart rate of 120
    B. White blood cell (WBC) count of 10.5
    C. Urine output of 75 mL/h
    D. Blood pressure of 160/80

4. What dose of Dilaudid IV is equivalent to the amount of oxycodone in a single Percocet tablet?

     A. 0.1 mg
     B. 0.33 mg
     C. 0.5 mg
     D. 1 mg

Answers

1. **Both A and C**. Toradol is an anticoagulant and can be nephrotoxic, so it should be avoided in patients with (or at risk for) bleeding or impaired renal function.

2. **C**. All of the other choices have either too high a dose (morphine 3 mg or Dilaudid 1 mg) or too short a lockout interval (2 minutes).

3. **A**. Tachycardia along with an abnormal amount of pain should alert you that a complication may have occurred.

4. **B**. Each Percocet tablet contains 5 mg of oxycodone, which is equivalent to 0.33 mg of IV Dilaudid.

A 72-year-old Man With Acute Confusion Postoperatively

Shamim H. Nejad, MD and Justin B. Smith, MD

Mr. Thompkins is an otherwise healthy 72-year-old man who was admitted after experiencing 15% total body surface area burns to his trunk, arms, neck, and face. He is now 2 days s/p excision and grafting of his injuries. His postoperative course was unremarkable until last evening when he became acutely confused. He stated that he was at the library and he was observed to be having conversations with people who were not there. The patient also began to pull at his lines and attempted to get out of bed. He required frequent redirection and reorienting by his nurse, which prompted a call to the night float resident. The nurse was particularly concerned that he may be in alcohol withdrawal as it was reported in his admission note that he consumed ethanol in "social situations."

The night float resident initially gave the patient lorazepam 2 mg IV to sedate him. He was then placed on lorazepam 1 mg IV every 4 hours standing, along with PRN lorazepam ordered "per signs of alcohol withdrawal." Despite these interventions the patient's mental status continued to worsen, and on rounds the following morning your team discovers that he now requires oxygen supplementation. You review the rest of his medications and note that the patient is also on a hydromorphone PCA, which the nurse tells you she has been activating "to keep him comfortable" as the patient is too confused to use the PCA himself.

On physical examination, his vitals are T: 99.9, HR: 115, BP: 150/90, R: 16, and O_2: 97% on 3 L of oxygen per nasal cannula. The patient is lying in bed with his eyes closed, although he can be aroused with loud verbal stimuli. He is oriented only to self and falls asleep repeatedly during the examination. When he is awake, he has difficulty maintaining focus and attention. Pupils are equal and reactive, and his cranial nerve examination is intact. Upper extremities are without cogwheeling, rigidity, or tremor. The patient displays a palmomental reflex bilaterally; however, no glabellar, snout, or plantar reflexes are noted. In addition, there are intermittent myoclonic jerks of the upper extremities and trunk.

Laboratory results are notable only for a WBC of 16,700 and a sodium of 129. A review of admission labs includes a normal MCV of 95, an ALT of 22, an AST of 28, and normal coagulation studies. A blood alcohol level along with a urine toxicology screen at the time of admission was negative.

1. **Based on the details given, does this patient meet the diagnostic criteria of delirium?**

2. **Is delirium life-threatening?**

3. **You've excluded any serious medical condition as the cause of his altered mental status (AMS). What else could be causing these changes?**

4. What is the first-line pharmaceutical agent for treatment of severe agitation?

5. What are the most common risks associated with this agent?

ALTERED MENTAL STATUS

Answers

1. In assessing mental status changes in the hospitalized patient it is important to distinguish delirium from other underlying psychiatric disorders. Delirium, as opposed to most other psychiatric disturbances, has an acute onset within hours to days, is caused by a medical condition, and is reversible. The cardinal sign of delirium is an altered level of consciousness accompanied by cognitive deficits that cannot be accounted for by a past or evolving dementia.

    In the case example, this patient's mental status changed acutely in the hours and days after surgery. The patient clearly demonstrated a continued disturbance of consciousness by falling asleep during the examination. In addition, he was disoriented and had difficulty maintaining focus and attention, all core features of delirium. He demonstrated cognitive deficits as noted by disorientation (thinking he was in the library, pulling out lines, requiring frequent redirection) and perceptual disturbances (having conversations with people who were not there).

2. Delirium is a medical emergency and the underlying cause must be identified and treated. While the delirium itself is not usually life-threatening, it can be the first sign of a more serious condition such as hypotension, hypoxia, anemia/bleeding, or infection. As such, you should respond immediately whenever you are paged about a patient with AMS.

    As you are evaluating the patient you should remember that there are seven states, designated by the mnemonic WHHHIMP (Table 24-1) that require immediate intervention to avoid death or permanent CNS damage.

    Simply evaluating the time of onset and course of the patient's symptoms can often lead to a preliminary diagnosis. But the diagnosis is not always so

Table 24-1. High-risk Causes of AMS

Wernicke encephalopathy
Hypoxia/hypoperfusion
Hypertensive encephalopathy
Hypoglycemia
Intracerebral hemorrhage
Meningitis/encephalitis
Poisoning (exogenous or iatrogenic)

simple—delirium can present in many different ways and psychiatrists refer to it as "the great imitator." After obtaining a history you should examine the vital signs closely. The most worrisome finding is any evidence that suggests the delirium is the result of end-organ hypoperfusion, that is, shock. You should also note the presence or absence of fever (suggesting infection) or hypoxia (which can cause delirium directly). After reviewing the vital signs, the clinical evaluation should proceed with a complete neurological examination. In assessing the patient's mental status you should evaluate the patient for paranoia or perceptual disturbances (either of which can cause patients to be quite agitated or even aggressive). Perceptual disturbances (most often visual hallucinations) are particularly notable as they are remarkably rare in primary psychiatric disturbances. While some patients are agitated, others may have a hypoactive delirium that goes unnoticed by staff because they are quietly confused. Physical examination should also include assessment for the presence of multifocal myoclonus, along with frontal release signs (palmomental, glabellar, and plantar reflexes). Positive findings are often associated with generalized encephalopathy (ie, frontal network syndrome caused by metabolic derangements, infection, or medications—opiates and benzodiazepines) and do not necessarily mean that there is an acute bleed or lesion. If there are any focal neurological deficits or you have any doubt as to the underlying etiology, then neurological or psychiatric consultation should be obtained.

In this patient, his level of consciousness was depressed and he required supplemental oxygen. These could be due to the medications he was being given (opiates and benzodiazepines) or could be the result of a pulmonary infection (note that his WBC is elevated). He also had both myoclonus and frontal release signs that suggest a nonfocal etiology such as medications, infection, or a metabolic cause. Looking at his labs, not only does he have the aforementioned leukocytosis but he also has a hyponatremia, one example of many possible metabolic causes of delirium.

The nurse was specifically concerned about alcohol withdrawal, an understandable concern given the timing of the AMS (alcohol withdrawal usually manifests 2-3 days after the last drink). However, prior to initiating *treatment* for alcohol withdrawal delirium it is mandatory to collect collateral history with regard to the patient's alcohol use, particularly given the fact that this patient's liver function tests, coagulation studies, and MCV were normal and the patient didn't exhibit any symptoms of tremor or diaphoresis. In short, alcohol withdrawal delirium is a diagnosis of exclusion and should be based on clinical findings, laboratory findings, and, if possible, collateral history.

3. If no medical cause can be identified (ie, you do not find evidence of one of the seven "high-risk" diagnoses, of infection, or of metabolic derangements), then the next step in management often involves simplifying the patient's medication list. Pharmaceutical agents are among the most common iatrogenic causes of AMS, and reducing or eliminating offending agents is often very effective.

Many classes of medications can contribute to delirium. Classic examples include anticholinergic medications such as diphenhydramine (Benadryl) or promethazine (Phenergan). Narcotics (such as hydromorphone) are also a common culprit for AMS. While the use of narcotics in surgical patients is often mandatory to obtain adequate analgesia, care should be taken to ensure that the patient receives the lowest effective dosage of medication to achieve pain control. Lastly, benzodiazepines (such as lorazepam) can also precipitate or contribute to delirium.

As an adjunct to simplifying the medication list, environmental interventions can also be helpful. You should ensure that the patient has his or her hearing/visual aids, instruct the nurses to provide frequent reorientation, and optimize the sleep/wake cycle by minimizing unnecessary overnight disturbances.

In addition, certain surgical conditions associated with inflammatory states (long bone fractures, burn injuries, pancreatitis, etc) often lead to AMS. These conditions and their associated inflammatory response states may result in a significant proinflammatory cytokine-mediated process that leads to fenestrations in the blood–brain barrier with resulting CNS dysregulation in the limbic cortices, resulting in encephalopathy. In burn patients, AMS will often persist until all wounds are excised, grafted, and fully closed. Furthermore, whether related to traumatic surgical intervention, unplanned surgery, or an elective surgery, *any* operation results in an expected inflammation-mediated process that usually peaks on postoperative day 2, coinciding with the time of the highest incidence of postoperative delirium.

4. The best option is to treat the delirium by treating the underlying medical cause. However, in some cases the underlying cause is not readily identifiable or rapidly reversible and pharmacologic treatment of the symptoms of delirium becomes necessary. This is particularly true for patients who are severely agitated and at risk of hurting themselves or others.

Dopamine antagonists are frequently used for the treatment of delirium. Haloperidol IV is the first-line agent for the treatment of agitated delirium, particularly in critical care settings given its relatively benign cardiopulmonary risk profile. It is also the primary agent for the treatment and management of severe agitation on the general care floor. When it is necessary to use an enteral formulation (due to preexisting hospital guidelines or attempting disposition to a rehabilitative facility), one may choose quetiapine (Seroquel) or olanzapine (Zyprexa). Quetiapine is generally preferred over olanzapine in patients with underlying neurodegenerative disorders due to its decreased affinity for dopamine blockage and less extrapyramidal symptom (EPS)–related side effects (see below). See Table 24-2 for dosing strategies for these medications for the treatment of agitation.

Caution is warranted in the use of benzodiazepines such as lorazepam because they carry the risk of *worsening* an underlying delirium and increasing morbidity and mortality. They are also associated with respiratory depression

Table 24-2. Dosing Strategies for Agitation

	Haloperidol (IV) (mg)	Olanzapine (mg)	Quetiapine (mg)
Mild	0.5-2	2.5-5	25-50
Moderate	2-5	10	50-100
Severe	5-20	20	100-200

Daily dose of olanzapine should not exceed 20 mg/day for elderly patients or 40 mg/day in nonelderly patients secondary to anticholinergic activity at higher doses. Daily dose of quetiapine should not exceed 500 mg in elderly patients or 800 mg in nonelderly patients secondary to increased anticholinergic activity.

and should be avoided in patients with respiratory compromise. Benzodiazepines should therefore be reserved for those cases of severe agitation that are initially refractory to escalating doses of IV haloperidol. Even then they should only be used sparingly, while other interventions are aggressively attempted.

5. While dopamine antagonists are relatively safe, it is important to understand their side effect profiles. The most significant risk associated with dopamine antagonists is their potential to cause EPS. This is particularly true of haloperidol. All dopamine antagonists also have QT prolonging effects and carry a theoretical risk of inducing *torsade de pointes*. To minimize the risk of QTc prolongation, potassium and magnesium repletion should be performed daily, avoidance and/or minimization of unnecessary QTc prolonging medications should be attempted, and a daily ECG should be performed to ensure it remains below 550 milliseconds. Sedation is also a side effect of the newer-generation dopamine antagonists, such as quetiapine and olanzapine, although this may actually be beneficial when treating a patient with delirium due to hyperarousal. Dopamine antagonists should be minimized in patients with Parkinson disease or other severe neurodegenerative disorders, and psychiatric consultation should be considered for assistance in management of these patients.

TIPS TO REMEMBER

- Delirium can be the first sign of a life-threatening medical condition.
- The first principle in managing delirium is to diagnose and reverse the underlying cause.
- A review of the entire medication list for offending agents should be completed. Medications including anticholinergic agents, benzodiazepines, and opiates are common contributors to delirium and should be reduced if possible.
- Dopamine antagonists (ie, IV haloperidol) are useful first-line pharmacologic agents for the treatment and management of delirium.

COMPREHENSION QUESTIONS

1. Which of the following is most helpful in securing a diagnosis of delirium as the cause of mental status changes?
    A. Paranoid delusions
    B. Altered level of consciousness with impaired cognition
    C. Agitation
    D. Perceptual disturbances
    E. Concurrent use of opiates and benzodiazepines

2. Of the following which would *not* be a first-line recommendation in the management of delirium?
    A. Provide visual/hearing aids.
    B. Reverse underlying medical etiology.
    C. Intravenous haloperidol PRN agitation.
    D. Diphenhydramine in the evening to optimize the sleep/wake cycle.

3. What risk factors does the patient in the vignette possess for the development of delirium?
    A. Anemia
    B. The second postoperative day
    C. Presence of leukocytosis
    D. Burn injuries
    E. Metabolic derangements
    F. All of the above

Answers

1. **B.** The core feature of delirium is an altered level of consciousness with impaired cognition. All of the other symptoms listed are associated with delirium but not necessary for diagnosis.

2. **D.** Although optimizing the sleep/wake cycle is important, diphenhydramine has strong anticholinergic properties and as such would not be a first choice in a patient with AMS.

3. **F.** Anemia, metabolic derangements, and the presence of leukocytosis all contribute to an increased probability of transitioning to delirium. In addition, as outlined above, burn-related injuries and postoperative states may result in a pro-inflammatory cytokine-mediated process that leads to CNS dysfunction, resulting in encephalopathy.

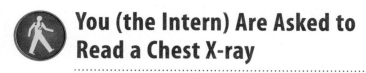

You (the Intern) Are Asked to Read a Chest X-ray

Alexander T. Hawkins, MD, MPH and Amy Robin Deipolyi, MD, PhD

You are in Tuesday morning trauma rounds after a night shift. The room is warm, and the senior's voice is monotonous. You begin to drift off to sleep when you hear your name called to go to the front of the room to read a chest x-ray. You know nothing about the patient. Where do you start?

1. **What is the first thing you should do with the chest x-ray?**
2. **What is an easy acronym you can use to recall all of the important parts of the chest x-ray?**
3. **What else do you need to look for on an ICU film?**

HOW TO READ A CHEST X-RAY

Answers

The key to reading a chest x-ray is to develop a system that you will be able to replicate time after time. This will ensure that you evaluate every important aspect of the chest x-ray consistently. If you are not looking for it, you are not going to see it! What follows is an example of such a system. It is by no means the only way to look at a chest x-ray, and you should develop your own system that works for you.

1. Make sure that it is hung (or displayed) correctly and that it is a chest x-ray of the correct patient. Sometimes images get mixed up or the side is incorrectly marked. Look for the heart on the left side of the chest (unless, of course, the patient has dextrocardia). Make sure that it has appropriate exposure and that you can see everything that you need to see (ie, apices of lungs, costophrenic angles). On a properly exposed film, the lungs are not too black and you can see the vertebral bodies through the heart. Ideally, patients are imaged straight on, rather than being rotated, which can distort the appearance of the mediastinum. Additionally, adequate inspiration is essential to good technique. In adults, approximately 9 posterior ribs should be identified. Low lung volumes mimic pulmonary edema.

2. Just like a trauma evaluation, ABCDE can be used to note each important part of the radiograph. This method takes advantage of the fact that all you want to

do when you look at a chest x-ray is look at the lungs—which is why it saves the lungs for last.

A—Abdomen. Look for free air under the abdomen on an upright film.

B—Bones. Examine all of the ribs, clavicles, and vertebrae for fractures or dislocations.

C—Cardiac. Trace the cardiac silhouette starting from the right base, along the right atrium, and examine the mediastinum for any tumors or deviation. Evaluate the aortic arch on the left and trace the silhouette down to the left ventricle. On a PA CXR you can measure the width of the heart and compare it with the width of the chest. A ratio greater than 1:2 is evidence of cardiomyopathy. This rule does not apply to a portable AP CXR, which magnifies the mediastinum and heart.

D—Diaphragm. This one is really about the pleura, but ABCPE does not really make sense. Start at the diaphragm and trace the pleura all the way around the thoracic cavity. Blunting of the costophrenic angles can indicate a pleural effusion. Increased lucency and/or lines where they don't belong can indicate a pneumothorax. Look especially hard in the apices of the lungs for this, although air can accumulate more inferiorly in patients who are supine. Look for a deep sulcus sign in supine patients, for example, in an ICU setting, which appears as a long pointed costophrenic angle.

E—Everything else. Now it is time to look at the lungs. Start with the trachea. Is it midline? Are any of the lobes opacified? Are there any tumors? Make sure you scan throughout the right and left lungs. Classic blind spots are the lung apices and lung behind the heart. Also note the pattern of an abnormal opacity. Is the process diffuse or localized? More central or peripheral? Hazy or linear? Does the opacity obscure a normal silhouette? For example, opacities that block the left or right heart borders represent an abnormality in the lingula or right middle lobe, respectively, whereas opacities obscuring either diaphragm are in the lower lobes. See Figure 25-1.

3. ICU patients are almost always imaged supine and are not able to take deep inspirations. Low lung volumes and portable technique significantly impair the ability to evaluate the lung parenchyma. Therefore, the most important function of the ICU chest x-ray is to identify tubes, lines, and drains and assure that they are in the proper positions. Three of the most important items you will use a CXR to assess include endotracheal tubes, esophagogastric tubes (including orogastric and nasogastric tubes), and central venous catheters (see Figure 25-2).

Endotracheal tubes: The ideal position for an endotracheal tube is in the mid-trachea, 3 to 5 cm from the carina when the head is neither flexed nor extended. The carina is the upside down V where the trachea splits into the left and right mainstem (see Figure 25-1). The minimum safe distance from the carina is 2 cm.

Esophagogastric tubes: Make sure the tube tracks down the esophagus and goes below the diaphragm into the stomach. A tube that does not make it all the way to the stomach should be advanced and the CXR retaken. A tube that makes a turn and stays above the diaphragm could be placed into the lung—you must replace the tube. Also check that the side hole is below the diaphragm. If it isn't, giving tube feeds can cause aspiration pneumonia as fluid may reflux back up the esophagus. In patients who are very tall it is often difficult to see the tip of the tube and a KUB may be necessary (see Figure 25-2).

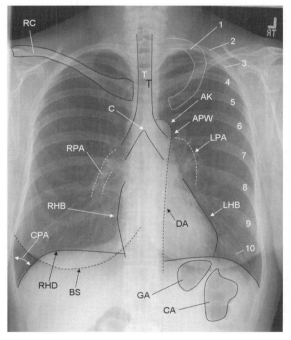

Figure 25-1. Structures seen on a posteroanterior (PA) chest x-ray. 1, first rib; 2–10, posterior aspect of ribs 2 to 10; AK, aortic knob; APW, aortopulmonary window; BS, breast shadow (labeled only on right); C, carina; CA, colonic air; CPA, costophrenic angle; DA, descending aorta; GA, gastric air; LHB, left heart border (*Note*: Most of the left heart border represents the left ventricle; the superior aspect of the left heart border represents the left atrial appendage); LPA, left pulmonary artery; RC, right clavicle (left clavicle not labeled); RHB, right heart border (*Note*: The right heart border represents the right atrium); RHD, right hemidiaphragm (left hemidiaphragm not labeled); RPA, right pulmonary artery; T, tracheal air column.

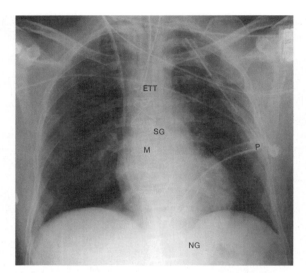

Figure 25-2. Frontal radiograph immediately after coronary artery bypass surgery shows typical lines and tubes encountered in the ICU. Endotracheal tube (ETT), nasogastric tube (NG), Swan-Ganz catheter (SG), mediastinal drain (M), and left pleural drain (P) are present.

Central venous catheter (CVC): Central venous catheters include those that terminate in the SVC or IVC. They may be placed through the neck/chest (internal jugular/subclavian veins), arm (PICC lines), or even lower extremities. They can be used to monitor central venous pressure, infuse large volumes of fluid, and infuse caustic medications that cannot be given through a peripheral vein. The optimal position for a CVC is for the tip to be right at the cavoatrial junction. As the right superior heart border is not a reliable determinant of right atrial position, the best way to confirm correct placement is to look for the tip to be at the junction of the right heart border with the right mainstem bronchus. Catheters should always go toward the heart: catheters inserted from the left should cross midline and end up on the right side near the right atrium. When right-sided catheters cross midline, intra-arterial rather than intravenous placement should be suspected (see Figure 25-3).

TIPS TO REMEMBER

● The best system for reading a chest x-ray is the one that you can remember easily and that helps you to remember to look for all important features.

● Be sure to identify all tubes, lines, and drains on an ICU film.

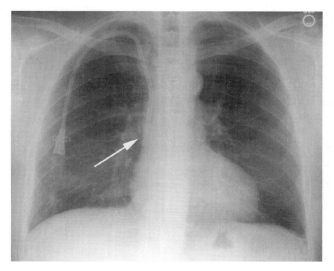

Figure 25-3. PA view of a patient whose tunneled central venous catheter placement is normal with its tip in the superior vena cava above the right atrium (arrow).

COMPREHENSION QUESTIONS

1. What is the most important system to read a CXR?
    A. The one that works best for you
    B. The one in this book
    C. The one you were taught in medical school
    D. The one the Chief of Radiology uses

2. Where should the tip of the endotracheal tube lie?
    A. Below the diaphragm
    B. Above the clavicles
    C. 3 to 5 cm above the carina
    D. Anywhere as long as the oxygen saturation is 100%

3. Which of the following does *not* represent a problem with central venous catheter placement?
    A. A right-sided pneumothorax after a right subclavian line placement
    B. A left subclavian line with the tip in the jugular vein
    C. A right-sided catheter that crosses midline
    D. A left-sided catheter that crosses midline

Answers

1. **A.** It is imperative that you develop your own system to consistently and accurately read chest x-rays.

2. **C.** The tip of the endotracheal tube should be positioned 3 to 5 cm above the carina. Any further and you risk the tube sliding into a mainstem bronchus with neck extension.

3. **D.** A left-sided catheter should cross the midline. The other choices represent serious problems with placement.

A 65-year-old Woman in Respiratory Distress

Alden H. Harken, MD and Brian C. George, MD

Ms. O'Sullivan is a 65-year-old woman who arrived in the PACU 30 minutes ago following a right colectomy. She was extubated in the operating room. Her vitals are: BP 140/90, pulse 120 (regular), respiratory rate 30, temperature 37.5°C, and finger oximetry 80%. She is anxious and agitated and says that she wants to "leave right now and go home."

1. **Until proven otherwise, what is the cause of agitation and/or disorientation in the postoperative recovery unit?**

2. **Explain several causes of postoperative hypoxemia.**

3. **What are the indications to intubate a patient?**

RESPIRATORY DISTRESS

If you are sitting comfortably reading this chapter, you are using about 3% of your energy in the work of breathing. Interestingly, the "driver" of this lung work is blood acidosis (actually CSF hydrogen ion concentration)—not oxygen. You are exquisitely sensitive to Pco_2/pH. If you hold your breath for a minute, at the end of that minute your only wish is for another breath—breathing is high on everyone's list of fun things to do. However, at the end of a minute of apnea, your Pco_2 has risen from 40 mm Hg to only about 48 mm Hg. Therefore, a relatively tiny decrease in arterial pH (or increase in Pco_2) translates into a profound stimulus to breathe.

Case Analysis

Mrs. O'Sullivan's respiratory rate has increased to 30. We could attribute this to her "agitation," but were we to check her arterial blood gas at this time, we would find:

Po_2: 55 mm Hg

Pco_2: 30 mm Hg

pH: 7.48

O_2 sat: 80%

She has a respiratory alkalosis and is actually "overbreathing." Her only abnormality is the drop in her hemoglobin saturation (O_2 sat) that confers a 20% (100% minus 80%) decrease in arterial oxygen content, which can be completely compensated by a 20% increase in her cardiac output, resulting in a rock stable systemic oxygen delivery. The patient's agitation has unquestionably pumped up her cardiac output at least the necessary 20%—so, what's the problem? You decide that "everything is fine," so you reassure the patient and the nurses and leave to check on another patient.

Answers

1. Fifteen minutes later you get a call that Mrs. O'Sullivan is climbing out of bed, making a lot of noise, and bothering the other patients (and the nurses)—so, "Can we sedate her?"

   Warning: if you depress this patient's respiratory drive with a sedative now, you will receive a follow-up call in 30 minutes that she just suffered a cardiac arrest. *Agitation/irritability/confusion in the PACU/ICU is hypoxemia until proven otherwise, and should be cause for alarm!* In most of us, the symptoms of hypoxemia are not an alteration in breathing volume/rate/pattern. Acute hypoxemia just makes a patient feel anxious and restless. Hypoxemia makes a patient want to get up, go out, and travel to someplace safer—and hypoxemic patients are very likely to announce this desire to everyone.

2. There are lots of reasons for hypoxemia in the early postoperative period. Atelectasis, aspiration, a touch of pneumonia, and even a pulmonary embolus are the most obvious reasons that ventilation doesn't match up with perfusion. More fundamental is that most inhalational anesthetics block hypoxic pulmonary vasoconstriction. Remember, this is the unique capability of the pulmonary arterioles to divert perfusion away from hypoventilated alveoli. When poorly ventilated lung is perfused, a shunt occurs that results in hypoxemia.

3. When you walk into any surgical ICU today, you have access to machines that can support almost all failing organ systems. The oldest, and arguably the best, of these devices is the ventilator. There are both hard and soft rules relating to when you breathe for your patient and when you can safely cut the patient loose (and the indices for starting and stopping are really the same criteria):

   A. Most importantly, the patient's mental status must be adequate to protect his/her own airway.

   B. Respiratory rate below 25 to 30. Again, breathing is a high priority for all of us. Although you and I are currently expending only 3% of our energy on "breathing," a big burn can exert 25% of energy expenditure on the "work of breathing" and leave little residual energy for "getting better."

   C. Your patient's lungs have got to be "working." Carbon dioxide excretion is a linear function of alveolar ventilation, so if patients can "breathe harder," they can rid themselves of CO_2. Oxygenation is not so simple. By the time hemoglobin crosses halfway across a ventilated alveolus, it is already fully saturated with oxygen. So, increasing the inhaled oxygen (in a patient with a shunt) won't help at all.

D. Strength is important, but it is hard to measure unless the patient is intubated. Negative inspiratory force (NIF) is an extubation parameter only. You and I can comfortably generate 100 mm Hg NIF. A patient who can only pull −25 mm Hg is solidly in the gray zone.

Putting It All Together

For the surgical intensivist, the following guidelines apply:

Intubation: After examining the aforementioned parameters, when *you* get frightened, intubate.

Extubation: After examining the aforementioned extubation criteria, when *you* are comfortable, extubate.

Tracheostomy: After living with your patient for 10 days, if you don't "feel" that he can fly, trach him.

Does anyone think this is science? It is art!

TIPS TO REMEMBER

- "Agitation" in the SICU/PACU represents a hypoxemic patient until proven otherwise.
- The "driver" of minute ventilation in the vast majority of patients is CSF pH—not oxygen.
- "Dyspnea" is a feeling—not a blood gas.
- Most inhalational anesthetics inhibit healthy hypoxic pulmonary arteriolar vasoconstriction.
- Increasing the inspired oxygen concentration in a patient with a shunt doesn't help.

COMPREHENSION QUESTION

1. You are called about an elderly patient who is in the PACU. He is extremely agitated and is trying to hit the staff. Which of the following is the correct answer(s)?
    A. Sedate him with a benzodiazepine (eg, lorazepam).
    B. Check his vitals.
    C. Check an ABG.
    D. Check an EKG.

Answer

1. **B, C, and D**. The important point is that answer A is wrong. In the acute post-operative period this patient's agitation most likely represents cerebral hypoxia. This could be due to several factors, including inadequate cardiac output or inadequate respiration. The vital signs are quick and easy to obtain and can help guide further workup. If they reflect inadequate oxygenation or are normal, then an ABG is indicated. An EKG is indicated if you suspect inadequate cardiac output, since this could be caused by a myocardial infarction or arrhythmia.

A Patient Who Is Postoperative Day 2 With New-onset Chest Pain

Alden H. Harken, MD
and Brian C. George, MD

You are in the middle of running the labs for all of your patients when you get a page. It says: Mr. Roberts is complaining of chest pain.—Pat MacDonald RN, phone 5-1234.

You remember that Mr. Roberts is on the exact other side of the hospital from where you are now. You pull out your cell phone and return the page as you are walking to the elevator. While you are on hold, you look at your list and see that Mr. Roberts is a vasculopath who is postoperative day 2 from a right below-the-knee amputation.

You get the nurse on the phone as you push the button for the elevator.

1. What is your first question to the nurse?

2. What diagnostic tests should you order over the phone?

3. Name 6 causes of chest pain that you must not miss.

CHEST PAIN

With disconcerting frequency you are going to be called to the emergency department, the recovery room (PACU), or the floor to see a patient who claims to have new-onset "chest pain." Frequently this will be "nothing." Sometimes it will be "something" and, occasionally, it will be "a really big deal."

Answers

1. "What are the vital signs?"

   This question determines your next response. Based on those vital signs you should initiate any needed supportive measures. Standard supportive measures include giving oxygen and pain control (both of which are protective if the patient is having an MI). If the patient is hypotensive, you should tell the nurse to call a code.

2. As you are going to see the patient, you can get a couple of things going so they will be available as soon as possible. An EKG is mandatory. Unless you are confident that the cause of the chest pain can be explained by some other benign process, you should also order a CXR.

3. In evaluating patients with chest pain, it is useful to relate the likely epidemiological frequency of the problem to (most importantly) *How Big A Deal If You*

Table 27-1. Causes of Chest Pain

Patient Presentation	Likelihood	HBADIYMI	First Screening Test
Acute myocardial infarction	+++	+++	12-Lead EKG
Pulmonary embolism	++	+++	Spiral CT
Aortic dissection	+	++++	TTE
Reflux esophagitis	++	+	Antacid
Leaking triple A	+	++++	Abdominal U/S
Costochondritis	+	+	ASA
Acute cholecystitis	+	+	GB ultrasound
Pneumonia	+	+	CXR
Tension pneumothorax	+	++++	Vital signs (not CXR!)
Pneumothorax	+	+	CXR
Cardiac tamponade	+	++++	Vital signs

Abdominal U/S, abdominal ultrasound; ASA, aspirin; CXR, chest x-ray; GB, gallbladder; leaking triple A, abdominal aortic aneurysm; TTE, transthoracic echo.

Miss It (HBADIYMI) (see Table 27-1). Note that there are 6 diagnoses with HBADIYMIs of 3+ or higher.

Acute myocardial infarction: In a 60-year-old cigar-chomping male, not only this happens, but also, in the perioperative period, the 30-day mortality increases by an order of magnitude (7% nonsurgical to 70% intraoperative in the Mayo Clinic series). Give an aspirin while obtaining a 12-lead ECG and cardiac enzymes.

Pulmonary embolism: In a 60-year-old patient soon following a pelvic operation for cancer, this is a frequent problem. If the patient is hypotensive, call for help. If the patient is stable, obtain a spiral CT. These studies are now so sensitive that they often pick up tiny PEs that are clinically irrelevant (but this decision is above your pay grade). It is OK to give 5000 U of heparin to a patient more than 48 hours, and lytic agents more than 8 days, following thoracoabdominal surgery.

Aortic dissection: The textbooks state that this presents as intrascapular back pain, but it can present as anterior chest/shoulder pain. The key is that it really hurts. Typically these patients are hypertensive, and urgent therapy includes aggressive blood pressure control. It is important to distinguish between ascending dissections (requires surgical intervention with a pump) and descending dissections (can be tucked away in your ICU with a *right* radial arterial line and intravenous antihypertensive drugs). This distinction can usually be made with a TTE or CT angiogram.

Reflux esophagitis: This is surprisingly common in the perioperative period, but it's OK if you miss it. Give an antacid.

Leaking triple A: This can be tricky because the stakes are high. Traditionally, when a previously hypertensive, elderly male presents with acute low back pain, the diagnosis is a "leaking triple A." If this patient is hypotensive, he should be taken directly to the operating room. A rapid ultrasound of the abdomen can be very reassuring. *Do obtain a 12-lead ECG.* If this patient is really having an acute MI, a midline abdominal incision will likely prove lethal.

Costochondritis: A diagnosis of exclusion, and it's OK if you miss it. Give anti-inflammatory Rx.

Acute cholecystitis: It seems unfair that this can masquerade as chest pain. In a fair/fat/fortyish female, it is more likely than myocardial ischemia. Obtain a RUQ ultrasound.

Pneumonia: This typically doesn't hurt unless the inflammation extends out to the exquisitely sensitive pleura—then it can hurt a lot. A chest x-ray should confirm the diagnosis.

Tension pneumothorax: This also usually doesn't hurt and presents as hypotension and tachycardia because the increased intrathoracic pressure decreases venous return—paradoxically, it is a volume problem (not respiratory). Do not wait for a chest x-ray. Obtain vital signs and listen to both sides.

Pneumothorax: Perhaps surprisingly, this can be completely painless. Unless this patient is hemodynamically unstable, there is no urgency. Confirm diagnosis with a chest x-ray.

Cardiac tamponade: This is a very rare cause of acute chest pain. The diagnostic and therapeutic urgency depends entirely on the hemodynamic status of the patient.

TIPS TO REMEMBER

- You can avoid unnecessary delay by initiating both treatment and the diagnostic workup prior to arriving at the bedside.
- Acute MI is both common and serious, but you must also not miss PE, aortic dissection, leaking AAA, tension pneumothorax, and cardiac tamponade.

COMPREHENSION QUESTION

1. Which of the following should *not* be ordered over the phone, before you have seen the patient?
> A. Sublingual nitroglycerin
> B. EKG
> C. CXR
> D. Oxygen

Answer

1. **A.** While nitroglycerin is indicated if there is evidence of myocardial ischemia, you don't yet know the diagnosis. In that case, nitroglycerin can actually make things worse—for example, in a patient with a tension pneumothorax.

A 65-year-old Woman With a New-onset Cardiac Arrhythmia

Alden H. Harken, MD

A 65-year-old female arrived in the postanesthesia care unit (PACU) 30 minutes ago following a sigmoid resection for adenocarcinoma. The operation went well, and there was minimal blood loss. She was extubated in the operating room. Blood pressure on arrival in the PACU was 130/80 with a heart rate of 90. Several minutes ago, her heart rate abruptly increased to 160 and her BP dropped to 90/60 mm Hg.

The nurse calls you, and when you arrive, you see a rhythm strip (see Figure 28-1):

1. **What is the most likely reason this patient is now hypotensive?**

2. **Is this patient hemodynamically unstable?**

3. **If you determine she is unstable, where would you place the pads for cardioversion?**

4. **How do you localize the anatomic origin of the dysrhythmia (ie, atrial or ventricular)?**

5. **Assume that, as in this case, the patient has atrial fibrillation (AF). What dose of what medication would you give to slow the heart rate?**

6. **What can you do to help prevent arrhythmias from occurring or recurring?**

SUPRAVENTRICULAR DYSRHYTHMIAS

Answers

1. The patient's current problem is a tachycardia. As we get older, our hearts become less compliant (stiffer) and therefore take more time to fill during diastole. This woman's left ventricle is not adequately filling during diastole, so her

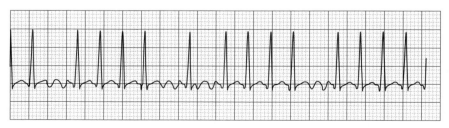

Figure 28-1. Rhythm strip of 65-year-old woman in the case above.

stroke volume is reduced and her cardiac output is down. This in turn results in hypotension.

2. This is a trick question because you don't have enough information. You must assess whether this patient is adequately perfusing her brain and heart (the only two organs that matter acutely). If the patient is diaphoretic and confused (ie, unstable) and she has a tachyarrythmia (eg, AF, ventricular tachycardia [VT], or ventricular fibrillation [VF]), proceed directly with external cardioversion. If the patient appears to be comfortable and you don't think that you need to shock her, examine the ECG rhythm strip more closely to try and determine the anatomic origin of the dysrhythmia.

3. Place one cardioversion paddle on in the right parasternal second intercostal space and the other in the posterior axillary line at the costal margin. If you want to be kind, you may push 20 mg etomidate IV for preshock anesthesia. Set the defibrillator on "sync" and 100 J and press the button. Keep pressing the button for 4 to 5 seconds. Remember that it will take the "quick-look" paddles four to five seconds to "time out" the rhythm so that it doesn't deliver the shock during the upstroke of the T wave and induce VF.

4. If the patient is stable, then examine the ECG rhythm strip and look at the width of the QRS. If the QRS is narrow (as in this case), the origin of the dysrhythmia must be supraventricular (above the AV node).

5. You can give drugs according to how long you want the A-V block to last. See Table 28-1.

    Remember, always give drugs intravenously to a hemodynamically unstable patient. Oral medications exhibit unpredictable absorption in a hypoperfused stomach. When a patient is in shock, a pill can rattle around in the stomach for hours.

6. Fluid and electrolyte shifts coupled with autonomic nervous system stressors conspire to make early postoperative cardiac dysrhythmias relatively common.

Table 28-1. Drugs Used to Slow the Heart Rate (A-V Blockade) and Their Length of Action

Drug	Dose	Duration	Comment
Adenosine	6 mg IV	Seconds	Give 6 mg twice or just give 12 mg
Diltiazem	20 mg IV q2min	Minutes	Begin a drip of 5 mg/h IV
Digoxin	0.5 mg IV q30min	Hours	Look up maintenance
Amiodarone	150 mg IV q10min	Days	Look up maintenance

After you have blocked the A-V node and the patient is stable again, you can do five things to make dysrhythmia recurrence less likely:

1. Check blood gases and provide face mask oxygen.
2. Check serum potassium and keep it above 4.0 mEq/L.
3. Check serum magnesium and keep it above 2.0 mEq/L.
4. Check the patient's prior medicines. Digoxin will block the A-V node, but makes the heart more excitable. Therefore, dysrhythmias are *more* likely, but less of a problem if they occur.
5. Pain stimulates the adrenals to produce catecholamines that cause dysrhythmias. Morphine 2 to 4 mg IV is a great antidysrhythmic drug.

TIPS TO REMEMBER

- If a patient is tachycardic and hemodynamically unstable, cardiovert.
- AV nodal blockers are first-line therapy for supraventricular tachyarrhythmias.

COMPREHENSION QUESTIONS

1. A 70-year-old patient arrives in the PACU following a peripheral vascular procedure. His blood pressure is 80/60 mm Hg, and you happen to glance at the monitor and note that, since leaving the OR, his heart rate has abruptly jumped to 160; he is diaphoretic and confused. Your therapeutic response depends on which of the following?

    A. Past medical history
    B. His current medical regimen
    C. His hemodynamic status
    D. His electrocardiogram

2. A 60-year-old woman arrives in the PACU following a hysterectomy. She is stable on arrival but abruptly develops a tachycardia of 160 with a BP of 110/70. She "feels" her heart beating, but she is alert. Your therapeutic response depends on which of the following?

    A. Past medical history
    B. Her current medical regimen
    C. Her hemodynamic status
    D. Her electrocardiogram

Answers

1. **C.** When patients are hemodynamically unstable, your goal is to recognize and treat their cardiac rhythms—nothing else matters. Usually a rhythm strip or the

monitor is adequate for these purposes, and waiting for a formal EKG can need-lessly delay treatment.

2. **D**. When a patient exhibits a tachydysrhythmia but is not symptomatic, you have time to determine whether the source of the problem is above or below the A-V node. If above (supraventricular), you have some pharmacologic options. A narrow complex QRS must derive from above the A-V node, and A-V nodal blockers should solve the problem. Remember, whenever in doubt (or just if you get frightened), you may always revert to cardioversion.

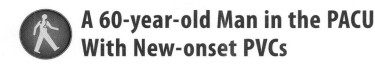

A 60-year-old Man in the PACU With New-onset PVCs

Alden H. Harken, MD

A 60-year-old male is admitted to the postanesthesia care unit (PACU) following an uneventful endovascular repair of an abdominal aortic aneurysm. On arrival, his BP is 140/90 and his heart rate is 110. Finger oximetry is 96%. He made 100 mL of urine during the previous hour. He is breathing comfortably with face mask oxygen. The nurse calls you because he is beginning to have a bunch of premature ventricular contractions (PVCs). When you arrive at the patient's bedside, the nurse hands you a rhythm strip (see Figure 29-1):

1. **Does this patient have a high or low risk of underlying cardiac disease?**

2. **What is the first thing you should ask the nurse to do?**

3. **Are the PVCs caused by a focal or diffuse myocardial process? How do you tell?**

4. **What are five things you can do to help to prevent the arrhythmia from progressing to ventricular tachycardia?**

5. **What is the therapy for a patient who progresses to ventricular tachycardia?**

VENTRICULAR TACHYDYSRHYTHMIAS

Answers

1. This is a patient with peripheral vascular disease and therefore likely coronary artery disease. He begins to throw multifocal (QRS morphology looks different) PVCs following a stressful, even if "uneventful," vascular procedure. Therefore, when evaluating this patient, your index of suspicion for myocardial ischemia should be relatively higher.

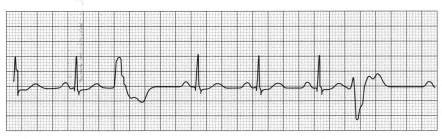

Figure 29-1. Rhythm strip which includes two wide complex beats that appear different (multifocal).

2. For any abnormal rhythm, your first step is to ask the nurse to obtain a 12-lead EKG to more fully characterize the rhythm, conduction, and repolarization of the myocardium. While you wait, you can begin by looking at the rhythm strip.

3. When all the PVCs look the same (monomorphic), the culprit is typically a small bit of myocardium on the edge of a previous myocardial infarction. This bit of ischemic muscle did not die and has become electrically unstable. However, all the impulses activate the ventricles along the same pathway and all the PVCs look the same.

   When the shapes (morphology) of the PVCs are different, the activation sites within the ventricles are also different, and something is making the whole myocardium electrically unstable/irritable.

   This patient's PVCs are polymorphic, and are therefore most likely related to a diffuse myocardial process.

4. The rhythm strip exhibits classical multifocal ventricular ectopy (extra beats from several sites). Most beats are sinus (NSR) with a "narrow" QRS (0.08 second, 80 milliseconds or two little boxes on the ECG paper) following an atrial "P" wave. But then two PVCs appear, each with a unique morphology. Each of them takes at least five little boxes or 0.2 second to completely activate the ventricles. This is termed "aberrant ventricular conduction." When an electrical impulse begins at the A-V node and travels down the high-velocity Purkinje fibers, the entire ventricles activate rapidly (0.08 second or a "narrow" QRS complex). When activation of the ventricles begins somewhere "ectopic" within the ventricular muscle, the impulse must travel along back dirt roads before it gets to the Purkinje superhighway. Activation of the ventricles takes a lot longer ("wide" QRS).

   One worst case scenario would be that the PVCs become more frequent and ultimately progress to ventricular tachycardia. In order to reduce the chance of that happening, we target the five "usual suspects" for PVCs:

   1. Regional hypoxemia: If this is due to fixed coronary disease, there is not much you can do acutely. Otherwise, you can place the patient on face mask oxygen. This won't hurt, and it might help.

   2. Hypokalemia: Make sure your patient's serum potassium is above 4.0 mEq/L.

   3. Hypomagnesemia: Make sure your patient's serum magnesium is above 2.0 mEq/L.

   4. Drugs: You can review the patient's medications. The estimate is that about 15% of antiarrhythmic drugs actually function to promote arrhythmias. Digitoxicity classically provokes multifocal PVCs.

   5. Pain: Discomfort promotes secretion of endogenous catechols, which causes multifocal ectopy (PVCs). Be liberal with a morphine 2 to 4 mg IV bolus.

5. Even if you do everything correctly, there are some patients who will still progress to ventricular tachycardia (see Figure 29-2).

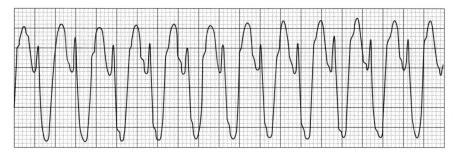

Figure 29-2. Ventricular tachycardia.

Note the "wide morphology complex" ventricular activation. All these QRS complexes look the same because the most irritable ventricular site has taken over the cardiac rhythm.

The therapy is electrical cardioversion. Some patients in ventricular tachycardia still have sufficient cardiac output to remain awake and even normotensive. If your patient remains conscious, it is kind to pretreat with 20 mg of etomidate IV. When a patient goes into ventricular tachycardia or fibrillation, everyone typically gets pretty excited. You can probably convert most patients with lower-energy cardioversions, but it is best when the first shock successfully restores sinus rhythm. Few people will criticize you for cranking the cardioverter up to maximum (typically 150 J biphasic or 200 J monophasic). You should "synchronize" (sync) the shock for all but ventricular fibrillation. When you do sync the shock, you will need to depress the button for 4 to 5 seconds before the machine discharges—these 4 to 5 seconds are when the machine is trying to determine the rhythm. If you do convert ventricular tachycardia to ventricular fibrillation, just shock the patient again, this time with sync turned off because in this case there is no rhythm with which the machine can synchronize.

When you have successfully restored the sinus rhythm, it makes sense in most instances to load with amiodarone in the following manner:

1. 150 mg IV over 10 minutes
2. Followed by 1 mg/min × 6 hours
3. Followed by 0.5 mg/min × 18 hours

TIPS TO REMEMBER

- PVCs result from electrically unstable ventricular myocardium.
- Initial treatment for PVCs is oxygen, electrolyte repletion, and pain control.
- Sustained ventricular tachycardia = cardioversion.

COMPREHENSION QUESTIONS

1. A 55-year-old male arrives in the PACU with multifocal PVCs. BP 140/80 and HR 80. Which of the following treatments is reasonable? (Choose all that apply.)
   A. Amiodarone load
   B. Diltiazem 20 mg IV
   C. Face mask oxygen
   D. 2 to 4 mg morphine IV

2. A 65-year-old male develops ventricular tachycardia during an open abdominal aortic aneurysmectomy. The appropriate therapy is which of the following?
   A. External cardioversion with 150 J
   B. Internal cardiac massage
   C. 100 mg lidocaine
   D. Amiodarone load

Answers

1. **C and D**. This patient is exhibiting a globally hyperexcitable myocardium. Amiodarone is better chronic therapy. Diltiazem will block the A-V route to no effect and probably also reduce the blood pressure. Both oxygen and morphine may reduce global myocardial hyperexcitability.

2. **A**. Electrical cardioversion will restore the cardiac rhythm most expeditiously. Once sinus rhythm is restored, both lidocaine and amiodarone make sense.

A 65-year-old Man With Bradycardia

Alden H. Harken, MD
and Brian C. George, MD

A 65-year-old gentleman arrives in your emergency department and is rapidly diagnosed with sigmoid diverticulitis and a free perforation. His BP is 80/60 with a heart rate of 120 and a temperature of 39°C. You initiate goal-directed therapy for septic shock with two boluses of 500 mL of Ringer's lactate and place a central venous line. As your catheter enters the right atrium, his heart rate drops to 30 and, to your surprise, this is a "sinus" bradycardia. You infuse 0.6 mg atropine for its vagolytic effect and his rate returns to 110.

Following successful resuscitation and within 45 minutes you are in the operating room with the patient. You are not surprised when, with intubation, he becomes bradycardic again. While you call for some additional medication, you double check to make sure that the pacing pads are placed appropriately.

1. What heart rate is "too slow?"

2. What is the most likely reason the patient became bradycardic a second time?

3. Besides atropine, what other drug could you give this patient (hint: it is chronotropic)?

4. Where exactly should external pacing pads be placed on a patient?

BRADYCARDIA

Your patient's heart is just a ball of muscle with some electrical wiring in it that tells it when to beat. If the heart rate is either too fast (traditional rule of thumb is 220 minus your patient's age) or too slow (by definition, less than 60), you should be able to improve cardiac output with better rhythm control. Problematic fast heart rates are much more common than problematic slow heart rates. This chapter will discuss what to do for patients whose heart rate is too slow. Other chapters will deal with the topic of heart rates that are too fast.

Answers

1. "Too slow" is not the same thing as bradycardia. Bradycardia is a definition; "too slow" is a clinical assessment. Bradycardia is defined as a heart rate less than 60, while "too slow" is any heart rate that does not adequately preserve cardiac output. Remember:

$$\text{Cardiac output} = \text{heart rate} \times \text{stroke volume}$$

An Olympic triathlete probably has a massive stroke volume and might be able to perfuse his or her end organs with a heart rate of 30. But a 95-year-old diabetic man with coronary artery disease, hypertension, and a dilated cardiomyopathy doesn't have a lot of inotropic reserve. Instead, he relies on his heart rate to increase his cardiac output—and even though 60 is not defined as bradycardia it might still be "too slow" for him. In the presented patient with freely perforated diverticulitis, a heart rate of 30 is both bradycardic and "too slow."

You can use your understanding of "too slow" when evaluating postoperative patients as well. For example, when a nurse calls you about a patient who has a heart rate of 55, the most important thing is not—surprise, surprise—the number. Instead, you must make a clinical assessment of the patient to determine if the heart rate is sufficient to maintain cardiac output. Is the patient symptomatic? Is the patient alert? Is this a dramatic change from baseline? If the patient is symptomatic, you should administer atropine and apply external pacemakers (as per the standard ACLS algorithm). If the patient is not symptomatic but this is a dramatic change, you should get an EKG to look for a new heart block.

2. You were ready for this to happen because you expected the intravenous atropine effect to last about 30 minutes.

3. Isoproterenol is the most chronotropic β-adrenergic agonist. You begin 5 µg/min and place external pacing patches (just in case this patient tries this again).

4. You know that the pads need to be placed so the heart is in between them. A typical position is one posteriorly, just to the right of T-10, and one anteriorly, just below the left nipple. A line drawn between these pads goes directly through the heart—which is also where the current will go.

External pacemakers are easy to place and rapid to initiate. Note that these types of pacemakers do stimulate both striated and cardiac muscle, and the patient will jump with each pacer stimulus. This is quite uncomfortable for the patient, but may be necessary regardless.

TIPS TO REMEMBER

- "Too slow" is not the same thing as bradycardia. The former demands immediate treatment; the latter demands immediate investigation.
- To speed up the heart you only need 2 drugs: 0.6 mg atropine IV push (lasts about 30 minutes) and isoproterenol 5 µg/min.
- Don't forget the external pacemaker.

COMPREHENSION QUESTIONS

1. What dose of atropine should you give for a patient with symptomatic bradycardia?
>   A. 0.2 mg
>   B. 0.6 mg
>   C. 1 mg
>   D. 10 mg

2. You are called about a 45-year-old patient who has a heart rate of 55. It was in the 70s for the past 24 hours. She is postoperative day 3 from a sigmoid colectomy, is asymptomatic, and has a BP 95/60. What information is the least useful?
>   A. The patient's heart rate as recorded in the preoperative H&P
>   B. EKG
>   C. Mental status
>   D. Urine output

Answers

1. **B**. Something to memorize: 0.6 mg atropine.

2. **D**. While urine output is a great measure of end-organ perfusion, it takes at least an hour to know whether the patient has become oliguric. Therefore, in the acute setting (ie, with newly discovered bradycardia), it is not as useful as the other items.

A 65-year-old Man With a Pacemaker Who Needs Surgery

Alden H. Harken, MD and Brian C. George, MD

A 65-year-old man arrives, again with a diverticular perforation, but this patient has an old median sternotomy incision and a lump just below his left clavicle. This patient's BP is 130/90 with a heart rate of 100. By ECG, it looks like the ventricle is being paced, but the atrium is not.

You tell the operating room circulating nurse that you would like to use the electrocautery during surgery. She suggests putting a magnet over the pacemaker.

1. What triggers a ventricular demand pacemaker to fire?

2. What does the magnet do?

3. Is it safe to use electrocautery?

PACEMAKERS AND ELECTROCAUTERY

Answers

1. The early pacemakers were all "fixed rate" and were programmed to emit one pulse/second, for a ventricular rate of 60. However, occasionally, even patients with complete 3° heart block will exhibit a spontaneous ventricular beat. When the repolarization of this spontaneous QRS (upstroke of the T wave) coincides with a fixed-rate pacer stimulus, ventricular fibrillation may result.

   So, the "demand" pacemaker was developed. This type of pacemaker is smart about how it fires. This can more easily be seen with an example. To make the math easier, we will pretend we have a demand pacer with a rate set at 60 beats/min. Every time this "demand" pacemaker senses a QRS complex it turns off and waits for one second. If, at the end of one second, it doesn't sense another QRS, it fires. So, the patient's ventricular rate can spontaneously rise above 60, but never below. The trick here is that the pacer can sense many electrical stimuli (like an electrocautery) as a QRS and will stop pacing, but only for as long as you use the cautery. So don't blast away for long periods.

   The ventricular demand pacer prevents the patient from dying; however, it does not increase its rate when the patient runs up stairs. Thus, an atrioventricular pacer coordinates electrodes in both the atrium and the ventricle. When this device "senses" an atrial P wave, it waits a short preset interval (say, 0.18 second), and if it senses a QRS, it turns off; if it doesn't detect a QRS, it paces one. This device can therefore track faster atrial rates and create atrioventricular synchrony (adds atrial "kick"). But if the sensed atrial rate ever drops below 60, the A-V pacer paces both the atrium and the ventricle.

2. Pacemakers are switched into a "fixed-rate" mode whenever a magnet is placed over it. Typically, the fixed ventricular rate is set to 60. If you place a magnet over this man's pacemaker to convert the pacer into its "fixed-rate" mode, his ventricular rate will actually slow down (from 100 to 60). This would probably be bad for his cardiac output.

3. Yes, but intelligently. The patient's demand pacemaker will sense the electro-cautery as the patient's heartbeat and transiently turn itself off. If you use it for too long, that means you've stopped the patient's heart. Therefore, you can use the electrocautery for very short bursts so that the patient will miss only one or two heartbeats during each cauterization. Of course, if you need to use electro-cautery for longer bursts, you can apply a magnet to induce a fixed rate.

TIPS TO REMEMBER

- Atrioventricular demand pacing preserves atrioventricular synchrony (ie, the "atrial kick") as well as tracks faster native atrial rates.

- A magnet converts a demand pacemaker to a fixed-rate pacemaker.

- Electrocautery effectively suppresses a demand pacemaker's firing—use it for only as long as the patient can tolerate asystole (typically one or two beats).

COMPREHENSION QUESTIONS

1. What does the magnet do to a pacemaker?
    A. Changes the mode
    B. Turns it off
    C. Makes it safe to use electrocautery
    D. All of the above

2. What type of pacemaker is most "physiologic?"
    A. Fixed ventricular
    B. Fixed atrioventricular pacing
    C. Demand ventricular
    D. Demand atrioventricular pacing

Answers

1. **A**. A magnet changes the pacemaker from a "demand pacing" mode to "fixed pacing" mode. While a magnet does prevent electrocautery from suppressing the pacemaker firing, it is not safer if the fixed rate is too slow to maintain cardiac output.

2. **D**. Look closely at the names of each type of pacing. The "atrio" part of "atrio-ventricular" means that the pacemaker coordinates ventricular pacing with the atrial beat (via the P wave). That coordination means the ventricular is paced just after the "atrial kick," which improves cardiac output. It also means that it paces the ventricle faster if the native atrial pacemaker is firing more rapidly. The "demand" part means that the pacemaker kicks in only if the heart doesn't produce its own beat—again, preserving normal physiologic function whenever possible.

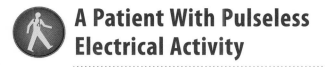

A Patient With Pulseless Electrical Activity

Alden H. Harken, MD
and Brian C. George, MD

You are in the operating room, in the emergency room, or maybe on the floor. Somebody says "I can't get a blood pressure."

You look at the cardiac monitor and there is still electrical activity apparent.

1. List the 6 H's and 6 T's.

2. Assume that you cannot rule out tension pneumothorax as the cause. Where and how should you decompress it?

3. Assume that you cannot rule out cardiac tamponade as the cause. What are the landmarks you use to do a pericardiocentesis?

4. Assume that you cannot rule out hypovolemia as the cause. When would you decide to stop treatment of the patient?

PULSELESS ELECTRICAL ACTIVITY

Answers

1. Pulseless electrical activity (PEA) has multiple causes, which you should memorize. During an emergency is not the time to be consulting a reference card (see Table 32-1).

   Regardless of cause, it doesn't make any difference whether the patient arrives in the emergency department (ED) with no blood pressure or whether your patient abruptly loses a blood pressure in the operating room—you start with the same "ABC" emergency protocol. You should automatically do the following:

   - Begin bag mask ventilation and start the process of intubating the patient. If the patient is already intubated (eg, in the OR), check the tube.

   - Check the monitor. While pulseless, PEA still implies a cardiac rhythm. If the rhythm strip displays ventricular fibrillation (VF), proceed directly to asynchronous cardioversion (see the Ventricular Tachydysrhythmia Chapter 29).

   - Place 2 large-bore IVs and give some crystalloid.

   From this point on, management diverges based on your index of suspicion for each of the possible causes. In general, however, if you cannot rule out a given possibility, then you should empirically treat *before* you've made the diagnosis—if you wait to be sure, you've waited too long.

   Let's continue the case for some of the more complex yet common scenarios.

Table 32-1. The Causes of PEA, Organized as the 6 H's and 6 T's

6 H's	6 T's
Hypovolemia	Toxins
Hypoxia	Tamponade (cardiac)
Hydrogen ions (ie, acidosis)	Tension pneumothorax (PTX)
Hyperkalemia or hypokalemia	Thrombosis (MI)
Hypoglycemia	Thrombosis (PE)
Hypothermia	Trauma (ie, myocardial contusion)

2. In this scenario, let's assume that your patient is a 70-year-old veteran with a 100-pack/year smoking history. He is undergoing a laparoscopic right colectomy for cancer. At the beginning of the case the anesthesiologist despairs of a peak inspiratory pressure of 45 mm Hg. The cancer is partially obstructing, so you decide to proceed anyway. Midway through the case, the patient loses his pressure. The monitor reveals a heart rate of 130. The tube looks OK. (With an open abdomen, you would feel the aorta in order to confirm hypotension.) You should give 500 mL of LR. Try to listen for breath sounds. Then insert a #18 needle directly up through the diaphragm (if the abdomen is open) or high in the midaxillary (*not* midclavicular) line. You don't need to connect the needle to anything. Your patient is already on positive pressure ventilation so you cannot produce a pneumothorax. This patient has bought himself a chest tube on the side that produces a gratifying "whoosh" of air.

3. Let's pretend you are stat paged to the cath lab where your cardiology colleagues have placed some stiff catheters into the right ventricle of a middle-aged man. The patient is under the sheets, and the only history you get is that the monitor reveals a heart rate of 120 and he abruptly lost his blood pressure. The cardiac silhouette has not gotten any bigger during fluoroscopy.

   After ensuring that the patient's airway is patent and that the patient is breathing (A and B), you should perform a pericardiocentesis. This is performed by inserting a long #18 (spinal) needle immediately below the xiphoid while aiming for the patient's left shoulder. If you get air, pull back and try again a little more medially. (If you are in the OR and already in the abdomen, you may more easily access the pleural and pericardial spaces directly across the diaphragm.) If you obtain blood, remove about 20 mL and squirt some on the sheets. If the blood clots on the sheets, you are in the right ventricle. If the blood does not clot, it represents defibrinated blood that was in the pericardial space.

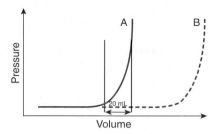

Figure 32-1. The pressure in the pericardial space remains low with increasing volume until the elastic limits of the pericardium are attained, at which point the pressure soars (A). Note that only a 20 mL volume difference produces a big increase in pressure at the elastic limit. A chronic pericardial effusion (B), however, can stretch gradually, with negligible increase in pressure.

Removing only 20 mL should make a huge hemodynamic difference (see Figure 32-1). Conceptually, let's take some impermissible physiological leaps: by removing 20 mL of pericardial fluid, you permit an additional 20 mL of ventricular end-diastolic filling. The augmented left ventricular end-diastolic volume (LVEDV) translates into 20 mL of additional stroke volume. An additional 20 mL SV × heart rate of 100 equals an increased cardiac output of 2 L! The good news is that you have helped your patient a lot. The bad news is your patient only needs to reaccumulate another 20 mL in order to get back into trouble.

4. In this scenario, let's pretend that the patient is a young, healthy-appearing biker who has rolled his bike at high speed on the interstate. Your crack paramedic team rings down: "No vitals in the field" on arrival in the ED. There is a big diagnostic fork in the road.

Fork A: The nurses slap on EKG leads, indicating a sinus tachycardia of 140 and no BP (PEA). On fast exam there is minimal or no ventricular motion. You should "call the code." A massive amount of epidemiological data confirms negligible "walkout of the hospital" survival following "blunt trauma with no vitals in the field."

Fork B: The fast exam reveals vigorous ventricular contractility and a belly full of blood. You should activate the massive transfusion protocol on the way to the operating room.

TIPS TO REMEMBER

● When you are stat paged, your destination determines your differential diagnosis. The most likely problems differ when you are called to the ED, the OR, the cath lab, or the dialysis unit.

- The three most common causes of PEA are hypovolemia, tension pneumothorax, and cardiac tamponade. All three respond to volume.
- The diagnosis of tamponade is not made by x-ray or ultrasound. Tamponade is not an "imaging" diagnosis.
- A "pericardial effusion" becomes "pericardial tamponade" when the patient can no longer compensate in order to maintain ventricular filling. Eventually such patients go into PEA arrest.
- Similarly, a "spontaneous pneumothorax" becomes a "tension pneumothorax" when the patient can no longer compensate, venous return falls, and once again the patient cannot maintain ventricular filling.

COMPREHENSION QUESTIONS

1. You are in the OR performing an open procedure when your patient goes into PEA arrest. The first thing you should do is which of the following?
    A. Obtain a rhythm strip.
    B. Decompress the bilateral chest through the diaphragm.
    C. Obtain a CXR.
    D. Check the ET tube position.

2. You are in the OR performing a laparoscopic procedure when your patient goes into PEA arrest. You decide to decompress the chest. You should place a #18 needle in which of the following positions?
    A. In the midaxillary line above the nipples
    B. In the midclavicular line as close to the clavicle as possible
    C. Through the diaphragm

Answers

1. **D.** ABC—airway comes first.

2. **A.** The diaphragm can be surprisingly high when a patient is supine—and especially when the abdomen is insufflated for a laparoscopic procedure. Don't place the needle in the midclavicular line as there is a risk of hitting the subclavian.

A 55-year-old Man Who May Require Perioperative β-blockade

Alden H. Harken, MD
and Brian C. George, MD

A 55-year-old banker is driving back to work following a three-martini lunch when he is T-boned by a cement truck. On arrival in the emergency department he is hemodynamically stable and alert. He prides himself on never having graced a physician's office and he is on no medications. FAST exam reveals fluid in the LUQ. During the next hour his blood pressure drifts down and you are forced to take him to the OR for a splenorrhaphy.

You are writing his postoperative orders using a template, and you arrive at the section with numerous possible options for postoperative β-blockade. As you write your postoperative orders, you wonder: "Should I put this guy on a β-blocker?"

1. **Should you put this patient on a β-blocker?**
2. **If he instead took metoprolol 25 mg PO twice a day at home, what dose would you give him of IV metoprolol while he is NPO?**

PERIOPERATIVE β-BLOCKADE

Answers

1. In 1999, Poldermans et al screened almost 800 high-risk vascular patients with dobutamine stress echocardiography. These investigations then culled approximately 200 very, very high-risk vascular patients formidably vulnerable to myocardial ischemia from the original high-risk group. Two weeks of β-blockade prior to the vascular surgical procedure cut the mortality from 34% (control) to 3.4% (β-blockers)—a huge difference.

   However, is it permissible to extrapolate from this very, very high-risk vascular surgical group to just high-risk or even moderate-risk patients? Mangano previously stoked the confusion by prospectively randomizing 200 surgical patients into β-blocker and placebo groups. The 30-day mortality was the same, but 2-year mortality statistically favored β-blockade. Taken together, it began to look like preoperative β-blockers were certainly good for very high-risk patients, probably benefited moderate-risk patients, and might be good for everyone. Extending the tenets of a great American philosopher (Mae West opined that "Too much of a good thing is wonderful") the PeriOperative ISchemic Evaluation (POISE) trial gave up to eight times the recommended dose of extended-release β-blockers to any patient with a heart rate over 60. In this huge study of 8351 patients in 23 countries (they could not talk any US investigators into participating), there was a reduction in myocardial infarction (5.7%-4.2%; $P <.0017$), but β-blocked patients with heart rates of 60 induced more strokes (0.5%-1.0%) and more deaths (2.3%-3.1%; $P <.03$). The investigators did not report whether they were surprised by the results of their pharmacological experiment.

Finally, Lindenaur et al retrospectively correlated cardiovascular events and in-hospital mortality with in-hospital β-blockers—another huge 663, 969-surgical-patient study in which β-blockers clearly benefited high-risk patients. Most low-risk patients were not on a β-blocker on hospital admission. This low-risk group did not receive a β-blocker until subsequent to their cardiovascular event, at which time they were statistically included in the β-blocker group. In fairness, this jaw-dropping experimental design flaw was emphasized in a companion editorial. From the flurry of studies examining perioperative β-blockade, several conclusions are permissible:

- Perioperative myocardial infarction, and probably death, is reduced by judicious use of low-dose, short-acting β-blockers (target a preoperative heart rate of 70 and a postoperative heart rate of 80).
- If your patient is on β-blockers on admission, do not stop them perioperatively.
- If your patient should have been on β-blockers preoperatively (ie, the patient had an indication such as hypertension, vascular disease, diabetes, etc), then start them as soon as possible.
- Overdosing any drug is bad, and overdosing long-acting β-blockers is associated with bradycardia, hypotension, CVA, and death.

2. You can figure this out by memorizing a single conversion. Note that both of these are the lowest doses normally used for each of these formulations:

$$12.5 \text{ mg PO q12h} = 5 \text{ mg IV q6h}$$

TIPS TO REMEMBER

- β-Blocker–naïve patients should be written for low-dose, short-acting β-blockers (ie, metoprolol 5 mg IV q6h with hold parameters).
- Continue any preoperative β-blockers (with appropriate conversion to IV as needed).
- Start low-dose β-blockers in those patients who should have been on them in the first place.

COMPREHENSION QUESTIONS

1. Do low-dose β-blockers reduce mortality?
   A. No, because they increase the rate of strokes.
   B. Unsure, the evidence is contradictory.
   C. Yes, because they reduce the risk of myocardial infarction.

2. What should you write for a patient on metoprolol 25 mg PO BID at home?
   A. No β-blockade
   B. 5 mg IV q6h
   C. 5 mg IV q12h
   D. 10 mg IV q6h
   E. 10 mg IV q12h
   F. 12.5 mg IV q6h
   G. 25 mg IV q12h

3. What should you write for a 65-year-old patient who is not on β-blockers at home and just underwent a right hemicolectomy?
   A. No β-blockade
   B. Metoprolol 5 mg IV q6h
   C. Metoprolol 10 mg IV q6h
   D. Metoprolol 10 mg IV q12h

Answers

1. **C.** The evidence suggests that low-dose β-blockers do indeed reduce the rates of MI and consequently of death. While the POISE trial showed an increase in mortality, the investigators in that study used doses of β-blocker that are higher than what is recommended.

2. **D.** Remember 12.5 mg PO BID equals 5 mg IV q6h, so twice that is 10 mg IV q6h.

3. **B.** This β-blocker–naïve patient should be given β-blockade only at the lowest dose, that is, at 5 mg IV q6h, and targeting a HR of less than 80. You should also be careful to write appropriate hold parameters (ie, HOLD for HR <60 or SBP <100).

SUGGESTED READINGS

Lindenaur PK, Pekow P, Wang K, Mamidi DK, Gutierrez B, Benjamin EM. Perioperative beta-blocker therapy and mortality after major noncardiac surgery. *N Engl J Med*. 2005;353:349.

Mangano DT, Layug EL, Wallace A, Tateo I. Effect of atenolol on mortality and cardiovascular morbidity after noncardiac surgery. Multicenter Study of Perioperative Ischemia Research Group. *N Engl J Med*. 1996;335:1713.

POISE Study Group, Devereaux PJ, Yang H, et al. Effects of extended-release metoprolol succinate in patients undergoing non-cardiac surgery (POISE trial): a randomised controlled trial. *Lancet*. 2008;371:1839.

Poldermans D, Boersma E, Bax JJ, et al. The effect of bisoprolol on perioperative mortality and myocardial infarction in high-risk patients undergoing vascular surgery. Dutch Echocardiographic Cardiac Risk Evaluation Applying Stress Echocardiography Study Group. *N Engl J Med*. 1999;341:1789.

A 65-year-old Man Who Is in Respiratory Distress 3 Days Postoperatively

Jahan Mohebali, MD

Mr. Jones is a 65-year-old man with a history of smoking, type 2 diabetes mellitus, and poorly controlled hypertension. He underwent an uncomplicated Whipple procedure 3 days ago and was transferred to the floor from the surgical ICU this morning. You are the night-float intern, and shortly after receiving sign-out, the nurse pages you to the patient's bedside stating that she is concerned about how he is doing. On arrival, you find him sitting up in bed and leaning forward. He states that he feels a bit anxious and is having trouble catching his breath. You ask the nurse to obtain a pulse oximetry reading that demonstrates an O_2 saturation of 88%. He is in obvious respiratory distress. You call for an EKG and CXR and proceed with your physical exam.

1. **What are the two most likely causes of this patient's acute decompensated heart failure?**

2. **Which findings in the patient's preoperative evaluation might suggest that he would be at increased risk of postoperative CHF?**

3. **What are typical physical exam findings seen in acute decompensated heart failure?**

4. **What laboratory and radiographic studies would be useful for confirming a diagnosis of heart failure and determining the underlying etiology?**

5. **What are the first two steps in managing acute postoperative heart failure?**

ACUTE POSTOPERATIVE HEART FAILURE

Answers

1. Like many other things in surgery and medicine, one of the best approaches to understanding and managing a clinical condition is to go back to the underlying physiology and basic science. In heart failure, one must think about the pathophysiology of cardiogenic shock that is essentially the result of inadequate cardiac output. Cardiac output is the product of stroke volume and heart rate. While heart rate is essentially dependent on autonomic tone and underlying rhythm, stroke volume is more complex and affected by preload, afterload, and contractility. In certain situations, rhythm may affect preload. Most causes of postoperative heart failure can be attributed to a problem or imbalance in one or more of these factors (see Figure 34-1).

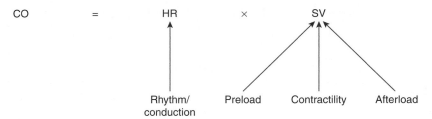

Figure 34-1. The relationship between the various parameters of cardiac output.

Preload: This should be thought of as the amount of volume in the heart at the end of diastole, right before the heart contracts. In the case of postoperative heart failure, too much preload can overdistend the myocardium and push cardiac function to the far end of the Starling curve (see Figure 34-2). The most common cause of this is overly aggressive fluid resuscitation in the immediate postoperative period. Often, patients undergoing large operations will have a postoperative systemic inflammatory response syndrome (SIRS) response that will result in third spacing of fluid. This fluid tends to "mobilize" back into the vascular space around postoperative day 3 resulting in sudden intravascular fluid overload. Rhythm can also affect preload. This is discussed separately in the section below.

The Frank-Starling relationship (see Figure 34-2): As preload increases, the myocardium stretches and cardiac output subsequently increases to a point where the myocardium becomes overstretched and stroke volume and cardiac output begin to decline. The #1 arrow represents the point on the curve where additional intravascular volume (preload) will augment cardiac output. The #2 arrow represents the equilibrium point, dependent on the specific patient's ventricular compliance where preload optimizes cardiac output. The #3 arrow represents postoperative fluid overload where

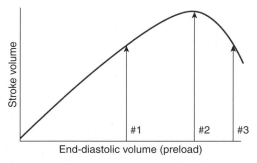

Figure 34-2. The Frank-Starling relationship, illustrating how increased preload results in increased stroke volume (and, hence, cardiac output).

too much preload overstretches the myocardium and actually decreases cardiac output resulting in heart failure.

Afterload: Afterload is perhaps best thought of as the pressure the heart has to pump blood out against. In most cases, it is directly related to the blood pressure and systemic vascular resistance. A common scenario is the patient with mild-to-moderate compensated heart failure and long-standing hypertension who develops a hypertensive crisis postoperatively, possibly secondary to pain, and discontinuation of home antihypertensives. The already weak heart is then forced to pump against a much higher afterload resulting in decreased forward flow and flash pulmonary edema.

Contractility/intrinsic pump function: Once preload and afterload are optimized, attention should be turned to contractility. The most concerning cause of decreased contractility is myocardial ischemia or infarction. As the myocardium becomes ischemic, it loses its ability to contract and force blood forward. Any time postoperative heart failure is encountered, one must ensure that it is not the result of myocardial ischemia. Another factor resulting in decreased intrinsic pump dysfunction and inability to move blood forward may be underlying valvular heart disease. Although a discussion of the intricacies of managing different types of valvular heart disease is beyond the scope of this book, it is important to consider this in one's workup, including the possibility of acute mitral regurgitation as a result of papillary muscle rupture in the setting of myocardial infarction.

Heart rate and rhythm: As mentioned, the second component of cardiac output is heart rate. Patients who develop heart block postoperatively with bradycardic underlying escape rhythms can also develop heart failure. It is important to remember that myocardial ischemia should also always be considered with new-onset heart block. Tachyarrhythmias represent a unique entity and they are discussed here as part of "rhythm disturbances"; however, their effects are actually on preload. Based on the equation defined above (Figure 34-1), it would seem that tachyarrhythmias should result in increased cardiac output because of increased heart rate. In the case of supraventricular tachycardias (SVT), and atrial fibrillation with rapid ventricular response, however, the result is often a drop in cardiac output. The mechanism for this phenomenon is a decrease in diastolic filling time that subsequently decreases end-diastolic volume (preload) and, therefore, cardiac output. Atrial fibrillation has the added effect of removing the "atrial kick" that can contribute anywhere from 20% to 30% to cardiac output because it augments ventricular filling. This augmentation is particularly critical for patients with long-standing hypertension and subsequent thickened myocardium with decreased ventricular compliance. When these patients suddenly flip into atrial fibrillation in the postoperative period, the result may be decompensated heart failure.

In summary, when thinking about the etiology of postoperative heart failure and its most common underlying pathophysiology, the following should be considered, in this order:

A. Too much preload—fluid overload, likely iatrogenic in the setting of aggressive postoperative resuscitation

B. Too much afterload—uncontrolled hypertension in the postoperative period

C. Decreased cardiac output (myocardial dysfunction)—most commonly from myocardial ischemia/infarction

D. Rhythm disturbance tachyarrhythmias such as atrial fibrillation, or bradyarrhythmias from new or chronic heart block

2. With regard to afterload, Mr. Jones has underlying hypertension suggesting that if his blood pressure is not adequately controlled in the postoperative period, he is at risk for a hypertensive crisis, subsequent heart failure, and flash pulmonary edema. With regard to contractility, the patient is a smoker and long-standing diabetic. These two factors alone significantly increase his risk of coronary artery disease making him vulnerable to myocardial ischemia in the postoperative period. Additionally, his long-standing history of poorly controlled hypertension not only increases his risk of coronary disease but also suggests that his left ventricle has been pumping against an increased afterload for many years. This typically results in some degree of left ventricular hypertrophy. As a result, he will likely have a stiff ventricle and some degree of diastolic cardiac dysfunction. Finally, with regard to rhythm, his increased left ventricular pressures will also likely have caused some degree of left atrial dilatation, placing him at increased risk for atrial fibrillation. Should he develop postoperative atrial fibrillation, he will be more likely to develop decompensated heart failure as he depends on his atrial kick to fill his left ventricle.

3. Returning to the underlying physiology of the disease process, one must keep in mind that all the physical exam findings seen in heart failure will be the result of the heart's inability to maintain forward flow of blood and perfusion to the body. As systemic perfusion decreases, one might expect to see cold and mottled extremities and perhaps decreased urine output. The cardiac exam may reveal an unusual rhythm or new murmur. Classically, an S3 gallop may also be heard. As left-sided failure results in pulmonary edema, the associated findings of basilar crackles and increased work of breathing will be seen. Hypoxemia is likely to result. When left-sided failure begins to result in right-sided failure, it is common to see distended neck veins, increasing peripheral edema, and perhaps RUQ pain and a hepatojugular reflex as the patient develops a congestive hepatopathy. If the patient is in an ICU and has a central venous or pulmonary artery catheter in place, one would expect to see elevated filling pressures (central venous pressure and wedge pressure) and a low cardiac output or index.

4. Again, our original framework can be applied to laboratory testing. A brain natriuretic peptide may be helpful in confirming fluid overload (too much preload). An EKG will help not only to evaluate for myocardial ischemia but also to elucidate any underlying rhythm abnormality. Troponins can also be sent to evaluate for ischemia. Serum electrolyte evaluation and appropriate repletion is crucial in the setting of arrhythmias. Patients often manifest decompensated heart failure with respiratory distress, and in those cases, a thorough workup with an arterial blood gas and CXR is often warranted to look for noncardiac causes of hypoxemia. Finally, once the patient is stabilized, an echocardiogram may provide insight into underlying myocardial and valvular function.

5. As always, the approach to stabilizing a patient should begin with the ABCs. Although these patients will typically not have airway issues, restoring ventilation and oxygenation should be a priority if there is a component of pulmonary edema. An arterial blood gas and CXR should immediately be obtained. As mentioned, an EKG will be useful in ruling out arrhythmias, conduction abnormalities, and ischemia as the cause of heart failure. If the patient is hemodynamically unstable, transfer to the ICU for inotropic support and invasive hemodynamic monitoring will likely be necessary and should be anticipated early. In the case of acute hemodynamic instability, the likely cause is an arrhythmia or ischemia. In the case of bradyarrhythmias, pacing pads should be placed and any nodal blockade should be reversed. Glucagon can be used to reverse the effects of β-blockers, and calcium can be used to reverse the effects of calcium channel blockers and improve myocardial contractility. Atropine or isoproterenol is also very effective for increasing heart rate. In the case of tachyarrhythmias with hemodynamic instability, the patient will need to be cardioverted and appropriate antiarrhythmics such as amiodarone and β-blockers started. If myocardial ischemia is suspected, an ACS protocol should immediately be instituted. In all of these cases, prompt evaluation by a cardiology service is beneficial. It is also important to note that a more senior resident should be notified of the patient's clinical status. Ultimately, the approach to managing postoperative heart failure begins by stabilizing the patient, thinking through the pathophysiology (ie, preload, afterload, contractility, and rate/rhythm), and then treating accordingly.

TIPS TO REMEMBER

- In most cases, postoperative heart failure is the result of one of the following four etiologies:
  - Too much preload—that is, fluid overload
  - Too much afterload—that is, uncontrolled hypertension
  - Poor contractility—likely related to ischemia resulting in decreased cardiac output
  - Bradyarrhythmias or tachyarrhythmias—resulting in decreased cardiac output

- Treatment is based on stabilizing the patient and treating the underlying cause or causes:
  - Preload—diuresis
  - Afterload—aggressive management of hypertension
  - Ischemia—ACS protocol, possibly inotropes, possibly invasive hemodynamic monitors, and emergent cardiology consult
  - Arrhythmias—pacing or appropriate nodal blocking agents ± cardiology consult

COMPREHENSION QUESTIONS

A 67-year-old man with long-standing hypertension is postoperative day 2 from a right upper lobe wedge resection for lung cancer. You are called by the nurse who tells you that his oxygen saturation has dropped into the mid-eighties and his heart rate is 134. He is hypotensive and his urine output has decreased significantly.

1. What two studies are likely to be most helpful during immediate initial evaluation in determining the cause of this patient's symptoms?
     A. An echocardiogram and a BNP
     B. Cardiac catheterization and a VQ scan
     C. An EKG and a CXR

2. This patient's heart failure is most likely related to which of the following?
     A. Too much preload
     B. Too much afterload
     C. Decreased contractility
     D. Loss of atrial kick

3. Assuming that the patient is hemodynamically unstable, you should be prepared to do which of the following?
     A. Obtain an echocardiogram.
     B. Give diuretics.
     C. Cardiovert.
     D. Give antihypertensives.

4. Every evaluation of a patient in potential heart failure should include which of the following studies at a minimum?
     A. CXR
     B. EKG
     C. Stress test

Answers

1. **C**. This patient has likely gone into atrial fibrillation, which occurs in 30% to 40% of patients undergoing thoracic surgery. An EKG will make the diagnosis. The hypoxemia is likely related to pulmonary edema as fluid from the left side of the heart backs up into the lungs as a result of a lost atrial kick and decreased diastolic filling time. However, given that the patient underwent a pulmonary wedge resection, a CXR is absolutely critical in ensuring that there is no other cause of hypoxemia such as a pneumothorax. An echocardiogram is a very helpful study, although there is little role for it during the immediate initial workup.

2. **D**. Loss of atrial kick (especially in patients with a stiff left ventricle) can result in a drop in cardiac output by up to 30%.

3. **C**. In a truly hemodynamically unstable patient with a tachyarrhythmia and a shockable rhythm, the first step is to attempt cardioversion.

4. **B**. Every evaluation of postoperative heart failure must include an EKG to rule out ischemia as this is the most serious, and in some cases, irreversible, cause of heart failure.

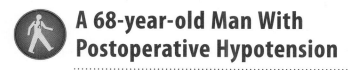

A 68-year-old Man With Postoperative Hypotension

Allan B. Peetz, MD and
Marie Crandall, MD, MPH

Mr. Patel is a 68-year-old, 90-kg male who underwent an exploratory laparotomy and lysis of adhesions 6 hours ago. You are on call and a nurse informs you that Mr. Patel's blood pressure is 92/43 and his heart rate is 102. He is completely asymptomatic and says he feels "fine except for the tube in my nose." You notice that his IVF bag is labeled "D5 0.45 normal saline" and is infusing at a rate of 125 mL/h.

1. Define hypotension.
2. What is the diagnosis of exclusion for all patients with postoperative hypotension?
3. What is the most likely cause of this patient's hypotension?

HYPOTENSION IN THE IMMEDIATE POSTOPERATIVE PERIOD

Postoperative hypotension is common and potentially serious, with a variety of underlying causes, including hypovolemia, cardiac failure, or sepsis. Because of the possibility of serious underlying pathology, the patient with postoperative hypotension should be rapidly evaluated and a diligent search for potentially life-threatening causes of hypotension should follow.

Answers

1. In general, a systolic blood pressure (SBP) less than 100 mm Hg or a mean arterial pressure (MAP) less than 65 mm Hg is considered hypotensive. That said, hypotension is best thought of as a *decreased blood pressure* rather than a *low blood pressure*—the difference between the patient's current and baseline blood pressures is the most critical factor. For example, a blood pressure measurement of 95/43 mm Hg after an uncomplicated laparoscopic appendectomy in an otherwise healthy 25-year-old female whose SBP is normally no greater than 105 mm Hg is probably not hypotension. On the other hand, a blood pressure of 125/64 mm Hg after an uncomplicated laparoscopic appendectomy in a 65-year-old, homeless male who has had many years of untreated kidney disease and whose preoperative blood pressure was 212/103 mm Hg probably *is* hypotension. While the blood pressure reading of 125/64 mm Hg is "normal"

in the conventional sense, the male patient's tissues and peripheral vasculature have probably compensated for a long history of hypertension and therefore this blood pressure may be too low to provide adequate oxygen delivery to his tissues.

2. Evaluation of the hypotensive patient starts with urgently ruling out hemorrhage as a cause of the patient's hypotension. If hemorrhage cannot be ruled out by history and physical exam, a workup including a CBC should be initiated while empiric treatment is begun.

   For those patients in whom you suspect hemorrhage, proper management includes infusion of 1 L of 0.9 NS or LR. The patient's blood pressure should respond soon after receiving the bolus, with an adequate response defined as a return to the patient's baseline blood pressure and/or improvement in urine output. If the patient's response is not adequate, a second 1 L bolus should be given, but suspicion for other, more life-threatening causes for the patient's hypotension should be high and rapid escalation of care should be initiated. This would include notifying the senior resident, possibly an ICU transfer, and a more extensive workup.

3. Hypovolemia is common in the postoperative patient and is a result of intraoperative fluid losses, ongoing sensible and insensible fluid losses, and fluid shifts. This is the most likely cause of Mr. Patel's hypotension. He has several factors contributing to an overall net negative fluid balance: inadequate maintenance fluids, NPO, and an open abdominal operation. The next step in managing Mr. Patel's hypovolemia should start with a 1 L bolus of resuscitative fluid—again 0.9% normal saline or lactated Ringer's solution. If the patient has congestive heart failure, then you should give fluid more judiciously, generally 250 to 500 cm^3 at a time. An adequate response should include resolution of tachycardia and a return to the patient's baseline blood pressure. If an adequate response is not seen after the first fluid bolus, a repeat 1 L bolus should be given. You may also consider raising the maintenance IV fluid rate.

   While hypovolemia is the most common cause of postoperative hypotension, analgesia is another common cause. Narcotics cause peripheral vasodilation and may also be accompanied by a depressed mental status and decreased sympathetic tone. Proper management of this patient depends on the severity of hypotension, but withholding additional narcotic administration until the patient's blood pressure returns to normal is the first step. In an emergency, reversal agents such as naloxone are also indicated. Epidural analgesia is another common cause of postoperative hypotension because it contains a solution of local anesthetic (eg, bupivacaine) by itself or mixed with a narcotic (eg, hydromorphone or fentanyl). These medications can anesthetize the efferent sympathetics of the spinal cord and cause peripheral vasodilation and therefore hypotension. Initial management includes decreasing or temporarily stopping the infusion of pain medication as well as judicious administration of IV fluids. You should alert your Anesthesia colleagues, who can readjust the infusion when the hypotension has resolved.

While less common, postoperative β-blockade can be yet another cause of postoperative hypotension. Note that, in contradistinction to hypovolemia and analgesics, β-blockers not only decrease blood pressure but also prevent normal reflex tachycardia. Once again, initial treatment depends on the severity of the hypotension. Options include a 1 L bolus and, in extreme cases, reversal of β-blockade with glucagon.

Lastly, you should consider a primary cardiac cause of hypotension—even if it is rarer than the other etiologies. Surgical procedures are associated with significantly increased cardiac demand, and patients with underlying coronary artery disease are at increased risk of myocardial infarction in the immediate postoperative period. If the heart attack is significant, the reduction in cardiac output will result in shock and most likely hypotension. If you suspect a cardiac cause of the hypotension, you should obtain an EKG while you begin treatment and notify your senior resident.

In summary, hypotension is a common issue in the postoperative patient and it will be something you will come across frequently. For severe cases, treatment and diagnosis should proceed in parallel, generally with the administration of fluid and collection of at least a CBC and an EKG. Most of the time, however, the cause of the hypotension will be nonhemorrhagic hypovolemia or a drug effect. In those cases, a 1 L bolus is both a therapeutic and a diagnostic maneuver and should be your initial response for all patients without underlying heart failure. You should follow up to ensure that the patient did indeed respond. If the patient's blood pressure does not respond to this intervention, you must broaden your differential, consider escalation of care, and notify your senior resident.

TIPS TO REMEMBER

- If the patient is critically ill, initiate CPR or ACLS per standard protocols.
- Be vigilant for signs of shock.
- Severe hypotension in a postoperative patient should prompt a call to someone senior to you (eg, senior resident, fellow, attending).
- In the absence of known or suspected heart failure, it is usually safe to give a 1 L bolus of resuscitative fluid (0.9% NS or LR).
- If giving boluses of IV fluids, it is also reasonable to increase the IV fluid rate.
- Adequately treating a hypotensive patient requires intervention (ie, boluses, increased infusion rates) *and* following for response.

COMPREHENSION QUESTIONS

1. You are paged to the bedside of a recent postoperative patient with a blood pressure of 100/83. Her preoperative blood pressure was 130/91. Which of the following exam findings is most concerning?
    A. Tachycardia
    B. Cold big toe
    C. Pallor
    D. Incisional tenderness

2. You are paged to the bedside of a recent postoperative patient with a blood pressure of 100/83. He is confused and oliguric. What is the first thing you do?
    A. Check a CBC.
    B. Check an EKG.
    C. Do a physical exam.
    D. Order a 1 L bolus of NS.

Answers

1. **C.** Pallor suggests that the patient is bleeding. Hypotension in this setting is particularly ominous and demands immediate attention.

2. **D.** While a physical exam and diagnostic tests are important, this patient is in shock and you should initiate empiric treatment while you begin your assessment. If during your assessment you determine that the patient does not need additional fluid, you can always turn it off with minimal negative consequences. Not giving fluid, however, has the potential for very large negative consequences if in fact the patient is hypovolemic.

A 57-year-old Man Who Is Postoperative With a Blood Pressure of 210/95

Eric N. Feins, MD

You are paged by the nurse in the postoperative recovery room about a 57-year-old man who underwent laparoscopic cholecystectomy 1 hour ago and is now hypertensive—BP 210/95.

On arrival to the recovery room you find the patient mentating normally. Temperature 98.5°F, HR 105, BP 190/92, RR 22, and O_2 98% on 2 L nasal cannula. He complains of 7 out of 10 abdominal pain, for which he has already received several doses of IV hydromorphone. He denies any headache, vision changes, chest pain, or difficulty breathing. He tells you that his systolic blood pressure normally runs in the 130s and that he took his prescribed metoprolol at home this morning. His cardiopulmonary exam is notable for mild tachycardia and clear lungs. He is obese, and his abdomen is soft with mild-to-moderate tenderness in his periumbilical region, right upper quadrant, and suprapubic region.

1. Name two possible reasons for his hypertension (HTN).

2. What is your next step in the management of this patient?

3. What blood pressure should be your goal for treatment?

4. List three medications that you could use to treat the patient's HTN.

POSTOPERATIVE HYPERTENSION

Answers

1. Postoperative HTN is a sympathetically mediated response that creates vaso-constriction and increased blood pressure. If left untreated, the acute rise in blood pressure can lead to endothelial injury and end-organ damage—hypertensive emergencies. These include neurologic (ie, hemorrhagic stroke, cerebral ischemia), cardiac (ie, ischemia/infarction), and surgically related problems (ie, failure of vascular anastomoses, surgical site bleeding). No absolute BP threshold exists for the occurrence of end-organ damage, and sometimes it is the rate of increase in BP that dictates organ damage.

   It is critical to consider postoperative HTN in terms of increased afterload. Acute HTN in patients with coronary artery disease (CAD), left ventricular dysfunction, and/or congestive heart failure (CHF) can be very serious. Increased afterload increases myocardial oxygen demand. This can lead to myocardia ischemia/infarction in patients with underlying CAD and limited oxygen supply. In patients with left ventricular dysfunction the acute increase in afterload is poorly tolerated by the heart, leading to worsening CHF and pulmonary edema.

There are multiple possible reasons why a patient can become acutely hypertensive from vasoconstriction following surgery. These include:

A. Pain and anxiety: When a patient is in pain and/or is anxious, his/her sympathetic nervous system is activated, leading to tachycardia, peripheral vasoconstriction, and therefore HTN.

B. Urinary retention: A common occurrence in postoperative patients (particularly males) that can lead to significant HTN if left untreated. The mechanism is partly related to the pain/discomfort caused by bladder distension.

C. History of HTN: This is a major risk factor for developing postoperative HTN. Patients with poorly controlled HTN are at particular risk. Additionally, patients who do not take their normal blood pressure medications prior to surgery are likely to develop HTN postoperatively. (This is common because patients who follow instructions to remain "NPO" will often avoid both food and their pills.)

D. Volume overload: Patients often receive a large volume of IV fluids during surgery, particularly in prolonged cases. The resultant volume overload can precipitate HTN postoperatively.

E. Hypothermia: This leads to peripheral vasoconstriction and HTN. Patients who are not adequately covered with blankets and kept warm in the immediate postoperative period can suffer from this.

F. Hypercarbia: This is typically due to hypoventilation in the immediate postoperative period (ie, the somnolent patient lacking respiratory drive) and can lead to blood pressure elevation.

G. Type of surgery: Vascular surgery (ie, carotid, abdominal aortic), cardiothoracic, and head/neck surgery are known to predispose toward postoperative HTN.

2. After noting that the patient has no neurologic or cardiopulmonary symptoms (ie, headache, vision changes, chest pain, shortness of breath), and before initiating antihypertensive pharmacotherapy, consider two common and easily treatable causes of postoperative HTN: *pain/anxiety* and *urinary retention*. It would be a shame to load up a patient with antihypertensive agents only to find out that the main reason for his/her HTN was an inability to void! Suprapubic fullness and discomfort on palpation, along with documentation that the patient had not voided since before surgery, would suggest urinary retention. If you are unsure, perform a bladder scan (quick, easy, and noninvasive) to confirm your suspicion.

In this patient, managing his pain with additional or alternative narcotic pain medication and assessing for urinary retention are appropriate first steps. If urinary retention is confirmed, then bladder catheter insertion is indicated. In some patients this can dramatically improve the blood pressure without ever having to give medication!

3. The goal in managing postoperative HTN is to avoid the potentially harmful consequences described above, while also not overshooting on blood pressure decrease. There is no absolute value for a blood pressure goal. When determining your goals of treatment, consider the following:

A. Baseline blood pressure: Find out the patient's blood pressure preoperatively. While it may seem intuitive to rapidly bring a patient's blood pressure down to "normal" (ie, 120/80), that may not be his/her baseline. If the patient's blood pressure is typically 150 to 160/90, then a BP of 110 to 120/50 would be low for him/her and put the patient at risk for coronary ischemia (relative hypotension, especially diastolic hypotension, leads to diminished coronary perfusion pressure and decreased oxygen delivery).

B. Rate of blood pressure decrease: The rate of blood pressure lowering is just as critical as the absolute value you aim for. Precipitous drops in blood pressure can lead to diminished end-organ perfusion.

   As a general guideline, aim to reduce the blood pressure by approximately 15% in the first hour of therapy. Aim to reduce the blood pressure by *no more than 25%* over several hours.

C. Type of surgery: Postoperative HTN can be a very serious problem after certain operations (ie, vascular surgery where an anastomosis is strained by elevated intraluminal pressure and wall tension, and cardiac surgery where the recovering heart experiences a higher afterload). Compared with noncardiac surgery patients, cardiac surgery patients should be treated more aggressively to maintain a BP less than 140/90. Knowing the type of operation and any salient operative details (eg, a tenuous vascular anastomosis) is important for guiding how aggressively you try to lower a patient's BP. Often in these types of surgery you will be given a specific blood pressure range to maintain, and this should be followed in the setting of postoperative HTN.

   The presented patient's past medical history is notable for HTN, for which he takes a β-blocker at home. He told you that his normal blood pressure is in the 130s and that he took his metoprolol the morning of surgery. Given his current BP in the 190s, and that he has undergone a low-risk operation, your target SBP should be in the 160s in the first hour, and the 140s over several hours. A β-blocker—which you know he tolerates—would be a good choice if he needs pharmacotherapy. See Figure 36-1 for a useful algorithm.

4. There are several medications used to treat postoperative HTN. There is no consensus on the "best" agent. Each has advantages and drawbacks. Three of the

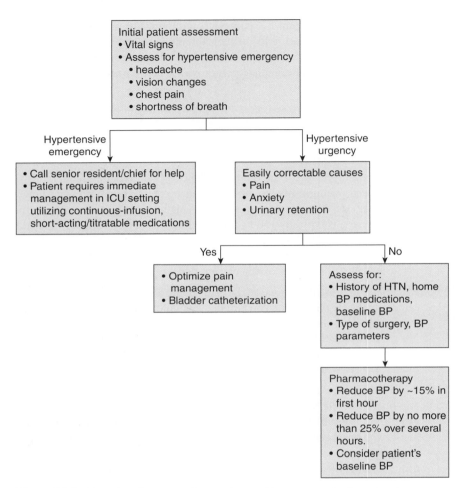

Figure 36-1. Algorithm for approach to patients with postoperative hypertension.

more commonly used medications are *labetalol, nitroglycerin,* and *hydralazine.* These are described as follows and summarized in Table 36-1:

A. Labetalol: Labetalol is an α-receptor and nonselective β-receptor blocker. It blocks vasoconstriction (α) and reduces inotropy and chronotropy (β). These actions reduce blood pressure and prevent reflex tachycardia. It is therefore a good agent for patients with CAD; they would benefit from afterload reduction as well as reduction of myocardial oxygen demand to prevent ischemia. While preventing reflex tachycardia can be advantageous, the negative chronotropic effect limits its use in patients with low-normal HR (ie, 50-60 bpm). Additionally, because it is a nonselective β-blocker, it can produce significant

Table 36-1. Pharmacologic Options for the Acute Treatment of Hypertension

Agent	Mechanism/Effect	Advantages	Drawbacks
Labetalol	α/β-Blocker	Good for CAD	Bradycardia
		No reflex tachycardia	Bronchospasm
			Long duration of action
Nitroglycerin	Nitric oxide, smooth muscle relaxant	Good for CAD	Reflex tachycardia
		Rapid onset, short duration, easy to titrate	Poor choice for patients w/ aortic stenosis or hypovolemia
			Can only give IV form as drip
Hydralazine	Direct arterial smooth muscle relaxant	—	Risk of myocardial ischemia/infarction → contraindicated in CAD
			Less predictable onset/ duration of effect

Before moving immediately to pharmacotherapy, consider any other potentially reversible/treatable factors that are known to cause postoperative HTN. In addition to poor pain control and urinary retention, also consider: hypoxia (ensure the patient's O_2 saturation is adequate [>90%]—a sufficient surrogate for Pao_2) and hypothermia with vasoconstriction (check body temperature and warm if necessary).

bronchospasm in patients with reactive airway disease. Its longer duration of action (3-5 hours) also can be problematic. IV form: dose—10 to 20 mg bolus, and then 10 to 40 mg every 10 minutes (can be given as continuous infusion in the ICU setting). Onset: within minutes. Duration: 3 to 5 hours.

B. Nitroglycerin: A vascular smooth muscle relaxant (veins >> arteries). Acts via release of nitric oxide. Relaxation of the vascular smooth muscle of the venous system increases venous capacitance and decreases preload. As a result, cardiac output and hence BP goes down. Nitroglycerin is another good agent for hypertensive patients with CAD who are at risk for myocardial ischemia. The smooth muscle relaxant effect enhances coronary perfusion; the decreased cardiac preload decreases myocardial oxygen demand. Additional advantages are its rapid onset and short duration of action—making it easy to titrate. There are several potential drawbacks of nitroglycerin. Since preload is reduced by nitroglycerin, patients who are "preload dependent" can experience dramatic, life-threatening blood pressure drops. This includes patients who are hypovolemic and those with aortic stenosis. Additionally, the decreased preload can lead to a "reflex tachycardia," especially in hypovolemic patients. Nitroglycerin can also cause headaches due to its vasodilatory effects. Lastly, while nitroglycerin comes in many different forms, it is the IV form that is typically used for perioperative HTN. The IV form must be administered as a continuous infusion, and therefore requires closer monitoring (ie, in the ICU). IV form: dose—5 to 300 µg/min. Onset: <1 minute. Duration: 5 to 10 minutes.

C. Hydralazine: A direct arterial smooth muscle relaxant, leading to decreased systemic vascular resistance (SVR) and blood pressure. This medication is ubiquitously used among interns and residents. However, this practice pattern is not supported by data. In fact, there are several risks with using hydralazine. Because of its effect on SVR, reflex tachycardia and increased cardiac output occur. Overall, the increased work by the heart without concordant increase in coronary blood flow puts the heart at risk for ischemia and infarction. This drug is therefore contraindicated in patients with known CAD or suspected ischemia. Another major drawback of hydralazine relates to its pharmacodynamics. IV hydralazine has a delayed onset and prolonged duration of action—not ideal when managing an acute condition. IV form: dose—5 to 20 mg q6h. Onset: 15 to 30 minutes. Duration: 4 to 6 hours.

TIPS TO REMEMBER

● When assessing a patient with postoperative HTN, first assess vital signs and for the presence of end-organ damage (neurologic, cardiopulmonary). Second, look for easily treatable/reversible causes of HTN (pain, urinary retention).

● When using pharmacotherapy, labetalol and nitroglycerin are good choices for patients with underlying CAD.

● Be careful using nitroglycerin in patients who are preload dependent (ie, hypovolemia, aortic stenosis).

● As a general guideline, aim to reduce the blood pressure by approximately 15% in the first hour of therapy. Aim to reduce the blood pressure by no more than 25% over several hours.

● Hydralazine—while used frequently by interns/residents—can be injurious to patients with CAD, and the onset and duration of its effects are hard to predict.

COMPREHENSION QUESTIONS

1. Which of the following comorbidities (one or more) would concern you most about a patient's ability to tolerate acute postoperative HTN?
    A. Emphysema/COPD
    B. CAD
    C. Systolic heart failure
    D. Hypothyroidism

2. Of the following, which is the most important to assess in a patient with acute postoperative HTN?

    A. Neurologic symptoms

    B. Home medication list

    C. Urinary retention

    D. Pain control

3. Which medication would be appropriate to use in a hypertensive patient who you think is hypovolemic and has a known history of CAD?

    A. Labetalol

    B. Nitroglycerin

    C. Hydralazine

Answers

1. **B and C**. A patient with CAD is at risk of demand ischemia due to the increased afterload. A patient with heart failure may not be able to maintain his/her already tenuous cardiac output with increased afterload.

2. **A**. While it is important to assess for treatable/reversible factors prior to pharmacotherapy, you must always first assess a patient's vital signs and whether he/she is experiencing symptoms of end-organ damage (ie, neurologic, cardiac, etc).

3. **A**. Labetalol is good for CAD and does not decrease preload, which is already low in a hypovolemic patient.

A 65-year-old Female Who Is 4 Days Postoperative With Nausea, Vomiting, and a Distended Abdomen

Ashley Hardy, MD and
Marie Crandall, MD, MPH

You are called to the surgical floor to evaluate a 65-year-old female who underwent a right hemicolectomy for colon cancer four days prior. For the last few hours the patient has had multiple episodes of nausea with vomiting and has yet to have flatus or a bowel movement since her procedure. Her vital signs are normal, her abdominal exam is notable only for distension, and labs obtained earlier that morning are unremarkable. Of note, the patient is still requiring use of her morphine PCA for postoperative analgesia. You order a KUB, as seen in Figure 37-1.

1. For this patient, name two key findings you should be looking for on the KUB.

2. How can you distinguish the small intestine from the colon on a KUB?

3. Given the patient's nausea and vomiting, you elect to place a nasogastric tube (NGT). What radiographic landmarks would you use to ensure the tube is properly positioned?

4. What findings on a KUB would warrant emergent surgical intervention?

READING AND USING A KUB

Answers

1. Although they stand for kidneys, ureters, and bladder, KUBs are more commonly utilized to assess for abnormal conditions of the gastrointestinal tract and to determine the position of various indwelling devices, including NGTs, Dobhoff (feeding) tubes, and ureteral stents. In a patient such as this one, with a history of recent abdominal surgery and several bouts of nausea and vomiting, it is important to assess for the presence of obstruction or evidence of anastomotic breakdown (as indicated by the presence of free intraperitoneal air). A KUB is quick, relatively inexpensive, and has a lower radiation dose than CT, making it a common initial diagnostic study.

When encountering any type of film, including a KUB, it is important to take a systematic approach to interpretation. Doing so ensures that key findings pertinent to making appropriate decisions regarding a patient's care are not missed. If previous films are available, it is helpful to compare the findings with those of the current study. After ensuring that you're viewing the film for the correct patient, determine the orientation (right vs left as indicated by a marker or using the gastric air bubble in the LUQ as a guide). Also determine

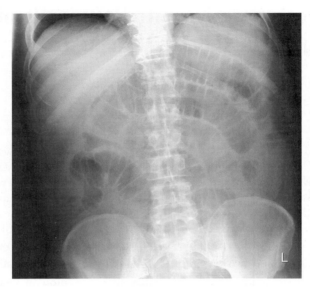

Figure 37-1. Small bowel obstruction. Supine film showing dilated loops of small bowel and no gas in the colon. (Reproduced, with permission, from Doherty GM. *Current Diagnosis & Treatment: Surgery*. 13th ed. New York: McGraw-Hill; 2010. Figure 29-5.)

if you're looking at a film that was obtained while the patient was supine versus erect as this will influence whether or not you're able to visualize the presence of air–fluid levels and free air under the diaphragm. Keep in mind that on plain radiographs high-density structures (generally those that contain calcium such as bone, gallstones, and kidney stones) are white. Similarly, soft tissue and fluid are light gray, while gas is black.

After orienting yourself to the image, be sure to look for the presence of extraluminal air. Then, turn your focus to the hollow organs. First try to locate the stomach within the LUQ. Note that its visibility is influenced by the presence or absence of gastric air and whether or not the film is erect versus supine—in a supine film the meniscus between the gas bubble and gastric contents will not be visible.

Next, locate the small intestine and the colon. You should assess the entire bowel for evidence of intestinal dilation, keeping in mind the "3/6/9 rule": the accepted upper limit of normal for the diameter of small bowel is 3 cm, for the colon 6 cm, and for the cecum 9 cm. Dilation of the small or large bowel usually represents either a functional obstruction (ileus) or a mechanical obstruction. The image in the case (Figure 37-2, copied from Figure 37-1 again here, with labels) is an excellent example of a KUB that demonstrates the uniform dilation of the small bowel often seen with either type of obstruction. Note there are no cutoff points or "coffee bean"–shaped loops of bowel that could represent a closed loop obstruction, something that would require immediate operative

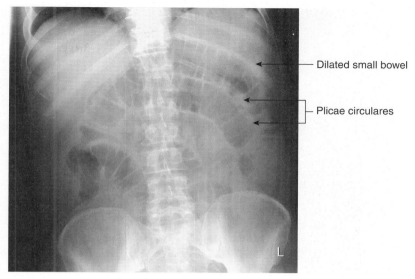

Dilated small bowel

Plicae circulares

Figure 37-2. The same supine film as presented in the case. Note the dilated loops of small bowel as well as what appears to be fluid between the small bowel walls. (Reproduced, with permission, from Doherty GM. *Current Diagnosis & Treatment: Surgery.* 13th ed. New York: McGraw-Hill; 2010.)

intervention. Furthermore, note that because it is supine, there are no air–fluid levels, although the boundaries between the loops of bowel are prominent and likely represent intra-abdominal fluid.

Figure 37-3, in contrast, is an upright film that shows air–fluid levels. You should note the very large gastric air bubble and the paucity of colonic air (normally seen deep in the pelvis, below the pelvic brim). Both of these elements suggest an obstruction. If you know approximately where the small and large bowels lie within the abdomen, the pattern of air–fluid levels can also suggest the location of the obstruction. For example, in the case of a small bowel obstruction, multiple air–fluid levels may be seen involving the small intestine only, whereas a large bowel obstruction may present with air–fluid levels within both the small and large intestines.

2. On a KUB, the small and large intestines are most easily distinguished from each other on the basis of position, diameter, mucosal markings, and gas patterns. As previously mentioned, the small intestine tends to lie within the midabdomen and has a normal diameter of less than 3 cm, whereas the colon usually courses along the periphery and is normally less than 6 cm in diameter. In terms of bowel markings, the circular mucosal folds (plicae circulares or valvulae conniventes) of the small bowel span the entire circumference of the wall. They are also closer in proximity to each other than are the haustra of the large intestine, which appear to cross only part of the large intestinal lumen (see Figure 37-2).

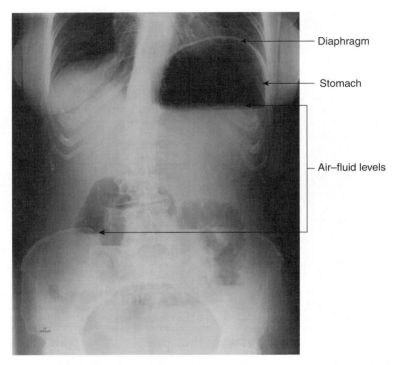

Figure 37-3. Upright film shows a distended stomach with a large gastric bubble. It also shows slightly dilated loops of small bowel with air–fluid levels and a paucity of colonic gas, both consistent with a small bowel obstruction. (Courtesy of Deborah Levine, MD.)

3. Using a KUB, one can follow the entire gastrointestinal course of an NGT and ensure its proper positioning beneath the left hemidiaphragm and well within the lumen of the stomach (see Figure 37-4).

   Postplacement imaging with a KUB can ensure that the tube is not erroneously placed within the patient's airway or that it ends too proximally within the esophagus.

4. The presence of extraluminal intraperitoneal gas or a pneumoperitoneum is a worrisome finding on a KUB and usually warrants emergent surgical intervention. Note that some extraluminal gas is to be expected after open and laparoscopic surgery, although it typically resolves over a period of 3 to 6 days and is not accompanied by concerning physical exam findings. The most common place to look for extraluminal gas is underneath the diaphragm. Because air is less dense than the intra-abdominal contents, it tends to rise, so extraluminal gas is most easily visualized on an erect or upright film. Note that it's best to look for air underneath the right hemidiaphragm as it may be difficult to distinguish

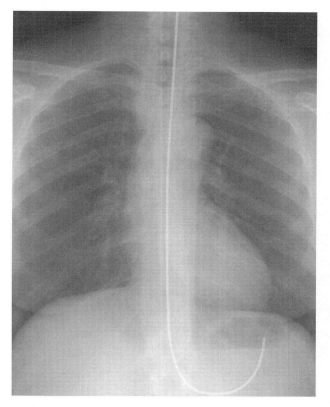

Figure 37-4. A feeding tube located below the diaphragm—note that in this image the tube is postpyloric. (Reproduced, with permission, from McKean SC, Ross JJ, Dressler DD, Brotman DJ, Ginsberg JS, eds. *Principles and Practice of Hospital Medicine.* Figure 119-4.)

the extraluminal air due to a perforation from the gastric air bubble on the left. Other potential locations for extraluminal gas include the bowel wall (pneumatosis intestinalis, which creates a "bubble wrap" appearance), the portal venous system (usually as a result of severe bowel ischemia), and within the biliary tree (usually following instrumentation or as a result of a biliary-enteric fistula).

TIPS TO REMEMBER

- Always take a systematic approach when interpreting a KUB.
- Dilated loops of bowel, a prominent gastric bubble or dilated stomach, air–fluid levels, and a paucity of colonic gas all suggest an obstructive process (either ileus or a mechanical obstruction).

- When trying to determine if bowel is dilated or not, remember the "3/6/9 rule" (small bowel, colon, cecum).
- The small and large intestines can be discriminated from each other by position (small intestine—central, large intestine—peripheral) and bowel markings (small intestine—markings span the *entire* wall circumference, large intestine—markings span only *part* of the wall circumference).
- Except in the acute postoperative period, the presence of free extraluminal intraperitoneal air usually warrants emergent intervention.

COMPREHENSION QUESTIONS

1. Which radiographic finding would most likely require emergent abdominal exploration?
>   A. Cecum dilated to 8 cm
>   B. Air–fluid levels within the small intestine
>   C. Air underneath the right hemidiaphragm
>   D. Radiopaque densities in the RUQ

2. Match each term with its radiographic characteristic:

A. Peripheral location	
B. Plicae circulares	a. Small intestine
C. Central location	b. Large intestine
D. Haustra	

Answers

1. **C**. Air underneath the right hemidiaphragm is an abnormal radiographic finding that suggests an intra-abdominal perforation, warranting emergent abdominal exploration. The upper limit of normal for cecal diameter is 9 cm, air–fluid levels within the small intestine suggest a bowel obstruction (which can often be treated nonoperatively), and radiopaque densities in the RUQ likely represent gallstones.

2. **A and D—b**. The colon tends to lie in a peripheral location within the abdomen and has haustra (bowel markings that cross only part of the intestinal lumen). **B and C—a**. The small bowel is identified radiographically by its central position in the abdomen and by the plicae circulares that span the entire circumference of the small intestinal wall.

A 30-year-old Woman With Postoperative Nausea and Vomiting

Abigail K. Tarbox, MD and Mamta Swaroop, MD, FACS

A healthy 30-year-old female undergoes an uneventful, elective ventral hernia repair under general anesthesia. She goes to the surgical floor, where she receives a hydromorphone PCA for pain control and is kept NPO until return of bowel function. She does well until postoperative day 2, when she develops nausea and vomiting. Her nurse calls you asking what to do. You evaluate the patient. When you arrive at her bedside, you find her sitting up in bed leaning over an emesis bin. She tells you she has been vomiting intermittently for the past 2 hours. Her incision looks benign and her abdomen is not distended. She has infrequent bowel sounds.

1. What is the best medication to give her to help with her symptoms?
2. Is this patient's nausea and vomiting likely due to the lingering effects of anesthesia?
3. Does this patient need an NG tube?

POSTOPERATIVE NAUSEA AND VOMITING

Answers

1. There are 3 types of afferent nerve inputs that ultimately result in vomiting—input from the vestibular complex, input from the viscera, and input from the chemoreceptor trigger zone in the base of the fourth ventricle. Numerous neurotransmitters are involved in these pathways, although dopamine and serotonin are the most clinically relevant. This is because visceral stimulation and stimulation of the chemoreceptor trigger zone are the most likely causes of nausea in postsurgical patients, both of which are mediated by these 2 neurotransmitters. This helps to explain why the most frequently used antiemetics following surgery target dopamine and serotonin.

   Metoclopramide (Reglan) and promethazine (Phenergan) are the most common dopamine antagonists. Promethazine is especially useful as it is available in both suppository and intravenous forms. Unfortunately, this entire class of medications may cause significant side effects, including orthostatic hypotension and excessive sedation. They can also cause extrapyramidal effects and are therefore strictly contraindicated in patients with Parkinson disease. In addition, promethazine can cause venous sclerosis at the site of administration, while metoclopramide has promotility effects and should not be given to patients with either confirmed or suspected bowel obstruction.

Due to their better side effect profiles, serotonin antagonists have become the primary treatment for a variety of causes of nausea. While side effects of serotonin antagonists are rare, they include headache, diarrhea, hypersensitivity reactions, and QT prolongation. The most common drug in this class is ondansetron (Zofran), which would be an appropriate first-line medical treatment for the case presented.

2. Nausea and vomiting are not uncommon in the postoperative period. Nausea and vomiting in the first 24 hours after surgery is defined as "early" postoperative nausea and vomiting (PONV), and is usually directly related to the effects of anesthesia. Early PONV occurs in 20% to 30% of patients, is more common in females, and is the number 1 reason for unexpected hospital admission following ambulatory surgery. Early PONV can often be prevented with appropriate chemoprophylaxis in people at high risk for PONV, and if it does develop, it usually resolves with antiemetic treatment alone.

When nausea and vomiting occur more than 24 hours after surgery, it is unlikely to be caused by the lingering effects of anesthesia. Frequent causes are medications (eg, opiates), electrolyte abnormalities (eg, hypokalemia), constipation (often also due to opiates), delayed return of bowel function (aka ileus), and mechanical bowel obstruction (ie, from an anastomotic stricture). However, more serious causes such as infection, acute myocardial infarction, and CNS disturbances can also cause nausea and vomiting and must be ruled out. Always think, "what could kill this patient?" and then rule out the most morbid diagnosis on the differential first. As with most situations, a careful history and physical exam will often guide you to the etiology. In your history, you should ask about the timing of the nausea and vomiting and relationship to meals or medications. Ask about the character of the emesis—if it is bilious, it indicates that duodenal contents have refluxed back through the pylorus and into the stomach. You will also want to know if the patient has passed flatus or had a bowel movement, if there is associated pain, and how many times the patient has vomited.

Next, assess the patient's vital signs and then examine the patient. Abdominal distension is frequently present in ileus and small bowel obstruction. Hypoactive or absent bowel sounds are characteristic of ileus on auscultation of the abdomen, whereas hyperactive bowel sounds are more likely in obstruction. Abdominal plain films will show global dilation of small and large bowel in the case of an ileus (see Figure 38-1). An obstruction, on the other hand, will have proximally dilated loops of bowel, with distal decompression and paucity of air in the colon or rectum (see Figure 38-2).

3. Treatment of PONV depends on the etiology. If you suspect an obstruction or ileus, if the patient has persistent vomiting no matter the cause, or if the patient is at high risk of aspiration, then you should strongly consider placing an NG tube. While uncomfortable and not without its own risks, an NG tube will reduce the chance of aspiration. If you are on the fence about whether

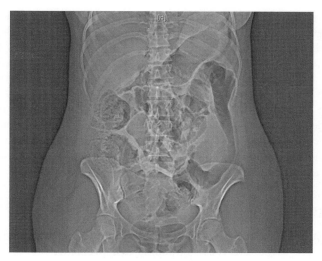

Figure 38-1. Postoperative ileus: radiograph from a patient with postoperative ileus shows gastric distention, distended small bowel loops, and air and stool throughout the colon.

or not an NGT is indicated, a plain film can be particularly helpful—dilated loops of bowel or a dilated stomach indicate that the patient is likely to continue vomiting. In that case, an NG tube would be of benefit. If you feel the patient would benefit from an NG tube, you should alert your senior resident prior to performing this routine but still invasive procedure.

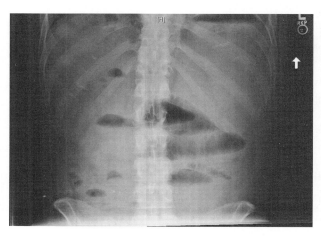

Figure 38-2. Upright radiograph of a small bowel obstruction shows dilated small bowel and multiple air–fluid levels.

If the symptoms always follow the administration of narcotics, try to minimize their usage and, when appropriate, use alternative pain relievers such as NSAIDs or Tylenol. Standing Tylenol (per rectum if necessary) is effective at reducing the total amount of opiates required, even if it can't replace them entirely. Antiemetics such as ondansetron can also be given concurrently with narcotics to prophylax against nausea.

While elucidating the diagnosis, a single dose of an antiemetic is often effective to help make the patient more comfortable. Make the patient NPO and remember to restart intravenous fluids or adjust the rate, if still infusing. If you haven't already checked the electrolytes that day, you should do so and then correct any abnormalities.

TIPS TO REMEMBER

- The first-line antiemetic is ondansetron given its superior side effect profile. Second-line agents are metoclopramide and promethazine, although they should not be used in patients with Parkinson disease.
- Early PONV is usually due to the lingering effects of anesthesia and can safely be treated with medications alone.
- Strongly consider nasogastric tube decompression in patients with persistent vomiting, small bowel obstruction, a large gastric bubble, or those at increased risk for aspiration.

COMPREHENSION QUESTIONS

1. Which antiemetic is a poor choice in a patient with a small bowel obstruction?
    A. Ondansetron (Zofran)
    B. Metoclopramide (Reglan)
    C. Promethazine (Phenergan)

2. Which is the greatest risk factor for development of *early* PONV in patients undergoing surgery?
    A. Long operative time
    B. Older age
    C. Female gender

3. Your patient is a frail 80-year-old male who is postoperative day 3 from a small bowel resection. You started him on clear liquids this morning, but in the past hour he has vomited twice. On exam he is distended. What is your next step?
    A. Get a KUB.
    B. Place an NG tube.
    C. Call your senior.

Answers

1. **B**. Metoclopramide (Reglan) is also a promotility agent that should be avoided in bowel obstruction—pushing against the obstruction only worsens the problem.

2. **C**. Female gender is the greatest risk factor.

3. **C**. This "frail" patient is at high risk of aspiration, the most likely diagnosis is ileus, and he has already vomited twice and so will most likely do so again. All 3 of these are independent reasons to place an NG tube, and a KUB would not change your management. But before you go ahead and perform this invasive procedure you should always make sure to notify your senior resident or attending.

A 79-year-old Man, Postoperative Day 3, Who has Not had a Bowel Movement in 4 Days

Anne-Marie Boller, MD and Joel M. Sternbach, MD, MBA

You are called to the bedside of a 79-year-old male patient for evaluation of his altered mental status. The patient is a nursing home resident, now POD 3 from a right total hip replacement, with complaints of abdominal distention and diffuse crampy abdominal pain for two days. There is no record of him having had a bowel movement since being admitted from his nursing home four days ago. A review of the patient's medication list reveals the addition of acetaminophen/ hydrocodone for pain control. He was started on a general diet and his home verapamil, furosemide, and clonidine today but was not given any of his home over-the-counter medications (including Miralax and Metamucil). There is no nausea or vomiting, vital signs are WNL and stable, and the patient has adequate urine output. He is passing flatus on a regular basis. On examination, his abdomen is distended but soft and mildly tender to palpation diffusely.

1. **What should be included in the initial evaluation of this patient?**

2. **What additional testing (labs, imaging) could help guide your management?**

3. **What are your options for treating constipation? Given their mechanisms, which would you choose for this patient?**

4. **You are concerned that the patient might have a fecal impaction. How do you diagnose and treat this condition? What prophylactic measures could have been taken to prevent this?**

CONSTIPATION

Constipation as described by individual patients varies widely but is generally defined by decreased frequency (less than 3 bowel movements per week) and/or symptoms such as straining, passage of lumpy or hard stool, sensation of blockage or obstruction, need for manual assistance (digitations or splinting), and sensation of incomplete evacuation (in >25% of stools).

Rome III criteria provide some standardization when enrolling patients in clinical trials.

Rome III Criteria for Functional Constipation

Diagnostic criteria (criteria fulfilled for the past 3 months with symptom onset at least 6 months prior to diagnosis):

1. Must include 2 or more of the following:
   A. Straining during at least 25% of defecations
   B. Lumpy or hard stools in at least 25% of defecations
   C. Sensation of incomplete evacuation for at least 25% of defecations
   D. Sensation of anorectal obstruction/blockage for at least 25% of defecations
   E. Manual maneuvers to facilitate at least 25% of defecations (eg, digital evacuation, support of the pelvic floor)
   F. Fewer than 3 defecations per week
2. Loose stools are rarely present without the use of laxatives.
3. Insufficient criteria for irritable bowel syndrome.

At-risk populations include the elderly, especially hospitalized or nursing home residents, and women, who are diagnosed 3 times more commonly than men. A western diet, low in dietary fiber, and inadequate fluid intake combined with prolonged immobility or a generally sedentary lifestyle all contribute to the development of constipation.

Other common causes of constipation include:

1. Medication side effects:
   A. Opiates—slow transit causing increased desiccation of stool
   B. Antihypertensives, especially calcium channel blockers (verapamil)
   C. Diuretics (furosemide)
   D. Anticholinergics (including antihistamines and many antidepressants)
   E. Iron supplements
   F. Antacids with calcium or aluminum, calcium supplements
   G. Antidiarrheal agents
   H. Long-term laxative use/abuse
   I. NSAIDs
2. Medical conditions:
   A. Hypothyroidism
   B. Diabetes
   C. Lupus
   D. Scleroderma
   E. Spinal cord injury

3. Structural abnormalities:

A. Prior abdominal surgery causing adhesions

B. Pregnancies or history of obstetric surgery

C. Colonic stricture due to cancer, IBD, or radiation exposure

Answers

1. The evaluation of the patient should start with a comprehensive history, focusing on establishing the onset and duration of symptoms. Constipation can be the first symptom and/or accompanying symptom of a bowel obstruction. Bowel obstructions must be thought of as organic in origin or functional in origin. Organic causes typically present acutely and can indicate the need for early imaging:

1. Hernia

2. Colorectal cancer

3. Diverticulitis

4. Sigmoid or cecal volvulus

5. Adhesions

6. Fecal impaction

7. Foreign body

Functional causes are typically more chronic and warrant a more extensive outpatient evaluation:

1. Normal-transit constipation

2. Slow-transit constipation

3. Outlet obstruction/constipation (pelvic floor dysfunction)

Alarm or "red flag" symptoms in addition to constipation include acute onset, nausea or vomiting, fever/chills, change in stool quality (caliber or consistency), inability to pass flatus (obstipation), severe abdominal pain and distention, unintended weight loss (>10 lb), rectal bleeding or melena, unexplained iron-deficiency anemia, or age >50 years with no prior screening for colorectal cancer with or without a family history of colon cancer. These "red flag" symptoms must be reviewed in the historical examination; they may indicate an organic cause for the patient's constipation.

After the history is complete, a thorough physical examination should include an assessment of the patient's general clinical condition and review of vital signs and should focus on an abdominal examination. All abdominal examinations should assess for distention, tenderness, or tympani, rule out hernias or masses, and evaluate for signs of peritonitis. Bowel sounds are generally decreased in

slow gut transit and increased or high-pitched in obstruction. External examination of the perianal region can identify anal fissures, hemorrhoids, abscesses,
or protruding masses. Results of a digital rectal examination should include the
following:

1. Description of the amount and consistency of stool in the rectum

2. Palpation for rectal masses

3. Identification of gross blood or stool leakage

4. Testing of the ability to contract/relax the anal sphincter voluntarily

2. Laboratory evaluation should include a complete blood count and basic chemistry panel to screen for anemia and identify hypomagnesemia, hypercalcemia,
and hypokalemia. Thyroid function tests for suspected hypothyroidism and
serum lead and iron levels are also useful in evaluating the patient.

   Early imaging may be considered in demented or delirious patients with
constipation, as the history and physical examination may not be adequate to
rule out obstruction. Plain films (KUB or acute abdominal series) may reveal
megacolon or megarectum in patients with stricture or obstructing mass and
can delineate the extent of fecal impaction. Evidence of bowel obstruction and
perforation may also be obvious on plain films (see Figure 39-1).

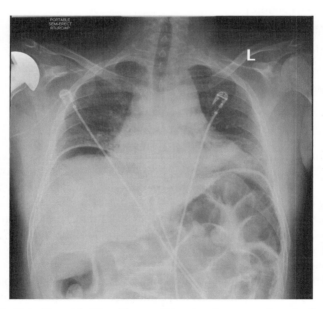

Figure 39-1. Plain film with dilated loops of bowel and, more ominously, free intraperitoneal air.

A water-soluble contrast enema with Gastrografin (diatrizoate meglumine) or Hypaque (diatrizoate sodium) can pass an impacted area and evaluate for a more proximal mass, stricture, or perforation. It can also be therapeutic in cases of fecal impaction.

A CT scan will assist in evaluation of any obstructing mechanical or inflammatory process. If these have been ruled out, it is most efficacious to get the patient's colon cleared of fecal debris and perform a colonoscopy, but this is not always possible in the patient with functional constipation.

3. The first step in almost all patient populations is optimizing modifiable dietary and lifestyle factors. These include:

   1. Increasing dietary fiber to a goal of 20 to 30 g daily

   2. Ensuring adequate fluid intake with at least 6 to 8 glasses (1.5-2 L) of water daily

   3. Encouraging ambulation/regular exercise

   4. Correcting underlying electrolyte/metabolic abnormalities (and determining their cause):

      A. Hypokalemia

      B. Hypomagnesemia

      C. Hypercalcemia

      D. Hypothyroidism

      E. Hyperparathyroidism

      F. Hyperglycemia (DM)

      G. Uremia

   5. Reviewing all medications for their constipation effects

   6. Reviewing all past and current medical/surgical problems for their possible constipating effects

   After optimizing dietary, lifestyle, and behavior factors, medications can often be helpful in addressing the problem of functional constipation. There are many different mechanisms and types of laxatives that are utilized in the treatment of constipation:

   Bulk laxatives—these work by colonic distention, triggering peristalsis:

   1. Psyllium (Metamucil) 1 tbsp BID—hygroscopic husks absorb water and become mucilaginous (jello-like).

   2. Methylcellulose (Citrucel).

   3. Calcium polycarbophil (Fibercon).

   4. Guar gum (Benefiber).

Osmotic laxatives—as a class, these act as hyperosmolar agents, drawing water into the lumen of the intestine as well as stimulating colonic activity via cholecystokinin:

1. Lactulose/70% sorbitol—poorly absorbed sugars:

   A. Sorbitol is sweeter than sucrose with ~1/3 fewer calories.

   B. Sorbitol is significantly less expensive than lactulose.

   C. Lactulose converts ammonia to nonabsorbable ammonium ion.

2. Magnesium salts:

   A. Magnesium ions stimulate the activity of nitric oxide (NO) synthase and increase levels of the proinflammatory mediator platelet activating factor (PAF) in the GI tract.

   B. NO may stimulate intestinal secretion via prostaglandin- and cyclic GMP–dependent mechanisms while PAF produces significant stimulation of colonic secretion and gastrointestinal motility.

   C. Can cause hypermagnesemia and hypocalcemia.

3. Sodium salts:

   A. Phospho-soda (OsmoPrep).

   B. Fleet Enema (sodium phosphate)—can cause hyperphosphatemia and hypocalcemia.

4. Polyethylene glycol 3350 (Miralax):

   A. Seventeen grams in 8 oz liquid once or twice daily.

   B. Safe in renal failure.

Stimulant laxatives—these alter water and electrolyte transport in the colon and increase colonic motility by causing low-grade inflammation in the colon through activation of prostaglandin/cyclic AMP and NO/cyclic GMP pathways:

1. Bisacodyl (Dulcolax)—diphenylmethanes inhibit water absorption in the small intestine and act via direct parasympathetic stimulation of mucosal sensory nerves, increasing peristaltic contractions.

2. *Senna* extracts (Ex-lax, Senokot)—anthraquinones act on enteric neurons and intestinal muscle to produce giant migrating colonic contractions in addition to stimulating water and electrolyte secretion.

3. Importantly, perforation and obstruction must be ruled out prior to giving stimulant laxatives!

Emollient laxatives—these act as stool softeners and are more effective in conjunction with stimulant laxatives:

1. Docusate sodium (Colace).

2. Glycerin suppository—exerts a hyperosmotic effect drawing water into the rectum; allows water and fat to penetrate the fecal mass.

3. Mineral oil:

   A. Poor oral choice.

   B. Aspiration causes lipoid pneumonia; depletes fat-soluble vitamins.

   C. Lubricates stool when given as an enema.

4. Soapsuds enema—should not be used due to irritation of the colonic mucosa and risk for hemorrhagic colitis.

Novel agents:

1. Methylnaltrexone (Relistor):

   A. Mu-opioid antagonist that does not cross the blood–brain barrier.

   B. Indicated only for opioid-induced constipation.

   C. Injectable.

   D. Expensive.

2. Lubiprostone (Amitiza)—bicyclic fatty acid, activates type II chloride channels in the apical membrane of the GI epithelium resulting in increased secretion of chloride and subsequently water:

   A. Contraindicated in pregnancy.

4. Fecal impaction: a firm mass of immovable stool in the rectum or distal colon; relatively common in the elderly, especially the bed-bound nursing home population. In one study, fecal impaction was found to be responsible for 55% of cases of diarrhea in hospitalized elderly patients (see Figure 39-2A and B).

   Steps in manual disimpaction:

   1. Consider analgesia and/or sedation.

   2. Position the patient in the lateral decubitus or dorsal lithotomy position.

   3. Soften impaction with mineral oil enema or glycerin suppository.

   4. Lubricate impaction.

   5. Break up impaction with scissoring motion of 2 fingers.

   6. Can follow with tap water or sodium phosphate enema.

   7. Start regular bowel regimen to prevent recurrence.

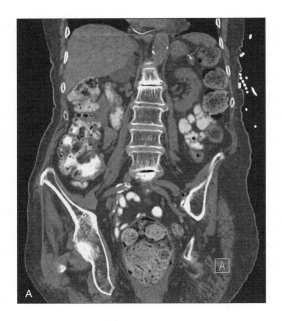

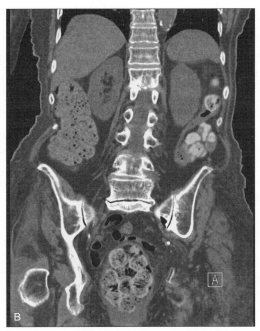

Figure 39-2. (**A** and **B**) CT images of a patient with fecal impaction and a hx of stercoral colitis.

Impaction of stool may be prevented by following a high-fiber, fluid-rich diet; getting regular exercise; limiting intake of constipating drugs; routinely using stool softeners or laxatives; and learning biofeedback and habit training.

TIPS TO REMEMBER

- More than 50% of patients taking narcotic pain relievers will develop dose-dependent constipation. A reasonable prophylactic regimen includes a combination of a bulking agent and a stimulant laxative.

- Plain films of the abdomen can reveal impacted stool, dilated proximal loops of bowel, air–fluid levels, and the presence of free intra-abdominal air (in the case of perforation). The normal maximal diameter of the colon is 6 cm and that of the rectum is 4 cm.

- Manual disimpaction involves softening, lubricating, and fragmenting the hardened stool.

COMPREHENSION QUESTIONS

1. Which of the following is contraindicated in patients with renal failure?
    A. Psyllium
    B. Sodium phosphate (Fleet Enema)
    C. Sorbitol
    D. Polyethylene glycol

2. Which of the following is not associated with constipation?
    A. Verapamil
    B. Furosemide
    C. Loperamide
    D. Metronidazole

Answers

1. **B**. Sodium phosphate can cause hyperphosphatemia. In high-risk patients, it can cause an acute nephropathy.

2. **D**. Although a treatment for diarrhea caused by *C. difficile* colitis, metronidazole is more commonly implicated in antibiotic-associated diarrhea itself.

A 70-year-old Postoperative Colectomy Patient Who Is Not Putting Out Much Urine

Brian C. George, MD and Alden H. Harken, MD

"Doctor, your postop colectomy patient isn't putting out much urine."

Mr. O'Flaherty is a 70-year-old gentleman who is two hours post left colectomy. His vitals are: BP 110/70, HR 110 (regular), respiration 18, and temperature 37.5°C. In the last hour he has made 15 mL of urine.

1. **List at least three clinical indicators of adequate peripheral perfusion.**

2. **What does a spot urine sodium of 12 mEq/L in a postoperative patient mean?**

3. **What does anuria usually represent?**

4. **In the vignette presented above, should you give the patient some furosemide to fix his oliguria?**

POSTOPERATIVE OLIGURIA

There are multiple possible causes of oliguria in the postoperative patient, although inadequate renal perfusion is the most common. Stress, acute kidney injury, and obstruction are other common causes (see Table 40-1). We will address each of these in turn.

Answers

1. As surgeons, we use multiple reassuring indicators of adequate cardiac output and hemodynamic stability, which include:

    Invasive indicators:

    A. Blood lactic acid

    B. Blood metabolic acid (pH >7.35 without respiratory compensation; so, $PaCO_2$ >35 mm Hg)

    C. Mixed venous O_2 sat >65% (requires a central venous or pulmonary artery catheter)

    Less invasive indicators:

    A. Stable BP (relative to preoperative)

    B. Stable heart rate

Table 40-1. The Most Common Causes of Oliguria

Prerenal	Inadequate perfusion Stress
Intrarenal	Acute kidney injury
Postrenal	Obstruction

C. Comfortable respiratory rate (when you are sick, or running up stairs, you breathe faster)

D. Big toe temperature (short of sepsis, if your big toe is warm, you're doing OK)

E. Urine output

The focus of this chapter is the last item on this list: urine output. Because the kidneys are exquisitely sensitive to changes in cardiac output, oliguria can indicate that your patient has compromised renal perfusion—usually but not always due to hypovolemia. Note that using urine output as a measure of end-organ perfusion is very similar to using goal-directed therapy (GDT) principles as described in the chapter on Shock.

Hypovolemia in the acute postoperative period is usually due to one of two causes. Most commonly it is the result of so-called third spacing, where leakage of plasma into the surgical field (and beyond!) results in depleted intravascular volume. However, hypovolemia can also be due to hemorrhage, which must always be in the back of your mind.

When treating an acutely postoperative patient who you believe is oliguric due to hypovolemia, a standard approach is to give a 500 mL to 1 L bolus of crystalloid. If the patient does not respond as expected within 30 minutes, then you should begin looking more carefully for other potential causes of inadequate cardiac output. This should include a CBC to evaluate for hemorrhage as well as a spot urine sodium (see below).

While hypovolemia is the usual focus of surgeons, it is important to remember that oliguria is also a normal response to stress. Stretch receptors in the left atrium, sensitive to low pressure, signal release of antidiuretic hormone (ADH or vasopressin) from the pituitary. Volume depletion, positive pressure ventilation, pain, nausea, and many other types of "stress" all provoke release of both ADH and mineralocorticoids (aldosterone). So, surgical stress promotes volume retention directly (via ADH) and less directly by renal retention of sodium (via aldosterone).

2. While oliguria may indicate reduced renal perfusion or increased ADH and aldosterone, it can also be because your patient has sick kidneys. In order to distinguish between those alternatives, you obtain a urine sodium. If the

urine sodium is less than 10 to 15 mEq/L, your patient's kidneys are working flat out (ie, beautifully) in response to stress. You can infuse some crystalloid and urine volume will increase. If, however, the urine sodium is elevated (say, 40–50 mEq/L), then your patient's kidneys are sick. Now, you have bigger trouble because there are no direct pharmacological agents that protect renal health. Do everything that you can to preserve kidney perfusion (be sure to still optimize cardiac output) and meticulously check for any nephrotoxic agents that your patient may inadvertently be receiving.

To sort out oliguria, you can calculate a fractional excretion of sodium (FENA). The FENA represents the percentage of sodium filtered by the kidneys that is excreted in urine. A kidney is a high-volume system, and in a healthy adult surgical resident, after dilution in the loop of Henle, approximately 20 L of hypotonic fluid reaches the collecting system each day. Thus, in the total absence of ADH (diabetes insipidus) a patient will put out 20 L of urine daily. The urine sodium depends on both renal water reabsorption and the health of the tubular sodium reabsorptive function. Mathematically, the formula looks like:

FENA = 100 × (urinary Na over plasma NA)
     × (plasma creatinine over urinary creatinine)

FENA <1% indicates hypovolemia.

FENA >3% indicates sick kidneys.

FENA between 1% and 3% indicates "I'm not sure."

Now, you can make these calculations even more inscrutable, but for all practical purposes, when you are confronted with an oliguric patient, you can usually just get a urine sodium.

A. If it's less than 15 mEq/L, try some crystalloid.

B. If it's higher than 40 to 50 mEq/L, you need to worry.

3. Whenever you are called about a patient with oliguria who has a Foley in place, you must convince yourself that the catheter is patent. Bladder distension and anuria should prompt you to have the Foley flushed. New anuria is highly specific for catheter obstruction—even sick or hypoperfused kidneys usually make a little urine.

4. The use of furosemide (Lasix) in an oliguric patient should not be initiated until it has been determined that the cause of the oliguria is not a lack of renal perfusion. In that case, diuresis reduces the circulating volume that in turn decreases preload and cardiac output, thereby worsening the situation. If, on the other hand, the cause of the oliguria is intrinsic, then one can argue that high-output renal failure is easier to manage than low-output renal compromise. The one circumstance in which furosemide is clearly indicated for oliguria is when a patient is hypoperfusing his or her kidneys due to congestive heart failure—in this case, diuresis can be predicted to improve cardiac output.

TIPS TO REMEMBER

● We use urine output as a "composite" indicator of a patient's hemodynamic stability.

● Oliguria is a normal response to stress.

● A stressed patient retains volume directly (via ADH) or less directly by renal retention of sodium (via aldosterone).

● A spot urine sodium less than 15 mEq/L means your patient's kidneys are healthy; give crystalloid.

● A spot urine sodium greater than 40 to 50 mEq/L means your patient's kidneys are sick; optimize renal perfusion and search for any nephrotoxic drugs your patient might be receiving.

● Lasix and low-dose dopamine may increase urine volume, but there is no evidence that they help the kidneys "bounce back" to health.

COMPREHENSION QUESTIONS

1. You are on night float and are called about an otherwise healthy patient who had a lysis of adhesions and small bowel resection during the day. The nurse tells you that the patient has made 20 mL of urine over the past two hours. You order a 1 L bolus after confirming that his vitals are normal and that he has no other evidence of hemodynamic instability. When you check back in an hour, you learn that the patient has only made an additional 5 mL of urine. You go to evaluate the patient. Other than a physical exam, your next step should be which of the following?
    A. Check a CBC.
    B. Order another 1 L bolus and reevaluate in 30 minutes.
    C. Order furosemide 40 mg IV.
    D. Flush the Foley.

2. A burn patient admitted 3 weeks ago has become progressively oliguric over the past six hours. She is now making just 15 mL/h and has not responded to 2 L of crystalloid. You ordered a urine spot protein. Which result would be most consistent with kidney injury (eg, ATN)?
    A. 3.2 mEq/L
    B. 10 mEq/L
    C. 25 mEq/L
    D. 50 mEq/L

Answers

1. **A.** The patient is at low risk of hemorrhage, so an empiric 1 L bolus was a reasonable first move. But since he didn't respond, it is important to rule out other

causes of inadequate renal perfusion. If the patient's oliguria is due to hypovolemia, furosemide will only make it worse. While a partially clogged Foley could be the cause, it is unlikely in the setting of low but nonzero urine output for three hours. While not listed as an answer, one can also check a spot urine sodium if there is any confusion about whether this is a prerenal or intrarenal problem.

2. **D**. Less than 15 mEq/L suggests a prerenal cause (hypovolemia, stress, shock), while more than 40 mEq/L suggests kidney dysfunction.

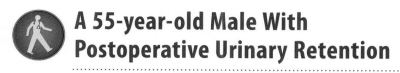

A 55-year-old Male With Postoperative Urinary Retention

Selma Marie Siddiqui, MD
and Marie Crandall, MD, MPH

A 55-year-old male with a history of diabetes mellitus underwent an uncomplicated hemorrhoidectomy under general anesthesia. No Foley catheter was placed. In the postanesthesia care unit, he complained of pain and was given IV narcotics.

The patient is admitted for observation. Six hours postoperatively, the floor nurse calls because the patient reports the urge to void but despite numerous attempts has been unable to do so. He is hemodynamically stable and mentating well, but does have distention and tenderness to palpation in the suprapubic area.

1. What additional history or physical examination findings would be useful in this patient? What are the most common risk factors for postoperative urinary retention (POUR)?

2. What are the most common etiologies of POUR? Which is most likely in this patient?

3. What is your next step?

4. In a patient with an indwelling Foley catheter removed on postoperative day #4 who is unable to void 6 hours later, what would be the best management plan?

5. When would it be appropriate to seek a Urology consult for POUR?

POSTOPERATIVE URINARY RETENTION

POUR is a common complication resulting in numerous pages to the PGY-1 on service. The process of socially appropriate voiding requires frontal cortex coordination with the pontine micturition center to control the spinal reflex arcs manipulating the delicate balance between the promicturition parasympathetic drive and the antimicturition sympathetic drive. The desire to void should normally present with 150 cm^3 of urine, with normal bladder capacity ranging between 400 and 600 cm^3. A clinical examination with a palpable bladder and dullness to percussion along with symptoms of lower abdominal discomfort are classic signs of POUR; however, a bedside bladder ultrasound should be obtained whenever possible to support clinical findings and estimate the degree of bladder distension.

Answers

1. Based on common risk factors, it is possible for the astute PGY-1 to anticipate which patients are likely to suffer from POUR. Risk factors include the following:

   - BPH or prior history of POUR
   - Age 50 years or more
   - Male gender
   - Neuropathy or neurologic disorders

   One can also stratify risk of POUR by type of procedure being undergone, anesthesia used, and postoperative analgesia delivered. Anorectal procedures are known for having a particularly high incidence of POUR, with studies demonstrating frequency of POUR after anorectal surgery to range between 16% and 50%, followed closely by inguinal herniorrhaphy. Spinal anesthesia, epidural anesthesia, and general anesthesia have higher incidences of POUR than local anesthesia. Opioid-based patient-controlled analgesia (PCA) has a slightly higher incidence of POUR compared with oral or IV push opioids due to the more constant inhibition of parasympathetic drives.

   The duration of the procedure indirectly increases the likelihood of POUR by dose-dependent effects of anesthetic/analgesic agents. The volume of IV fluids received intraoperatively in the absence of a Foley catheter can also affect POUR as higher volumes may lead to overdistention of the bladder with possible subsequent cystopathy.

2. Etiologies of POUR are broken down into 3 major categories:

   - Drug effect
   - Obstructive
   - Neurogenic (increased sympathetic activity)

   The most common of these categories encountered in the surgical patient tends to be retention secondary to drug effects from anesthetic and narcotic agents.

   In the patient presented above—a 55-year-old male with diabetes—drug effect, obstructive, and neurogenic causes are all plausible. This patient underwent general anesthesia and therefore has a high risk of a drug effect cause of his retention. BPH is the most common obstructive cause in male patients and can easily be assessed for with a digital rectal examination or review of medications taken to search for an α-blocker. Pain and anxiety, often caused by concern over being unable to void, can cause increased sympathetic tone that can further suppress micturition arcs. Furthermore, diabetes and the sequelae of neuropathies that accompany severe disease can also include diabetic cystopathy. Other neurologic disorders such as stroke, multiple sclerosis, mass effects, etc, can cause similar neurogenic bladder symptoms and can be exacerbated by stress in the postoperative state.

3. The most appropriate next step here is to immediately obtain a bedside ultrasound estimate of intravesicular volume. Bedside bladder scanners are commonly used and a nurse can easily obtain this value. Typically, 3 scans of the bladder with an average of the 3 values are used for clinical decision making.

After obtaining a bladder ultrasound demonstrating a volume at or above normal limits (thus ruling out postoperative oliguria), it is appropriate to proceed with single intermittent catheterization. Given that this is likely a drug effect in the majority of patients, single intermittent catheterization allows the bladder to avoid damage secondary to significant distention and allows the central and peripheral nerve centers to regain function. If a patient is still unable to void an additional 6 to 8 hours later and bedside ultrasound again supports clinical evidence of a significant volume of urine in the bladder, it is appropriate to repeat intermittent catheterization.

After 2 intermittent catheterizations, if the patient is still unable to void, placement of an indwelling catheter is appropriate to prevent possible urethral trauma and overdistention of the bladder. It would also be appropriate to allow for regular intermittent catheterization if the patient or nursing staff can perform catheterization in an aseptic manner and the patient has an uncomplicated urethral tract.

In the event of urine volumes above 600 cm^3 on intermittent catheterization, there is potential for significant distention-induced dysfunction of the detrusor muscle and the patient may require bladder rest for an extended period of time. Use clinical judgment with large-volume outputs from intermittent catheterization and consider 1 or more days of bladder rest with indwelling Foley catheters before repeating a voiding trial. Patients with a history of obstructive pathology may tolerate a larger volume of distention without developing dysfunction compared with others.

4. The appropriate next step would be to obtain a bladder ultrasound to verify a volume of urine sufficient to stimulate the micturition reflex arcs. If greater than 150 cm^3 of urine is present in the bladder, but less than 300 cm^3, it would be appropriate to allow the patient additional time for the coordination of the multiple signals controlling physiologic micturition. If a volume of urine greater than 300 cm^3 is present on bladder ultrasound, single intermittent catheterization should be performed. If the patient is unable to void a second time with a significant bladder volume, either the patient may have an indwelling catheter placed with a plan for a repeat voiding trial subsequently or the patient can continue with aseptic intermittent catheterization until physiologic micturition function normalizes.

5. Urology consultation may be considered when failure to void has occurred multiple times and there is unlikely to be persistent drug effect. In these patients the possibility for neurogenic or obstructive pathology must be considered and urologic evaluation is appropriate.

In a patient who presents with probable obstructive pathology causing retention, it is appropriate to initiate α-blockers (as long as the patient does not have any contraindications to this class of medications). It is appropriate to proceed with outpatient urologic evaluation for obstructive pathology that improves with α-blockers and to continue the patient on these medications postoperatively until further evaluation can be obtained.

TIPS TO REMEMBER

● Bladder ultrasound is the most sensitive and specific noninvasive method for assessing intravesicular volume. If the volume exceeds 300 cm³, the bladder should be drained with intermittent catheterization.

● An initial failure to void after anesthesia is likely a drug effect. A second or third failure should raise suspicion for obstructive or neurogenic pathology, especially in patients with additional risk factors.

COMPREHENSION QUESTIONS

1. Which of these patients is at highest risk of developing POUR?
   A. A 40-year-old hypertensive male undergoing systemic analgesia for wide local excision of a forearm melanoma.
   B. A 22-year-old female who is 10 weeks pregnant undergoing general anesthesia for a laparoscopic appendectomy.
   C. A 70-year-old female with well-controlled diabetes undergoing spinal anesthesia for left greater saphenous vein radio-frequency ablation and stab phlebectomy.
   D. A 65-year-old male with BPH undergoing general anesthesia with epidural analgesia for a laparoscopic right inguinal hernia repair.

2. Which of the following is true?
   A. The first step in evaluation of POUR is to obtain an intermittent catheterization.
   B. In a patient with POUR who has a known urethral stricture and hematuria after initial intermittent catheterization, it is appropriate to proceed with intermittent catheterizations until physiologic micturition normalizes.
   C. After obtaining a bladder scan with 400 cm³ intravesicular volume 6 hours postoperatively, a single intermittent catheterization is the appropriate first step.
   D. A volume of 1000 cm³ urine output on intermittent catheterization is unlikely to cause detrusor dysfunction in a patient with no prior history of urinary obstruction.

3. Which of the following is most sensitive and specific for determining the initial presence of POUR?

    A. Patient complaint of low abdominal pain and failure to void

    B. Clinical examination of a palpable bladder with dullness to the umbilicus

    C. Bladder ultrasound

    D. Bladder catheterization

Answers

1. **D.** This patient has obstructive pathology, is advanced in age, is male, and is receiving general anesthesia for a procedure with a high risk of urinary retention.

2. **C.** Parasympathetics trigger detrusor contractions and relax the internal urethral sphincter. Sympathetics relax the detrusor and tighten the internal urethral sphincter. In the immediate postoperative period there is excess sympathetic tone. A little extra time can be all that is required for that balance to normalize and allow the patient to recover the ability to urinate. In other words, don't rush to place a catheter for a problem that may resolve on its own in another few hours.

3. **C.** Bladder ultrasound is noninvasive and can provide an estimated volume of urine being retained to guide further management choices.

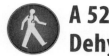

A 52-year-old Female Who Is Dehydrated Postoperative Day #1

Aisha Shaheen, MD, MHA and Marie Crandall, MD, MPH

During your morning pre-rounds you see Ms. Yang, a 52-year-old female who is POD #1 from a small bowel resection for a high-grade obstruction. Ms. Yang states her pain is well controlled with medication but she feels tired and a little light-headed. In checking her postoperative orders you note she is NPO, her naso-gastric tube should be attached to continuous wall suction, and she should have IV fluids running. Although the NGT is in place and appears to be functioning properly, you notice on closer inspection her IV fluid tubing is disconnected. The patient tells you the tubing was bothering her while she was sleeping, so she disconnected it during the night. Her vitals reveal her to be mildly tachycardic and hypotensive with a heart rate of 103 and a blood pressure of 98/70. As you examine her, you notice her mouth and lips are dry and she is clearly dehydrated.

Her wound dressings are clean, dry, and intact, and her exam is otherwise unremarkable. You realize the patient needs to be given fluids.

1. What type of intravenous fluid is most like plasma?

2. For each of the following types of fluid loss, what type of crystalloid solution is most appropriate and why?
   A. Gastric losses
   B. Pancreatic/biliary/small bowel losses
   C. Large intestine (diarrheal) losses

3. What effect do crystalloids have compared with colloids on plasma volume expansion? On mortality?

4. Estimate the patient in this vignette's maintenance fluid requirement. Assume she weighs 80 kg. Now adjust this estimate based on a 24-hour NGT output loss of 600 cm³.

5. If another patient, Ms. Bradford, was a cardiac patient with an ejection fraction of 31%, what precautions would need to be taken in administration of her maintenance fluid?

6. If Ms. Bradford was diabetic, should her maintenance fluid contain dextrose?

IV FLUIDS

Answers

1. Table 42-1 summarizes the ion concentrations in the 2 most common types of crystalloid fluids—normal saline (NS) and lactated Ringer's (LR). Note that the

Table 42-1. The Concentration of Ions in Common Crystalloid Fluids Compared With Plasma

Electrolyte Composition	NS	LR	Plasma
Na	154	130	140
Cl	154	109	103
K	—	4	4
Ca	—	2.7	5
Bicarbonate	—	28	25

composition of LR most closely approximates that of plasma and is commonly used for surgical patients. However, because of the addition of calcium and lactate (bicarbonate) to this solution, it should not be used in certain clinical scenarios. For example, the calcium in LR can bind to certain drugs including amphotericin, ampicillin, and thiopental and reduce their effectiveness. Preclinical studies have also shown that calcium can bind to the anticoagulant in donor blood and promote clot formation; therefore, in clinical practice many centers do not infuse LR simultaneously with red blood cell transfusions.

There are no clear contraindications to the use of NS. However, it is important to know that the high chloride concentration of this solution can lead to a non-anion gap (hyperchloremic) metabolic acidosis if large volumes are infused.

Understanding the tonicity of various crystalloid fluids is important when deciding what to use for resuscitation and for maintenance. Both NS and LR are isotonic fluids, meaning the osmolar concentration of these solutions is the same as that of the interstitial space. Infusion of isotonic fluids into the vascular space results in diffusion of the fluid until it is evenly distributed among all of the fluid compartments of the body. About 1/3 of the total volume of infused isotonic crystalloid stays within the vessels. Isotonic solutions can be used for resuscitation or for maintenance. Hypotonic solutions (eg, 0.45% NS), in contrast, have a lower osmolar concentration than the intracellular and interstitial space. As a result, more of the water leaves the intravascular space in order to achieve osmolar equilibration with the interstitium. Because the water in hypotonic crystalloid leaves the intravascular space more rapidly than isotonic solutions, hypotonic solutions are never used for resuscitation. They are commonly used for maintenance fluid administration, as the insensible losses they are meant to replace are typically hypotonic in nature (ie, more water is lost than solutes).

2. The most appropriate crystalloid to use for losses from the gastrointestinal tract depends on the area of the loss—each portion of the GI tract has a different electrolyte composition. Replacement should be chosen to match, as closely as possible, the composition of those losses (see Table 42-2).

Table 42-2. Fluid Losses and Recommended Replacements

Site of Loss	Replacement Fluid
Salivary	NS + potassium
Gastric	NS + potassium
Pancreatic/biliary/small bowel losses; ileostomy losses	LR + bicarbonate
Large intestine (diarrheal) losses; colostomy losses	LR + potassium

3. Crystalloid fluids are those fluids that contain only water and dissolved salts. Colloids are fluids that contain water and larger molecules or even cells (eg, albumin, packed red blood cells). Crystalloid fluid contains only small molecules, and they distribute freely throughout the extravascular space. As discussed above, when crystalloid fluids are administered, the interstitial volume expands more than the intravascular plasma volume. In contrast, the large molecules and/or cells in colloid fluids do not diffuse readily between body fluid spaces and remain intravascular. This creates an osmotic pressure that attracts water and thereby preferentially expands the intravascular plasma volume. For this reason, conventional teaching suggests 3 L of crystalloid solution is required to obtain the same incremental increase to plasma volume obtained with just 1 L of colloid solution. For those situations in which a patient cannot tolerate large volumes of fluid, colloids (albumin in particular) are widely used.

While the theoretical basis for this practice may be sound, there are no clinical trials that have demonstrated any difference in outcomes when using crystalloid or the most commonly used colloid, albumin. For example, the Saline versus Albumin Fluid Evaluation (SAFE) study showed that the type of fluid administered (colloid vs crystalloid) conferred no survival benefit in critically ill patients. The uncertain evidence combined with the significantly higher costs of colloid solutions suggests that crystalloid solutions should continue to be preferred over albumin for most routine clinical situations.

4. The "4-2-1 Rule" is a quick way to estimate volume replacement (see Figure 42-1). Using this rule for Ms. Yang gives us:

$$\text{IV fluids (cm}^3\text{/h)} = (4 \text{ cm}^3\text{/kg/h} \times 10) + (2 \text{ cm}^3\text{/kg/h} \times 10)$$
$$+ (1 \text{ cm}^3\text{/kg/h} \times [80 \text{ kg} - 20 \text{ kg}]) = 120 \text{ cm}^3\text{/h}$$

In clinical practice the maintenance fluid requirement is then often adjusted based on the estimated quantity of other losses. For example, patients with high NGT outputs often receive 1 cm³ : 1 cm³ replacement for their NGT fluid losses in addition to their maintenance fluids. For Ms. Yang, this would

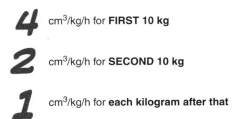

Figure 42-1. 4-2-1 Rule for estimates of maintenance fluid requirements.

mean receiving a 600 cm³ bolus in addition to her 120 cm³/h maintenance fluid rate. The 600 cm³ loss can also be added incrementally over 24 hours (600 cm³/24 hours = 25 cm³/h + 120 cm³/h = 145 cm³/h maintenance fluid rate). It is important to note that the "4-2-1 Rule" provides only an estimate and that estimate should be used for initial maintenance fluid administration, not to calculate resuscitation requirements.

When the formula is used to calculate initial maintenance rates, adequate volume replacement must still be continually reassessed. The goal of adequate volume replacement, as discussed in the chapter on Shock, is to optimize pre-load and thereby optimize cardiac output and end-organ perfusion. For this reason, urine output (a measure of renal perfusion) is often used to determine when adequate volume replacement has been achieved. It should be maintained at least to 0.5 cm³/kg/h.

5. Certain patient populations require special attention when being resuscitated postoperatively or when calculating maintenance fluid requirements because they have increased risks for volume overload. Patients with poor cardiac function or patients on dialysis are especially susceptible to this complication. Oftentimes in clinical practice these patients receive fluids based on ideal body weight (IBW) that adjusts body weight based on height.

One of the first signs of volume overload is weight gain. The excess fluid can also cause swelling in the extremities manifested as peripheral edema. Excess fluid can also enter the air spaces of the lungs and compromise oxygenation leading to shortness of breath. This can manifest as crackles on physical exam. Finally, when fluid overload is significant, there may be cardiac compromise in the form of arrhythmias such as atrial fibrillation or the development of congestive heart failure.

6. Diabetic patients are another patient population requiring special caution when IV fluids are being administered. Because this patient population receives exogenous insulin to control blood glucose levels, extra care must be taken to avoid hypoglycemia when patients are NPO. Adding dextrose to the maintenance fluid of diabetic patients ensures they do not "bottom out" their blood glucose

levels. Furthermore, just as with nondiabetic patients, small amounts of dextrose help prevent the diabetic patient who is NPO from going into "starvation mode" and entering a catabolic state.

TIPS TO REMEMBER

- Both NS and LR are isotonic crystalloid solutions. LR solution is similar to plasma in electrolyte composition (ie, it includes potassium, bicarbonate, and calcium).
- Isotonic solutions are used for resuscitation.
- Hypotonic solutions should only be used as maintenance fluids.
- Crystalloid solutions redistribute more into the interstitial and intracellular space, and colloid solutions remain in the intravascular space.
- The "4-2-1 Rule" is used to estimate maintenance fluid requirements.
- Care must be taken to avoid volume overload in susceptible patient populations such as cardiac and dialysis patients.
- Dextrose should be added to the maintenance fluid for diabetic patients who are NPO to avoid hypoglycemia.
- Urine output is 1 indicator of adequate cardiac output and hence of adequate volume replacement.

COMPREHENSION QUESTIONS

1. Which acid–base disturbance can occur with large-volume infusions of NS?
    A. Anion gap metabolic acidosis
    B. Metabolic alkalosis
    C. Respiratory acidosis
    D. Non-anion gap metabolic acidosis

2. What is the appropriate solution to use for large intestine (diarrheal) losses?
    A. LR with potassium
    B. LR with bicarbonate
    C. NS with chloride
    D. NS with bicarbonate

3. To obtain the same theoretical increase in plasma volume, what ratio of crystalloid to colloid solution is needed for 0.45 (ie, 0.5) NS compared with albumin?
    A. 1:1
    B. 3:1
    C. 6:1
    D. 10:1

Answers

1. **D.** Non-anion gap metabolic acidosis results from the large infusion of chloride ions.

2. **A.** The large intestine has a high potassium concentration and so this is the electrolyte that needs to be replaced with diarrheal losses. LR contains potassium, but NS with added potassium can also be used.

3. **C.** 0.45% NS is also known as 0.5 NS. Since it is half the tonicity of 0.9% NS, you must double the 3:1 ratio described above.

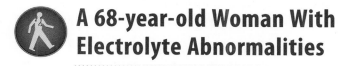

A 68-year-old Woman With Electrolyte Abnormalities

Molly A. Wasserman, MD
and Mamta Swaroop, MD, FACS

Ms. Jones is a 68-year-old female with a past medical history significant for hypertension and hyperlipidemia, now 2 years status post open sigmoidectomy for recurrent diverticulitis. She presents with a 3-day history of crampy abdominal pain, nausea, and 5 episodes of nonbloody, nonbilious emesis. She also reports a gradual onset of abdominal distension with obstipation. Her last bowel movement was 4 days ago and was normal. She has had associated anorexia and subjective fevers. Her medications include furosemide and atorvastatin.

On physical exam, her vitals are as follows—T: 101.5; HR: 120; BP: 140/90; RR: 16; O_2: 99% on RA; and weight: 70 kg. Abdominal exam reveals absent bowel sounds, abdominal distension with diffuse tympany, and tenderness in the left upper and lower quadrants with no rebound or guarding. The remainder of the exam is normal. Labs are notable for a sodium level of 130, potassium of 2.8, and magnesium of 1.5.

1. Why are Mrs. Jones' electrolytes abnormal?

2. What are the risks associated with leaving her sodium and potassium uncorrected?

3. What orders would you write to replete her potassium?

ELECTROLYTE ABNORMALITIES

The ability to anticipate electrolyte abnormalities is of paramount importance in the treatment and management of the surgical patient. It will also be one of your primary responsibilities as a surgical intern. You will be expected to take care of all but the most severe abnormalities. It is important to know when and how to replace electrolytes, and when to alert the senior on service in the case of a severe and potentially life-threatening abnormality.

Answers

1. Fluids and electrolytes can be lost most commonly from the gastrointestinal tract (emesis, diarrhea, nasogastric tubes, enterocutaneous fistulas), from the genitourinary system (renal disease), from the skin (sweat, burns, fever), and from fluid shifts (third spacing, postoperative open abdomens, vacuum-assisted wound closure devices, hemorrhage). Electrolyte abnormalities may be worsened by a patient's NPO status and the administration of intravenous fluids that

Table 43-1. Symptoms and Signs of Electrolyte Abnormalities

Hypernatremia	Lethargy, weakness, irritability, **confusion**, **seizures**, **coma**
Hyponatremia	Lethargy, anorexia, nausea, emesis, weakness, fatigue, **confusion**, **seizures**, **coma**
Hyperkalemia	Nausea, emesis, abdominal pain, areflexia, confusion, paralysis, **cardiac hypoexcitability**, **and asystole**
Hypokalemia	Fatigue, weakness, **ileus, cardiac arrhythmias**
Hypermagnesemia	Sedation, areflexia, diarrhea, paralysis, **coma**, **cardiac arrhythmias**
Hypomagnesemia	Weakness, abdominal cramping, hyperreflexia, **cardiac arrhythmias**, **refractory hypokalemia, and hypocalcemia**
Hyperphosphatemia	Muscle cramps, perioral tingling, paresthesias, **ventricular** arrhythmias
Hypophosphatemia	Confusion, weakness, seizures, **respiratory failure**, heart failure

are insufficient to meet the patient's metabolic demands. Predicting losses and repleting the patient early is the best way to thwart electrolyte abnormalities. In the case above, this patient has had both diarrhea and emesis, most likely has not been able to replete her losses secondary to anorexia, and will be made NPO and receive a nasogastric tube as part of her initial treatment. All of these factors compound each other to cause this patient to be at high risk of having severe electrolyte abnormalities. Additional consideration must be given to the patient's medications. As an example, loop diuretics (eg, furosemide) put the patient at risk of hypokalemia.

2. Table 43-1 depicts the common symptoms and signs of electrolyte abnormalities. As shown below, electrolyte disorders have a wide range of symptoms. Common among these are a delayed return of bowel function, muscle weakness and fatigue, cardiac dysfunction and dysrhythmias, seizures, and failure to wean from a ventilator.

3. It is important to memorize how to treat each of the most common electrolyte abnormalities.

   Hyponatremia: Hyponatremia is defined as a serum sodium concentration <135 mEq/L. There are a variety of causes of hyponatremia in the surgical patient. ADH is elevated as a part of the normal stress response, and activation of inflammatory and stress cytokines (IL-1, IL-6, TNF-α) further increases ADH release. Fluid overload, high-output enterocutaneous fistulas, and aggressive diuresis may also result in hyponatremia. Initial treatment of hyponatremia involves determination of the sodium deficit and overall volume status:

$$Na \text{ deficit} = TBW \times (140 - \text{serum Na})$$

where TBW = $0.6 \times$ (weight in kg) for male and TBW = $0.55 \times$ (weight in kg) for female.

In treating hyponatremia, it is important to determine the overall fluid status of the patient. Hypovolemic, hyponatremic patients can often be treated by rehydration with normal saline or Lactated Ringer's solution. Conversely, euvolemic or hypervolemic patients who are asymptomatic are best initially treated with free water restriction. Symptomatic patients require administration of hypertonic saline. Overly aggressive treatment of hyponatremia will result in central pontine myelinolysis and possible permanent spastic quadriparesis and pseudobulbar palsy. As such, serum sodium should be repleted at a rate of ≤ 8 mEq/kg/day or 0.25 mEq/L/h.

Hypernatremia: Hypernatremia is defined as a serum sodium concentration of >145 mEq/L. It is less common in the surgical patient but may be seen in patients with increased insensible water losses (burns, tracheostomies), major GI losses (NG tube suction, diarrhea, emesis), administration of sodium (TPN, sodium bicarbonate infusion), and when hypotonic losses are replaced with isotonic solutions (eg, post resuscitation). As with hyponatremia, the initial step in the treatment of hypernatremia is determining the free water deficit:

$$\text{Free water deficit} = \frac{\text{serum Na} - 140}{140} \times 0.6 \text{ (weight in kg)}$$

Patients with severe (Na >160 mEq/L) or symptomatic hypernatremia should be treated with D5W or D5 0.45 NS to correct at a rate of less than 0.5 mEq/L/h. Once the free water deficit is calculated, the first half of the total deficit should be administered over the first 24 hours, and the second half over the subsequent 24 hours. Overly rapid correction may result in cerebral edema and brainstem herniation.

Hypokalemia: Potassium is the dominant intracellular cation, and only 2% of total body potassium resides in the serum. Potassium balance is controlled by the renin–angiotensin–aldosterone axis. Hypokalemia is defined as a serum potassium concentration <3.5 mEq/L. Total body potassium levels may be depleted by decreased potassium intake, increased loss from the GI tract (NG tube, emesis, diarrhea), renal disease, catecholamine stimulation, and certain medications (insulin, diuretics). Signs and symptoms of hypokalemia include gastrointestinal ileus, generalized fatigue and

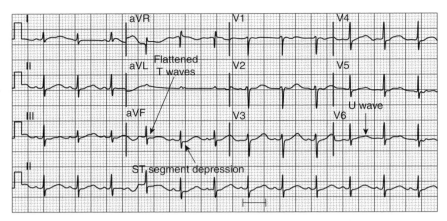

Figure 43-1. ECG abnormalities seen in hypokalemia. (Modified, with permission, from Longo DL, Fauci AS, Kasper DL, Hauser SL, Jameson JL, Loscalzo J. *Harrison's Principles of Internal Medicine*. 18th ed. New York: McGraw-Hill; 2012. Figure e28-24. <www.accessmedicine.com>. Copyright © The McGraw-Hill Companies, Inc. All right reserved.)

weakness, cardiac arrhythmias, and renal insufficiency. ECG abnormalities include flattened T waves, depression of ST segments, prominent U waves, and prolongation of the QT interval (Figure 43-1).

Treatment of hypokalemia consists of oral or parental potassium supplementation. Oral formulations are preferred if the patient is able to take medications orally or is undergoing active diuresis. Intravenous potassium can be administered to patients unable to take po or those with severe hypokalemia (<2 mEq/L) at a rate of 10 mEq/h at a concentration no greater than 40 mEq/L. If repleting through a central line, it is permissible to replete at 20 mEq/h. Potassium can also be added to maintenance intravenous fluids at a concentration of 20 mEq in 1 L of fluid. As a general rule, administration of 10 mEq KCl, in either IV or po formulation, will increase the serum potassium level by 0.1.

It is important to note that hypomagnesemia antagonizes correction of hypokalemia. As such, if the patient is concomitantly hypomagnesemic, correction with magnesium supplementation must occur before potassium supplementation will correct hypokalemia.

Hyperkalemia: Hyperkalemia is defined as a serum potassium concentration >5.5 mEq/L. Common causes of hyperkalemia include renal disease and a decreased ability to excrete potassium, crush injuries, rhabdomyolysis, ischemia–reperfusion injuries, adrenal insufficiency, succinylcholine administration, β-receptor agonists, digitalis, and excessive administration of intravenous fluids containing potassium. Early identification and

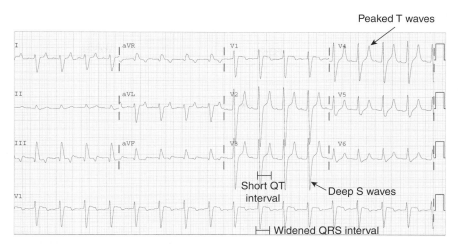

Figure 43-2. ECG abnormalities of hyperkalemia. (Reproduced, with permission, from Knoop KJ, Stack LB, Storrow AB, Thurman RJ. *The Atlas of Emergency Medicine.* 3rd ed. New York: McGraw-Hill; 2010. Figure 23.45A. Photo contributor: R. Jason Thurman, MD. <http://www.accessmedicine.com>. Copyright © The McGraw-Hill Companies, Inc. All right reserved.)

treatment of hyperkalemia is imperative, as hyperkalemia has life-threatening consequences including cardiac arrhythmias and neuromuscular weakness leading to flaccid paralysis. EKG abnormalities include peaked T waves, QRS widening, shortened QT intervals, deepening of the S wave into a sinusoidal pattern, and ventricular ectopy followed by hypoexcitability presenting as asystole (see Figure 43-2). It can less commonly also lead to ventricular fibrillation.

Treatment of hyperkalemia consists of early stabilization of the myocardium and a temporary shift of potassium intracellularly, followed by elimination of potassium into the stool or urine. Initial temporizing treatment includes administration of 1 ampule of calcium gluconate, which acts to antagonize myocardial depolarization. Another temporizing treatment is the administration of sodium bicarbonate, especially if the patient is acidotic. Both measures antagonize the effects of hyperkalemia on the membrane potential and also facilitate the intracellular shift of potassium. Additionally, 10 U of insulin is given to shift potassium intracellularly. This is followed by 1 ampule of D_{50} to thwart the impending insulin-induced hypoglycemia.

While the above measures will help reduce the serum potassium level, the effects are only transient. More definitive correction requires that potassium be excreted from the body. This is facilitated by administration of a loop diuretic (furosemide) or a sodium–potassium exchange resin (Kayexalate). Refractory hyperkalemia may ultimately require hemodialysis. A common mnemonic to remember how to treat hyperkalemia is "C-BIG-K-D," or "See BIG Potassium Drop":

C: Calcium gluconate

B: Bicarbonate (if acidotic)

I: Insulin

G: Glucose

K: Kayexalate

D: Dialysis

Hypomagnesemia: Magnesium is an intracellular cation that serves as a cofactor in enzymatic reactions and is essential for protein synthesis, energy metabolism, and calcium homeostasis. Hypomagnesemia occurs when serum magnesium levels are <1.6 mg/dL. In the surgical patient this most commonly occurs secondary to hemodilution, but may also occur with chronically poor po intake, steatorrhea, biliary and enteric fistulas, or chronic use of loop diuretics. Severe hypomagnesemia places the patient at risk for lethal ventricular arrhythmias. Magnesium repletion should be considered if the magnesium level falls below 2.0. This may be done orally with magnesium citrate if the patient is able to take it. However, large doses will result in diarrhea and thus po repletion is generally neither necessary nor recommended in the acute hospital setting. Intravenous administration of magnesium sulfate is a better route of repletion for patients with severe hypomagnesemia and those unable to tolerate po.

Hypermagnesemia: Hypermagnesemia is defined as a serum magnesium concentration >2.8 mg/dL. It is rare if the patient has normal kidney function, but may be seen in patients with burns, crush injuries, or those who require chronic hemodialysis. It may also be seen in pregnant women who are being administered magnesium sulfate as a tocolytic agent. Treatment starts with elimination of magnesium-containing medications. Calcium infusion at 5 to 10 mEq is administered to stabilize the myocardium, followed by normal saline to expand the intravascular compartment. Loop diuretics and hemodialysis may also be used to eliminate excess magnesium.

Hypophosphatemia: Phosphorus is an important molecule in energy metabolism and ATP generation. Hypophosphatemia is defined as a serum phosphate concentration <2.5 mg/dL. It can be the result of renal failure and excessive renal losses, GI losses, diuretic use, major hepatic resection, or intracellular electrolyte shifts as occur in refeeding syndrome. Symptoms are related to ATP depletion and include cardiac and respiratory failure. Repletion should be considered when levels fall below

2.0 mg/dL, and this may be administered as $NaPO_4$ or KPO_4 (depending on the potassium level).

Hyperphosphatemia: Hyperphosphatemia is defined as a serum phosphate concentration of >5.0 mg/dL. This is a rare postoperative occurrence but may be seen in renal failure, rhabdomyolysis, and tumor lysis syndrome. Treatment options include expanding the plasma volume with normal saline, administration of phosphate binders (aluminum-containing antacids), or, if severe and associated with renal failure, hemodialysis.

TIPS TO REMEMBER

- Surgical patients are at risk for a variety of electrolyte disorders based on the pathophysiology of their disease states (emesis, diarrhea, NG tubes, fistulas, burns, trauma, wounds, etc) and anticipation of these abnormalities will greatly enhance treatment and management of these patients.

- It is important to know the volume status in the hyponatremic patient, as treatment differs based on whether the patient is fluid overloaded or dehydrated.

- Repletion of magnesium to normal levels is necessary before the patient will respond to potassium repletion.

- Calcium rapidly stabilizes the myocardium in the hyperkalemic patient.

COMPREHENSION QUESTIONS

1. In the case presented above, what are Ms. Jones' anticipated electrolyte abnormalities?
   - A. Hypernatremia, hyperkalemia
   - B. Hyponatremia, hyperkalemia
   - C. Hypernatremia, hypokalemia
   - D. Hyponatremia, hypokalemia

2. Ms. Jones' chemistry panel revealed a serum sodium level of 130. How would you replete her deficit?
   - A. High-sodium diet
   - B. 2.5 L of 3% hypertonic saline over 48 hours
   - C. 2.5 L of NS over 24 to 48 hours
   - D. Free water restriction

3. Which of the following is the initial treatment of severe hyperkalemia?
   - A. Insulin 10 U
   - B. Calcium gluconate 1 ampule
   - C. Kayexalate
   - D. Hemodialysis

Answers

1. **D**. Ms. Jones is hypovolemic and hyponatremic secondary to her GI losses. As a result, her renal plasma flow and GFR will be low, ultimately resulting in increased sodium reabsorption by the kidneys in exchange for potassium.

2. **C**. In order to replete her sodium, it is imperative to determine her actual sodium deficit. Using the equation for Na deficit (0.55 [weight in kg] × [140—serum Na]), her total Na deficit is 385 mEq. Using 0.9% NS for repletion (which has 154 mEq of Na per liter), she would require 2.5 L (385/154) to make up for her sodium deficit.

3. **B**. Calcium gluconate is the initial treatment of acute hyperkalemia. It stabilizes the myocardium, but is temporizing with effects lasting only 30 minutes. Insulin is also a rapid-acting and temporizing measure, but is second line. Both Kayexalate and dialysis are definitive treatments for hyperkalemia, and should be instituted as soon as the hyperkalemia has been acutely corrected with more rapid measures.

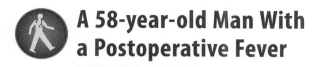

A 58-year-old Man With a Postoperative Fever

Jahan Mohebali, MD

You are paged about a fever of 101.8°F in a 58-year-old man who is postoperative day 3 from a colostomy reversal. He is normotensive, his heart rate is 110, and while he is oxygenating well, he is breathing at 22 breaths/min. His past medical history is notable for COPD and his preoperative medications include 4 mg of oral prednisone taken daily. This is the first fever that he has had since the operation and his nurse is requesting that you order Tylenol. When you evaluate the patient at the bedside, he states that he "doesn't feel too well."

1. **Based on the timing of the patient's fever, would you be surprised if he is ultimately diagnosed with a pneumonia?**

2. **What history and physical exam findings will help to confirm the diagnosis?**

3. **What are the initial steps in the workup of postoperative fever?**

4. **Other than pneumonia, what other factor may be responsible for the patient's tachypnea and fever?**

5. **What are the initial steps in empiric treatment of this patient's fever?**

6. **Should the patient receive acetaminophen (Tylenol)?**

POSTOPERATIVE FEVER

A surgical fever is defined as a temperature greater than 101.5°F or 38.5°C. The major etiologies for postoperative fever that should always be considered include atelectasis, pneumonia, urinary tract infection, intra-abdominal infection or leak, wound infection, and deep venous thrombosis. Other processes such as malignant hyperthermia, superficial thrombophlebitis, *C. difficile* colitis, endocarditis, and line infections should also be considered given the appropriate circumstances.

It is often helpful to categorize these various etiologies by the postoperative day on which they are *most likely* to occur (see Table 44-1). It is, however, important to note that any of these processes can occur on any postoperative day.

POD 0 to 1: There are multiple possible causes of fever on POD 0 and 1, including malignant hyperthermia, necrotizing wound infection, systemic inflammatory response syndrome (SIRS), and atelectasis. While atelectasis has traditionally been considered the most common cause of fever on postoperative day 1, it is a diagnosis of exclusion and more serious etiologies should be ruled out. These include malignant hyperthermia that is most likely to manifest in either the operating room or the PACU, and a severe necrotizing wound infection. Therefore, even if atelectasis is suspected, the patient should be examined and the dressing should be removed in order

Table 44-1. Most Likely Fever Etiology by Postoperative Day

Time	Cause of Fever
POD 0	SIRS response, atelectasis, malignant hyperthermia, necrotizing soft tissue infection
POD 1	Atelectasis
POD 3-4	Pneumonia, urinary tract infection
POD 5	Deep venous thrombosis
POD 7-10	Intra-abdominal abscess

to inspect the wound. Within the first 48 hours post surgery the dressing removal should be done in a sterile fashion.

If more serious causes have been ruled out, the fever is most likely due to a postoperative SIRS response or atelectasis. If you suspect the latter, then treatment is simple and consists of aggressive incentive spirometry, encouraging coughing and deep breathing, and ambulation.

POD 3 to 4: Classically, this is the time that urinary tract infections and pneumonias first manifest. Again, however, it should be noted that this time frame is not absolute. For example, an aspiration pneumonia related to intubation will probably present earlier, and a patient may present to the hospital already having a UTI. Nonaspiration pneumonias typically result from inadequate pulmonary toilet, and postoperative UTIs are often secondary to Foley catheter insertion or failure to remove the Foley catheter as early as possible. A final etiology that should always be considered in patients who have undergone abdominal surgery is an anastomotic leak that can manifest as fever as early as POD 3.

POD 5: Deep venous thrombosis. Surgery increases the risk of deep venous thrombosis. These clots can be a nidus for inflammation and infection.

POD 7 to 10: Intra-abdominal abscess. It takes a while for the bacteria to multiply and for the body to react.

It is important to remember that any source of infection can lead to bacteremia, or sepsis. Although a full discussion of the SIRS response and sepsis is covered in other chapters, the astute clinician should always be looking for systemic signs of infection whenever presented with a patient with postoperative fever.

Answers

1. The patient in the case above is experiencing a fever on postoperative day 3. Given his concomitant tachycardia and tachypnea, there should be concern for pneumonia or a more serious infection with systemic effects. In this case, given

his specific operation and his preoperative steroid use, there should also be a higher-than-usual suspicion for an anastomotic leak.

2. The junior surgical resident will often encounter postoperative fever when paged by a member of the nursing staff. Although it may be tempting to simply order Tylenol and address the issue later, particularly if the page occurs in the middle of the night, the patient should always be evaluated at the bedside. A brief history focusing on symptoms such as dyspnea, sputum production, worsening abdominal pain, leg pain, diarrhea, or urinary frequency and burning should quickly be obtained. A physical exam should include auscultation of the lungs, an abdominal exam, an exam for leg edema or pain with passive motion (Homans' sign), and palpation of the calves for "cords" suggestive of DVT. Finally, the patient's primary dressing should be removed in order to evaluate the wound.

3. After a brief history and physical exam, a diagnostic workup should be initiated based on the postoperative day as well as any other patient-specific factors (see Figure 44-1). Often, no additional workup is needed in the first 24 hours in an asymptomatic patient assuming that the serious causes of fever in this time period have been ruled out as mentioned above. After the first 24 hours, minimal workup should include a complete blood count with differential, urinalysis, chest x-ray, and 2 sets of blood cultures drawn from separate sites. Depending

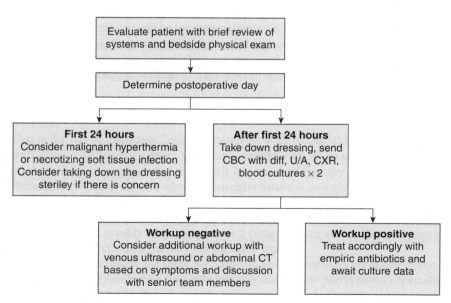

Figure 44-1. Algorithm for evaluating postoperative fever.

on the patient's symptoms or chest x-ray findings, a sputum culture and duplex venous studies may also be obtained. In general, the decision to obtain additional imaging such as an abdominal CT scan to look for an anastomotic leak or intra-abdominal abscess should be made in conjunction with the senior resident or attending.

4. Although respiratory symptoms such as tachypnea may simply indicate an underlying pulmonary process such as pneumonia, they should also raise concern for a severe infection or impending sepsis. A portable chest x-ray is very useful to help differentiate among the possibilities.

5. If you suspect an infection, workup should proceed as above with the goal of identifying a target for possible antibiotic treatment. If no target can be identified (ie, the patient has a fever of unknown origin), then a decision must be made regarding initiation of empiric treatment. That decision will be made in consultation with either your senior resident or attending, and will typically integrate factors such as patient symptoms, hemodynamics, and overall risk of complications.

   In this case, the patient is 3 days into a hospital course, has COPD, and is on prednisone suggesting that broad-spectrum coverage for pneumonia should be employed. A good regimen would be vancomycin, Zosyn, and levofloxacin.

6. Although acetaminophen (Tylenol) is beneficial for the symptomatic treatment of postoperative fever, its downsides are 3-fold. Most seriously, high doses of acetaminophen are hepatotoxic. More subtly, it is often clinically useful to follow a patient's fever curve as a marker of adequate source control, and the use of acetaminophen can obscure these data. Lastly, fevers are a physiologic response to infection that change the temperature of the culture medium (ie, the patient) for bacteria that are adapted to reproduce best at normal body temperatures. Medically "correcting" this mild hyperthermia therefore is of benefit mostly to the bacteria—it is unlikely to augment either the doctor or the patient's ability to resolve the infection.

   For all of these reasons it is best to avoid reflexively treating a fever with acetaminophen, but instead reserve it for those cases where the patient is dangerously hyperthermic or if the fever is especially symptomatic.

TIPS TO REMEMBER

- The etiology of postoperative fever is often related to the specific postoperative day on which the fever occurs:
  - POD 0 to 1: atelectasis:
    - Less common causes include malignant hyperthermia and severe necrotizing wound infections.

- POD 3: UTI, pneumonia, or anastomotic leak
- POD 5: Deep venous thrombosis
- POD 7 to 10: Intra-abdominal abscess

● Basic initial workup of postoperative fever should include a CBC with differential, 2 sets of blood cultures, a urinalysis, and a chest x-ray. Additional studies such as CXR, sputum sample, venous duplex studies, or CT scan may be necessary in certain circumstances.

● Acetaminophen (Tylenol) can be used to symptomatically treat fever. Downsides include suppression of the adaptive and normal physiologic response to infection, an inability to accurately follow a patient's fever curve, and the possibility of hepatotoxicity.

COMPREHENSION QUESTIONS

1. A 25-year-old female experiences a fever of 101.6°F on postoperative day 1 after a laparoscopic cholecystectomy. On evaluation, she looks and feels quite well. The most likely cause of her fever is which of the following?
      A. Deep venous thrombosis
      B. Urinary tract infection
      C. Atelectasis

2. All of the following are appropriate *immediate* first steps in the workup of a postoperative fever except which one?
      A. Blood cultures
      B. Abdominal CT scan
      C. Urinalysis
      D. Removal of the primary dressing

Answers

1. **C.** A fever on postoperative day 1 is most likely the result of atelectasis. This is even more likely in a patient who has undergone an operation that will result in diaphragmatic irritation and subsequent shallow breathing.

2. **B.** In most cases, the initial reflexive workup for a postoperative fever should include removal of the patient's dressing to inspect the wound, 2 sets of blood cultures, and a urinalysis. Additional studies such as an abdominal CT should be obtained after discussion with a more senior member of the surgical team.

A 42-year-old Woman 4 Hours Postoperative With a Fever and Extreme Pain

Michael W. Wandling, MD
and Mamta Swaroop, MD, FACS

You arrive at the bedside of a 42-year-old woman to perform a postoperative check four hours after she underwent a gastric bypass operation. Before you enter the room you note that she currently has a temperature of 102.3°F. She tells you her abdominal incision is excruciatingly painful, and on exam you are surprised by the unusual degree of tenderness in the region under and around her dressing.

1. What is your next step?

NECROTIZING SOFT TISSUE INFECTION

Answer

1. You should remove the dressing and examine the wound for any signs of necrotizing fasciitis.

   The term necrotizing fasciitis was coined in 1951 to describe all gas-forming and non–gas-forming necrotizing infections, both of which shared the common feature of fascial necrosis. Recently, the term necrotizing soft tissue infection (NSTI) has replaced the older terminology, as this encompasses all infections regardless of the depth of tissue involved.

   Patients who are most at risk for NSTIs include individuals with diabetes mellitus, obesity, peripheral vascular disease, chronic kidney disease, and alcohol abuse. NSTIs present with pain out of proportion to the physical exam, anxiety, and diaphoresis within 48 hours of bacterial inoculation in a wound. Other classic findings include erythema, pain or tenderness beyond the margins of erythema, woody edema, crepitus, bronzing of the skin, grayish, or "dishwater" discharge from the wound, skin necrosis, bullae formation, induration, fluctuance, fever, and hypotension. For examples of these skin findings, see Figure 45-1. Unfortunately, many of these distinctive features are late findings that are indicative of severe, life-threatening infection. You should therefore have a high index of suspicion for this type of infection, especially in a patient who has an otherwise unexplained fever in the acute postoperative period. In those cases it is incumbent on you to take down the dressing and, using sterile technique, examine the wound and surrounding skin.

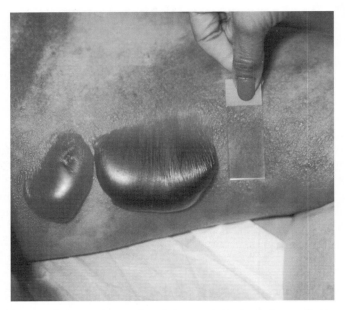

Figure 45-1. Images of several examples of characteristic physical exam findings of NSTI. Variations in the appearance of bullae overlying NSTIs. (Reproduced with permission from Knoop K, Stack L, Storrow A, et al. *Atlas of Emergency Medicine.* 3rd ed. New York: McGraw-Hill Education; 2010. Figure 12.8. Photo contributed by Lawrence B. Stack, MD.)

Diagnosis

One of the hallmarks of NSTIs is a rapid progression of symptoms that can lead to death within hours. Delays in diagnosis and debridement are associated with a nine times greater mortality rate. It should be clear that any consult for a potential NSTI must be seen quickly, taken seriously, and be escalated to more senior residents or attendings should any suspicion of NSTI exist.

When evaluating a patient for an NSTI, it is essential to remember that the more dramatic physical exam findings associated with NSTIs are often not seen at the time of presentation, which can make differentiating them from non-necrotizing infections difficult. Edema and erythema are almost always present, but are very nonspecific. You should at a minimum mark out the boundaries of the erythema in order to characterize the rate of spread of the infection.

While the physical exam can be nonspecific or even misleading, there are other features characteristic of NSTIs that can aid in making an early and potentially life-saving diagnosis. A basic set of labs can be key and should not be overlooked. A white blood cell count of >15,400 cells/mm^3 or a sodium level <135 mmol/L on admission to the hospital has an 80% positive predictive value and, if not present, an 80% negative predictive value, respectively, for NSTI.

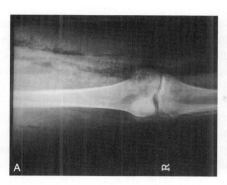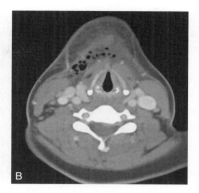

Figure 45-2. Radiographic evidence of necrotizing soft tissue infections. (**A**) Plain radiograph that demonstrates gas in the soft tissue of the right lower extremity. (Courtesy of Susan Dufel, MD.) (**B**) CT scan demonstrating gas within the soft tissue of the neck as well as fat stranding that crosses fascial planes. (Reproduced, with permission, from Tintinalli JE, Stapczynski JS, Ma OJ, et al. *Tintinalli's Emergency Medicine.* 7th ed. New York: McGraw-Hill; 2011. Figure 241-5.)

Imaging studies may be useful but only in those instances where the patient is not decompensating and the diagnosis remains equivocal. Plain radiographs may show gas within soft tissues, although this is only present in one third of patients and a negative study cannot rule out NSTI. There are some data that suggest CT scans, with or without contrast, may be helpful in identifying characteristic features of NSTIs such as soft tissue gas and inflammatory changes. Although CT scans may have a role in diagnosing NSTIs, this has not yet been adequately studied. MRI has been shown to have a sensitivity of 90% to 100% in diagnosing NSTIs, but a specificity of only 50% to 80%. Because MRIs take such a considerable amount of time to obtain, the risks associated with delaying treatment drastically limit the utility of MRI in the evaluation of NSTIs. For examples of imaging studies that demonstrate NSTIs, see Figure 45-2.

The gold standard in the diagnosis of NSTI is operative exploration. Operative findings consistent with necrotizing infection include tissue necrosis, lack of bleeding, foul-smelling discharge, and loss of normal fascial resistance to finger dissection. When there is any level of concern for NSTI and especially if a patient is showing signs of rapid clinical deterioration, the patient should be emergently taken to the operating room for exploration. The consequences of not doing so are far more severe than those associated with a negative exploration.

Treatment

The treatment of NSTIs is based on four key principles: (1) immediate surgical debridement; (2) fluid resuscitation and correction of electrolyte and acid–base abnormalities; (3) antimicrobial therapy; and (4) support of failing organ systems.

Early surgical debridement, as previously discussed, is the mainstay of treatment and has been shown to increase survival. Fluid resuscitation with crystalloids is necessary, as nearly all patients with NSTIs have intravascular volume depletion. Lactated Ringer's solution is the crystalloid of choice since it is common for these patients to be acidotic. Electrolyte abnormalities should be corrected in the usual fashion. Antimicrobial therapy should be started immediately in cases of NSTI. Although they do not penetrate necrotic tissue and thus are not curative, they do decrease the systemic symptoms of infection and are an important adjuvant therapy. Given the rapid progression and extremely high morbidity and mortality associated with NSTIs, initial antibiotic coverage should be broad until culture results are available. Clindamycin should also be included in the initial antibiotic regimen, as it decreases the toxin production by *Staphylococcus aureus*, hemolytic *Streptococcus*, and *Clostridium* infections. Lastly, providing support for failing organ systems is essential in the ICU setting.

In summary, if you have any suspicion that a wound infection might be an NSTI, you should examine the wound closely, removing the original operative dressing if necessary. If you remain concerned about an NSTI, you must immediately notify your senior resident or attending in order to expedite the diagnostic workup and/or the possible emergency operation. While you wait for the resident or attending to call you back, you should start IV fluids and a broad-spectrum empiric antibiotic regimen that includes clindamycin.

TIPS TO REMEMBER

- NSTIs can widely vary in presentation. Concerning findings include pain out of proportion to the exam, diaphoresis, woody edema, crepitus, bronzing of skin, dishwater discharge, skin necrosis, bullae formation, unexplained fever, and hypotension.

- A white blood cell count of >15,400 cells/mm^3 or a sodium level <135 mmol/L on admission to the hospital has an 80% positive predictive value and, if not present, an 80% negative predictive value in individuals with NSTI.

- Early operative debridement is the mainstay of NSTI management and is associated with decreased mortality rates.

- If there is any suspicion of NSTI, it is imperative to notify senior members of the surgical team immediately.

COMPREHENSION QUESTIONS

1. You are performing a postoperative check on a trauma patient who just underwent an exploratory laparotomy after a motorcycle crash. He tells you that he is having severe pain in his right leg, where there was a "road rash" that was previously cleaned and dressed. You remove the bandage on his thigh and discover that

the previously minor wound now has 2 to 3 cm of surrounding erythema. On palpation, you notice he has extreme tenderness beyond the margins of the erythema and you notice some crepitus. You suspect NSTI. What should be your next step?

    A. Send a BMP to check his serum sodium level.

    B. Wake up your senior resident and inform her of your findings.

    C. Come back and reevaluate the wound in 2 to 3 hours.

    D. Culture the wound.

    E. Order a stat MRI of the right lower extremity.

2. Which of the following are key principles in the management of NSTIs?

    A. Immediate surgical debridement

    B. Supporting failing organ systems

    C. Fluid resuscitation

    D. Correction of electrolyte and acid–base abnormalities

    E. Antimicrobial therapy

    F. A, C, E

    G. All of the above

Answers

1. **B.** Any time that an NSTI is suspected, it is essential to notify senior members of the surgical team immediately. NSTIs are surgical emergencies and should be approached with the same level of urgency as a trauma or an acute abdomen. Cultures would not be immediately useful in this case, as NSTI is a clinical diagnosis that must be debrided before cultures would have time to come back. Although MRI can aid in the diagnosis of NSTIs, it is time consuming and is not justified—a negative operative exploration is perfectly acceptable in this case.

2. **G.** All of these options are key principles in managing NSTIs.

A 35-year-old Man With Crohn Disease Who Needs Postoperative Orders

Roy Phitayakorn, MD, MHPE (MEd)

You are taking care of a 35-year-old man with Crohn's disease. His symptoms were somewhat controlled with 30 mg of oral prednisone daily, but he developed a chronic, long-segment ileal stricture that required an open ileocolectomy with primary anastomosis. You are writing his postoperative orders.

1. **What is the mechanism of acute adrenal insufficiency?**
2. **Should you have given him a "stress" dosage of steroids at the start of the case? Why or why not?**
3. **How do you determine how much steroids to give for stress dosages?**
4. **How much steroid should he have postoperatively and how fast can you taper this stress dose?**
5. **Are there any risks to using steroids perioperatively?**

PERIOPERATIVE CORTICOSTEROIDS

Answers

1. In patients who are glucocorticosteroid dependent, insufficient amounts of corticosteroids or cortisol resistance during critical illness may lead to secondary adrenal insufficiency with eventual hypotension, shock, and death. The pathophysiological mechanism for this hypotension cascade is not entirely clear, but is likely due to enhanced prostacyclin production and its subsequent vasodilatory effects leading to hypotension and shock.

2. As a general rule of thumb, any patient who has received at least 20 mg of prednisone or its glucocorticoid equivalent (see Table 46-1) for greater than 5 days is at risk for hypothalamus–pituitary–adrenal (HPA) axis suppression. Inhaled glucocorticoids may or may not cause HPA suppression. Patients who are on lower dosages of glucocorticoids may require at least a month to develop HPA suppression. Following tapering of glucocorticoid therapy, it may take patients a year or longer to resume normal HPA axis responses with pituitary function being the first to normalize. If you are uncertain and time permits, these patients are often referred to an endocrinologist for an ACTH stimulation test to see if they secrete normal amounts of cortisol in response to ACTH.

   Because this patient was chronically on 30 mg of prednisone, he should receive stress dose steroids postoperatively.

3. Although the actual incidence of adrenal insufficiency due to lack of exogenous glucocorticoids is likely low, it is a highly preventable cause of morbidity/mortality.

Table 46-1. Equivalent Dosages of Glucocorticosteroids

Hydrocortisone	20 mg
Prednisone	5 mg
Prednisolone	5 mg
Methylprednisolone	4 mg
Dexamethasone	0.75 mg

The risk of secondary adrenal insufficiency in glucocorticoid-dependent patients is directly related to the duration and severity of the surgical procedure. Relatively minor procedures that are less than 1 hour long or can be done under local anesthetic have a low degree of physiological stress. A dose of hydrocortisone of 25 mg or its equivalent is a sufficient "stress dosage" for minor procedures. For moderate-stress procedures such as peripheral bypass surgery or a straightforward small bowel resection and anastomosis a dose of 50 to 100 mg of hydrocortisone should be given intravenously prior to or at the time of skin incision. Finally, for high-stress procedures such as a total proctocolectomy or cardiac bypass procedure, a stress dose of 100 mg of hydrocortisone should be given at the start of the procedure.

4. For minor procedures, the patient should take his or her normal dosage of steroids the morning of surgery and then resume the normal home dosage postoperatively. For moderate-stress procedures, patients should receive 25 mg of hydrocortisone intravenously every 8 hours for 24 hours and then rapidly taper to the home dosage. For high-stress procedures, patients should receive around 50 mg of hydrocortisone intravenously every 8 hours after the initial stress dose for the first 2 to 3 days after surgery and then taper dosage by half each day until you reach the home dosage.

5. Patients who receive steroids perioperatievly are at increased risk for delayed wound healing (increased friability of the skin and vessels), infectious complications (anastomotic leak, abscess, superficial surgical site infections, etc), and gastrointestinal hemorrhage (an antacid protocol is a customary adjunct) with resulting increased length of hospitalization and need for readmission. Also, there is a normal leukocytosis with steroid administration, which may disguise normal markers of infection (fever, tachycardia, abdominal pain, etc). Finally, it is important to remember that hydrocortisone has mineralocorticoid activity at dosages above 100 mg, which can lead to unwanted fluid retention/edema and hypokalemia. Therefore, if large dosages of hydrocortisone are required beyond the initial stress dose, it is wise to use methylprednisolone as it lacks any mineralocorticoid activity.

TIPS TO REMEMBER

- Any patient who has been on 20 mg or more of prednisone (or its corticosteroid equivalent) for 5 or more days should be considered to receive "stress dose" steroids prior to any procedure more complicated than an in-office "minor" procedure.

- These stress dose steroids can cause significant postoperative complications and should be weaned to chronic dosage levels within 48 hours post surgery.

COMPREHENSION QUESTIONS

1. Which patient is most *un*likely to have perioperative acute adrenal insufficiency?
   - A. A 40-year-old woman taking 5 mg of prednisone daily for the last year for her rheumatoid arthritis
   - B. A 20-year-old man taking 20 mg of prednisone daily for the last 2 weeks for a recent Crohn's flare
   - C. A 55-year-old woman who has received 40 mg of prednisone daily for the last 3 months to control her recently diagnosed autoimmune hepatitis
   - D. A 67-year-old man taking high-dose inhaled corticosteroids for his COPD

2. Which of the following is the correct "stress dosage" of hydrocortisone intravenously for a patient undergoing a right hemicolectomy (to be given just prior to surgery)?
   - A. 5 mg of hydrocortisone
   - B. 25 mg of hydrocortisone
   - C. 100 mg of hydrocortisone
   - D. 200 mg of hydrocortisone

3. How long should "stress dose" steroid levels be given postoperatively?
   - A. Less than 3 days
   - B. For 5 days postoperatively
   - C. For 10 days postoperatively
   - D. Until the patient has completely healed his or her surgical wounds

4. A patient is POD #1 from a CABG and is receiving 50 mg of hydrocortisone every 8 hours. The patient is at risk for all of the following complications secondary to the hydrocortisone *except*?
   - A. Hypothyroidism
   - B. Hypokalemia
   - C. Sternal wound infection
   - D. Leukocytosis

Answers

1. **A**. Patients taking less than 20 mg of prednisone daily (or its corticosteroid equivalent) are unlikely to develop perioperative acute adrenal insufficiency.

2. **C**. A right hemicolectomy would be considered a "moderate-stress" procedure, so 100 mg of hydrocortisone is more than an adequate stress dosage.

3. **A**. Stress dosage levels can be rapidly titrated down to home corticosteroid dosage levels within 48 hours postoperatively.

4. **A**. Hypothyroidism is not a recognized complication of hydrocortisone therapy.

A 65-year-old Man With Diabetes Needing Postoperative Orders

Roy Phitayakorn, MD, MHPE (MEd)

You are taking care of a 65-year-old man with Type 1 diabetes, which is well controlled using an insulin pump. Unfortunately, he was recently admitted with his second attack of diverticulitis and is now on your service for an elective sigmoidectomy. His surgery is uncomplicated, but now you have to write his postoperative orders.

1. **Is glycemic control really that important for patients after surgery? Why or why not?**

2. **What types of insulin does a surgical patient require?**

3. **How would you handle the insulin requirements of this Type 1 diabetic?**

4. **What if the patient is a Type 2 diabetic who uses insulin at home?**

5. **What if the patient is a Type 2 diabetic who is non–insulin dependent at home, but now requires insulin as an inpatient to maintain proper glycemic control?**

PERIOPERATIVE INSULIN

Answers

1. Diabetes is very common in hospitalized patients and inpatient hyperglycemia has been associated with an increase in overall infection rate, morbidity, mortality, and length of stay in surgical patients. These complications are probably because hyperglycemia triggers phagocyte and endothelial cell dysfunction, as well as increased vascular inflammation, platelet activation, and oxidative stress. Exogenous insulin administration not only decreases blood glucose levels but may also have a direct anti-inflammatory effect on vascular endothelial cells. However, overaggressive glycemic management can lead to hypoglycemia with possible coma, neurological injury, and death. In short, while hypoglycemia is more dangerous than hyperglycemia, both are bad. Therefore, it is essential that you understand how to properly manage perioperative insulin dosages.

2. In broad terms, the easiest way to think about insulin requirements is the concept that inpatients require a basal or baseline amount of insulin and then a prandial or nutritional requirement (see Figure 47-1). The baseline amount is the quantity of insulin that patients need to avoid unchecked gluconeogenesis and ketogenesis. The prandial amount is the quantity of insulin needed to cover meals, dextrose in intravenous fluids, enteral feeds, and/or TPN. If the patient is eating, then ideally the prandial amount is given as a correction-dose therapy

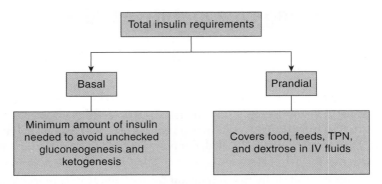

Figure 47-1. Components of total insulin requirements.

before or between meals. Sliding insulin scales are substandard for this purpose since the dosage of insulin is given without regard to meals and after hyperglycemia has already occurred. If the patient is NPO and on a continuous infusion of intravenous fluids that contain dextrose, then sliding insulin scales may be sufficient to cover nutritional insulin requirements, although they should be adjusted daily until optimal glycemic control is achieved.

3. By definition, these patients are insulin deficient and therefore require a constant basal supply of insulin to avoid entering diabetic ketoacidosis. Adult Type 1 diabetics are frequently very familiar with how much insulin their bodies require and are very comfortable recognizing sensations of hyperglycemia or hypoglycemia. Often these patients will be able to subcutaneously administer insulin to themselves via an insulin pump that lets them control the precise dosage of insulin administered to their bodies. In my experience, it is best to work/ negotiate with these patients and let them control their own insulin delivery. If they are eating, these patients should be on a long-acting insulin (such as NPH or lente) that they administer in the morning or evenings. In addition, a bolus of short-acting insulin (such as lispro or aspart) is given before or after eating to cover carbohydrates that will be or were consumed. If Type 1 diabetics are not eating, it is essential that they still receive their basal insulin requirements! For many patients, the basal insulin requirement will not change even when they are NPO. If you are unsure or the patient is particularly brittle, you can start at half of the basal insulin requirement and increase accordingly. Fluctuations in blood glucose levels secondary to dextrose in intravenous fluids or TPN should be covered by a sliding insulin scale. Note that patients who had a recent pancreatectomy or who have severe pancreatic dysfunction may now be considered Type 1 diabetics.

4. Unlike Type 1 diabetics, these patients have a problem with insulin resistance. Initially, Type 2 diabetics have high levels of basal insulin secretion, but may

need additional prandial insulin to defeat this resistance. When eating, these patients should be on all of their insulin sensitizers and secretagogues (such as metformin, sulfonylureas, glitazones, exendin-4, etc) in addition to their basal and nutritional insulin requirements to maintain glucose levels less than 180 mg/dL. Over time, these patients may lose some of their insulin production capacity and therefore require supplemental basal insulin as well. Interestingly, the glycemic profile of Type 2 diabetics is frequently diet related and their total insulin needs typically decrease when they are NPO even without their normal oral diabetes agents. Therefore, Type 2 diabetics who are NPO may only require a correction dosage or sliding-scale coverage. However, it is important to remember that these patients still have insulin resistance so their overall insulin requirements may still be quite high.

5. Often, these patients were precariously close to requiring insulin at home, but either did not have regular glucose checks or the stress of surgery has pushed them into requiring insulin. Patients may also receive postoperative corticosteroids that can exacerbate preexisting poor glycemic control. Starting de novo insulin treatments may seem daunting to new resident physicians, but is actually quite straightforward.

First, check a HbA1C to get a rough idea of preoperative glycemic control and then multiply the body weight in kilograms by 0.4 U of insulin (0.3 if very elderly, 0.5 if morbidly obese) to get a total daily insulin requirement. Give half of the daily requirement as glargine at night or in divided NPH dosages every 12 hours. If the patient is able to eat, give the other half as short-acting insulin divided into 3 equal correctional dosages shortly before meals. The patient should also be restarted on his or her oral diabetic agents. The patient's nurse should be asked to record the patient's blood glucose levels prior to giving all insulin injections. A glucose reading ≤70 mg/dL indicates that the patient is receiving too much insulin and the dosages should be adjusted accordingly. Patients should be appropriately counseled that it is unlikely they will go home on insulin, but may require insulin therapy in the future if their diabetes worsens. If the patient will be NPO for long periods of time and therefore requires TPN or PPN, insulin should be calculated based on your institution's protocols and included directly with the TPN. Any exogenous basal or prandial insulin should be used with caution in patients on TPN/PPN as these infusions are frequently disrupted and the patient could become quickly hypoglycemic.

TIPS TO REMEMBER

- Surgical patients require good glycemic control to avoid many types of postoperative complications.
- A useful framework to think about insulin replacement therapy is that each patient needs both basal and prandial insulin. Basal therapy consists of

long-acting insulins given in the morning, nighttime, or both. Ideally, prandial therapy should be given before or between meals.

● Sliding-scale insulin coverage is a substandard, reactive form of prandial therapy, but may be sufficient in surgical patients who are NPO.

COMPREHENSION QUESTIONS

1. Prolonged hyperglycemia in diabetic patients has been associated with all of the following *except*?
    A. Phagocyte dysfunction
    B. Endothelial cell dysfunction
    C. Platelet activation
    D. Vascular inflammation
    E. Increased catecholamine production

2. You are going to start insulin therapy on a 55-year-old man with Type 2 diabetes who weighs 200 kg. What are his estimated total daily insulin needs?
    A. 40 U of insulin
    B. 60 U of insulin
    C. 80 U of insulin
    D. 100 U of insulin
    E. 120 U of insulin

3. Which of the following complications will most likely occur if you do not give an insulin-dependent diabetic (Type 1) his or her basal amounts of insulin?
    A. Diabetic ketoacidosis
    B. Stroke
    C. Myocardial infarction
    D. Wound infection
    E. Pulmonary insufficiency

Answers

1. **E.** Increased catecholamine production has not been linked to prolonged hyperglycemia in diabetic patients.

2. **C.** His estimated total daily insulin requirement is approximately 0.4 U/kg × 200 kg = 80 U of insulin.

3. **A.** Lack of insulin in Type 1 diabetics leads to ketoacidosis that features ketonemia, hyperglycemia, and an anion gap metabolic acidosis. This condition can be fatal if not recognized early.

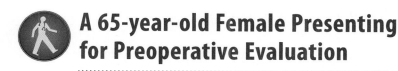

A 65-year-old Female Presenting for Preoperative Evaluation

Jahan Mohebali, MD

A 65-year-old female with a PMH notable for paroxysmal atrial fibrillation and recent coronary stent placement presents to your office for preoperative evaluation for repair of a ventral hernia. She has had the hernia for many years; however, it has recently begun to cause some occasional discomfort after she stands for prolonged periods of time. The hernia has always been easily reducible, and she has had no previous episodes of bowel obstruction related to it. With regard to her cardiovascular history, in addition to the paroxysmal a-fib, she reports poorly controlled hypertension, diabetes, and a transient ischemic attack a few years ago. Since that time, she has been taking warfarin. One month ago she underwent cardiac stress testing that demonstrated ST changes in the inferior leads resulting in cardiac catheterization and deployment of a drug-eluting stent. An echocardiogram demonstrated an ejection fraction of 35%. Plavix was added to her medical regimen and she has been doing quite well since that time. She denies any ongoing chest pain or dyspnea on exertion.

1. Should this patient's hernia repair be delayed?
2. If the patient undergoes an elective hernia repair 12 months later, should Plavix and warfarin be held?
3. How many days before an operation should antiplatelet medication be held?
4. If the decision is made to stop the patient's warfarin, how many days prior to the operation should it be held?
5. What is the patient's CHADS2 score, and what score typically suggests that a patient should receive bridging therapy with heparin?
6. On what postoperative day should you restart her antiplatelet and anticoagulation medications?

PERIOPERATIVE ANTICOAGULATION AND ANTIPLATELET DRUGS

Perioperative management of anticoagulation and antiplatelet drugs can often be overwhelming for the junior resident since improper decision making can have serious consequences. Moreover, this area of perioperative medicine has been involved in the highest number of litigation events. These facts are only stated to emphasize that a multidisciplinary approach should be encouraged in dealing with perioperative anticoagulation. Typically, the decision should at a minimum include the patient, the surgeon, and the patient's primary care physician or cardiologist. That being said, there is no reason for this subject to cause intimidation as there is an algorithmic and methodical way to go about dealing with it.

The first question that should always be considered is whether or not the procedure is elective or emergent, and if elective, whether the procedure should be delayed. Regardless of whether or not anticoagulants will be held, the timing of an operation can have a significant impact on the risk of postoperative thrombotic complications. For example, patients who have experienced venous thromboembolism are at the highest risk for recurrence within the first three months. Likewise, patients who have experienced an arterial embolic event from a cardiac source have a risk of recurrence of 0.5% per day in the first month. Finally, in the case of antiplatelet agents that were started for coronary stent placement, it is recommended that these medications be continued through the perioperative period if the stent was placed less than six weeks prior for bare metal stents, or less than 12 months prior for drug-eluting stents. Stopping antiplatelet agents within these windows may otherwise lead to a devastating stent thrombosis. Given these considerations, sometimes the best option is to simply delay an elective operation.

Answers

1. The patient underwent coronary stent placement one month ago. Because of this, the American College of Cardiology and the American Heart Association guidelines recommend that her antiplatelet therapy not be discontinued for a minimum of six weeks in the case of a bare metal stent, and a minimum of 12 months for a drug-eluting stent. In general, patients who undergo placement of a drug-eluting stent will be started on two antiplatelet agents. (This patient was only started on Plavix because she was already taking warfarin.) Current guidelines advise continuing both agents for a minimum of 12 months. In very rare cases, it is reasonable to stop one of the agents; however, aspirin should typically be continued. The exact guidelines continue to evolve and some studies now suggest that antiplatelet agents may be stopped as early as six months following drug-eluting stent placement. Operating on this patient within the 12-month window would mean continuing her Plavix and subsequently, significantly increasing her bleeding risk. Although her hernia has become mildly symptomatic, there is no evidence of strangulation, incarceration, or previous obstruction to suggest that she meets criteria for an emergent repair. Her operation should therefore be delayed until antiplatelet therapy can be safely held in the perioperative period to avoid the risk of bleeding and catastrophic coronary stent thrombosis. Because of the complex and evolving nature of guidelines related to the use of antiplatelet agents in patients with coronary stents, consultation with a cardiologist is always recommended. This will also serve the medicolegal purpose of protecting the surgeon, should an adverse event related to the stent occur.

2. The next question in the algorithm is to determine whether or not the patient's anticoagulation needs to be held for the surgical procedure being considered.

A consideration of all surgical procedures is beyond the scope of this chapter; however, for the average junior surgical resident, the literature suggests that minor dermatologic excisions and many GI endoscopic procedures can be performed without holding warfarin. In the case of dermatologic excisions such as the removal of actinic keratoses, basal and squamous cell cancers, and premalignant or cancerous nevi, the literature suggests a three-fold increase in bleeding risk if the procedure is performed while the patient is on warfarin. However, most bleeds were self-limiting. It is important to note that in the case of GI procedures, the addition of a biopsy or sphincterotomy generally requires correction of coagulopathy prior to the procedure. Any other major surgical procedure is likely to require that warfarin or antiplatelet medications be temporarily held. Therefore, once the patient in the above case is ready to undergo an elective hernia repair, both her Plavix and her warfarin will need to be held.

3. In order to determine the timing of antiplatelet therapy cessation prior to an operation, the mechanism of action of the medication must be considered. While NSAIDs *reversibly* inhibit cyclooxygenase, aspirin *irreversibly* inhibits the enzyme. As a result, the effect of aspirin does not wear off until new platelets are synthesized, a process that takes approximately 7 to 10 days. Therefore, aspirin should be held 7 to 10 days prior to an operation, assuming there is no contraindication. Thienopyridines such as Plavix work by inhibiting ADP-mediated platelet aggregation. Some are short-acting and may be discontinued 24 hours before surgery, but in the case of Plavix, which is long-acting, the medication should be held for 7 days prior.

4. Again, determining the timing of medication cessation is based on the mechanism of action of the specific medication and the associated pharmacokinetics. Warfarin works by inhibiting vitamin K–dependent carboxylation of factors II, VII, IX, and X. Therefore, in order for the effects of the medication to wear off, new coagulation factors have to be synthesized. The literature suggests that, in general, warfarin should be held five days prior to surgery. This number comes from a series of studies demonstrating an average preoperative INR of 1.2 after warfarin was held for five days, and from the fact that five days is approximately two half-lives of factor II—enough time for the levels to become adequate for proper hemostasis.

To summarize, the steps in the algorithm so far have been to first ask if the patient's operation should be delayed for any reason such as venous thromboembolism within the last three months, coronary stent placement in the last six weeks or 12 months depending on the type of stent, and whether there has been an episode of arterial thromboembolism in the last month. Assuming there is no contraindication to proceeding with surgery, the next step is to determine whether there is even a need to hold anticoagulation—this might be true if, for example, the patient is undergoing a procedure at low risk of significant bleeding. If anticoagulation (ie, warfarin) is going to be held, we arrive at the next point in the decision tree: should bridging therapy be used?

5. The decision of whether or not to bridge the patient ultimately depends on the bleeding risk balanced against the risk of arterial and venous thromboembolism. The risk of thromboembolism varies based on the severity of the underlying disease, and can be classified as high, moderate, or low. The criteria used to classify the most common reasons for anticoagulation—mechanical heart valve, atrial fibrillation, and venous thrombosis—are listed below.

For patients with a mechanical heart valve:

High-risk patients include those with any type of mechanical valve in the mitral position, anyone with an older model of mechanical valve in the aortic position (ie, ball and cage valve), or anyone with a stroke or TIA related to the valve in the past six months.

Moderate-risk patients include those with bicuspid aortic valves plus one of the following: atrial fibrillation, prior stroke or TIA, hypertension, diabetes, heart failure, or patients who are older than 75.

Low-risk patients are those with bileaflet aortic valves without atrial fibrillation and no other risk factors for stroke.

For patients with atrial fibrillation (AF), the risk is based on the CHADS2 score that is calculated in Table 48-1.

High-risk patients with AF include those with a CHADS2 score of 5 or 6, a recent stroke or TIA within the last three months, or those with rheumatic valvular heart disease.

Moderate-risk patients include those with a CHADS2 score of 3 or 4.

Low-risk patients include those with a CHADS2 score of 0 to 2.

For patients with previous venous thromboembolism:

High-risk patients are those with a recent venous thromboembolism within the last three months, or those with a severe thrombophilia.

Table 48-1. Calculation of CHADS2 Score

	Condition	Points
C	Congestive heart failure	1
H	Consistent hypertension, or use of antihypertensive medication	1
A	Age ≥75 years	1
D	Diabetes	1
S2	Prior stroke or TIA	2

Moderate-risk patients include those with a venous thromboembolism within the last 3 to 12 months, those with recurrent venous thromboembolism, those with active cancer, or those with a nonsevere thrombophilic condition such as factor V Leiden deficiency.

Low-risk patients include those with a single venous thromboembolism within the past year, and no other risk factors.

In most cases, patients at high risk should undergo bridging therapy with intravenous unfractionated heparin (IVUH) or low-molecular-weight heparin (LMWH). Patients at moderate risk may or may not need bridging depending on their individual circumstances, and patients at low risk may not require bridging at all. It is important to emphasize that the patient should be included in the discussion about whether or not to bridge as many patients are more concerned about the possibility of a stroke than a bleeding event. This is a reasonable concern given that recurrent venous thromboembolism is fatal in 5% to 10% of cases and that arterial thromboembolism is fatal in 20% of cases. In cases where arterial thromboembolism is not fatal, it causes permanent disability at least 50% of the time. This is in contrast to major bleeding events that, while fatal 9% to 13% of the time, rarely cause permanent disability.

Our patient in the case above has diabetes, hypertension, CHF, and a history of a TIA a few years ago. Therefore, her CHADS2 score is 5 placing her at high risk for an event. She should therefore undergo bridging therapy at the time of hernia repair.

In general, bridging therapy should be started approximately 36 hours after the last dose of warfarin. The time at which bridging therapy should stop is based on the half-life of the medication used for bridging, generally five elimination half-lives prior to the procedure. The half-life of LMWH is approximately five hours, and if it is dosed BID, the last dose should be given 24 hours before surgery. If LMWH is dosed once daily, then the dose given 24 hours prior to surgery should be 50% of the therapeutic dose. The half-life of IVUH is approximately 45 minutes and, therefore, unfractionated heparin should generally be held four hours prior to a procedure.

6. No clinical data support a definitive regimen for when to resume bridging, antiplatelet, or anticoagulation therapy in the postoperative period. As a result, the timing is, in practice, highly variable. The lack of clear recommendations does not diminish the importance of these decisions, as bleeding is more than a theoretical risk—for example, evidence suggests that there is a 5- to 6-fold increased rate of major bleeding in patients who receive full (ie, therapeutic) dose LMWH or IVUH in the immediate postoperative period. As a general guide, one should wait approximately 24 hours, and perhaps 48 to 72 hours if there is concern for major bleeding. These time frames are based on the physiology of hemostasis and the time required for the platelet plug to form and stabilize.

While antiplatelet medications and bridging anticoagulation therapy have a rapid onset of action, warfarin typically requires more time to deplete the vitamin K–dependent clotting factors. For this reason there are some circumstances in which the first postoperative dose can be given on the evening after surgery, or on the morning of postoperative day 1. If bridging is employed, IVUH or LMWH should be continued until the target INR is achieved.

The timing of restarting antiplatelet therapy is more variable and the decision should be a multidisciplinary one involving the patient's cardiologist or antiplatelet medication prescriber. More broadly, any decisions with regard to the resumption of antiplatelet or anticoagulation medications should obviously involve discussion with the primary surgeon.

TIPS TO REMEMBER

- Elective cases should be delayed in the following situations:
  - VTE within the last 3 months
  - Bare metal stent placement within the last 6 weeks
  - Drug-eluting stent placement within the last year
  - Stroke or TIA in the past month in the setting of AF or a mechanical valve
- The decision to bridge begins by categorizing the patient into high-, moderate-, or low-risk groups for a thromboembolic event. Patients in the high or moderate groups should generally receive bridging therapy.
- The ultimate decision of whether or not to bridge should include a discussion between the surgeon, patient, and the patient's cardiologist, hematologist, and/or primary care physician.
- In general, warfarin should be held 5 days prior to the operation.
- When bridging is employed, it should be started 3 days prior to the operation.
- IVUH should be held for a minimum of 4 hours before the case. If a patient is receiving twice-daily LMWH for bridging, the last dose should be given 24 hours prior to surgery. If daily dosing is used, then the last dose should be given 24 hours prior to surgery at 50% of the regular dose.
- Bridging should generally be resumed within 24 to 72 hours post surgery, after there is evidence of adequate hemostasis.
- Warfarin can generally be resumed on postoperative day 1 as it will not have an effect for a few days.
- In general, Plavix should be held 5 to 7 days prior to surgery.

COMPREHENSION QUESTIONS

1. A 75-year-old female with factor V Leiden deficiency and atrial fibrillation presents to your clinic after she was referred for a cholecystectomy by her PCP. Further questioning reveals that she also has poorly controlled hypertension and

diabetes. She has been on warfarin for many years. With regard to her hypercoagulability, she states that she developed a left ileofemoral DVT two months ago. Which of the following facts in the patient's history suggests that her elective cholecystectomy should be delayed?

A. Her poorly controlled hypertension
B. Her CHADS2 score of 2
C. Her recent DVT
D. Her factor V Leiden deficiency

2. A 42-year-old female with a past medical history of endocarditis requiring placement of a mechanical bileaflet aortic valve, currently anticoagulated with warfarin, is scheduled to undergo a small bowel resection for a gastrointestinal stromal tumor. This will require holding her anticoagulation for approximately 24 hours. She is otherwise healthy and has no other comorbidities. Should she receive bridging therapy?

A. Yes, because her valve is in the aortic position and she is at high risk for a stroke.
B. No, because her valve is in the aortic position and therefore there is a decreased risk of thrombus formation.
C. Yes, because any mechanical heart valve requires bridging.
D. No, because mechanical valves do not require bridging.

Answers

1. **C**. The risk of recurrent DVT is highest within the first three months. This patient's operation is elective and should therefore be postponed. The other risk factors will not improve with time, and therefore these are not indications for delay.

2. **B**. Any mechanical valve in the mitral position requires bridging because of slower flow rates and stasis around the valve. Aortic valves only require bridging if the valve is an older model (ie, ball and cage type), or if the patient has other comorbidities such as hypertension, CHF, or diabetes.

A 33-year-old Woman Who Needs Postoperative Orders for DVT Prophylaxis

Brian C. George, MD and Alden H. Harken, MD

Ms. Wang is a 33-year-old female who just underwent a left mastectomy. As the attending is leaving the room she stops to ask if you know how to write "the normal postoperative orders for DVT prophylaxis."

1. Why is DVT prophylaxis indicated in this patient?

2. What kind of DVT prophylaxis would you write for?

3. When using pharmacologic DVT prophylaxis, should you use heparin or low-molecular-weight heparin and why?

DVT PROPHYLAXIS

Deep venous thrombosis is frighteningly prevalent, especially in some pelvic and oncological surgical subgroups—approaching 50% of patients in some studies. While the data are less robust, an NIH consensus development panel has established the logical link between DVT and pulmonary embolism.

Answers

1. When deciding whether to write a patient for standing postoperative DVT prophylaxis, you should think about the patient's risk profile. The most commonly encountered high-risk populations include those with cancer, patients who are not ambulatory, trauma patients, pregnant women, those with a history of a hypercoaguable disorder, and those who are older (increasing risk after age 40). The risk of DVT, however, must be balanced against the risk of bleeding, and the risk of side effects, as well as patient discomfort with multiple subcutaneous injections per day. Furthermore, patients who are at risk of a major bleeding complication (eg, neurosurgical patients) are usually not started on prophylaxis in the immediate postoperative period.

   In summary, if the patient is low risk (and especially if the patient is expected to be ambulatory), then DVT prophylaxis is not necessary. If, on the other hand, the patient is at moderate or high risk for DVT, then the patient should always be written for DVT prophylaxis.

2. The Cochrane database has examined intermittent pneumatic leg compression and pharmacologic prophylaxis individually and together. Interestingly,

pneumatic compression works by diminishing venous stasis, but also works because it promotes fibrinolysis (so you can even put the leg squeezers on the arms). The Cochrane review concludes that pneumatic compression plus pharmacologic prophylaxis (2500 U heparin 2 hours preoperatively and 12 hours postoperatively) is more effective than either strategy alone. Surprisingly, multiple studies report no increase in bleeding with this regimen.

3. While heparin is the oldest agent, it has a significant risk of causing heparin-induced thrombocytopenia (HIT) (2.6% in one meta-analysis). This contrasts with low-molecular-weight heparin (eg, enoxaparin or dalteparin) with a 10-fold decreased incidence of HIT in a population that consisted mostly of postoperative orthopedic patients. So, in general, it is better to use enoxaparin when you can—but you need to know, of course, when you cannot. There are only two common reasons that you might choose heparin. First, low-molecular-weight heparin is cleared renally, and so it can accumulate and lead to bleeding if given to a patient with renal insufficiency. Second, the half-life of low-molecular-weight heparin is longer than that of heparin and it cannot be easily reversed—both of which mean that heparin is preferred when the risk of bleeding is greatest. This is most commonly seen with epidurals, which the anesthesiologists are reluctant to remove when low-molecular-weight heparin is being used.

TIPS TO REMEMBER

● DVTs are a serious and common postsurgical complication—and you will be responsible for ensuring that every patient is on appropriate prophylaxis.

● Low-risk patients don't need DVT prophylaxis, especially if they are ambulating.

● Use low-molecular-weight heparin in most patients, except those who may need rapid reversal, those who are going to undergo another procedure in the near term (including removal of an epidural), or those with renal failure.

COMPREHENSION QUESTIONS

1. A 23-year-old male is in a motor vehicle crash and has a closed femur fracture. His postoperative DVT prophylaxis regimen should include which of the following?

      A. Sequential compression device (SCD) on the contralateral leg only
      B. Heparin 2500 U × 1 + SCD
      C. Heparin 5000 U TID + SCD
      D. Enoxaparin 30 mg SQ q12h + SCD

2. A 54-year-old female just underwent an abdominoperineal resection (APR) for rectal cancer. Her pain is being controlled with an epidural and she has both an

NG tube and Foley in place. Her postoperative DVT prophylaxis regimen should include which of the following?

A. Nothing
B. SCDs only
C. Heparin 2500 U × 1 + SCDs
D. Heparin 5000 U TID + SCDs
E. Enoxaparin 30 mg SQ q12h + SCDs

3. A 55-year-old male is being admitted for an SBO that is being managed nonoperatively. Your admission orders should include which of the following?

A. No DVT prophylaxis but instructions to the RN to help the patient walk three times per day
B. Heparin 5000 U TID + SCDs
C. Enoxaparin 30 mg SQ q12h + SCDs

4. A 65-year-old female who is on the kidney transplant list undergoes a right colectomy for colon cancer. Her pain is being controlled with dilaudid IV. Her postoperative DVT prophylaxis regimen should include which of the following?

A. No DVT prophylaxis but instructions to the RN to help the patient walk 3 times per day
B. Heparin 5000 U TID + SCDs
C. Enoxaparin 30 mg SQ q12h + SCDs

Answers

1. **D**. He is a trauma patient with an orthopedic injury that will prevent him from ambulating. He is therefore at high risk of DVT and should be started on both pharmacologic and mechanical (SCD) prophylaxis. He is at low risk of serious bleeding complications, and so the risk of HIT associated with unfractionated heparin (choices B and C) is not justified.

2. **D**. She is at high risk (cancer, unlikely to ambulate well given the operation and the epidural). Heparin is more appropriate because she has an epidural.

3. **A**. If the patient is able to ambulate and he is otherwise at low risk of DVT, then it is reasonable to avoid the injections and side effects of pharmacologic DVT prophylaxis. SCDs are an option, although not strictly indicated—and if the patient is walking, he probably won't wear them much anyway.

4. **B**. This patient is at high risk of DVT but has renal failure. Low-molecular-weight heparin is therefore contraindicated.

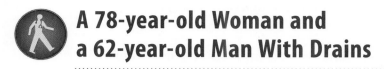

A 78-year-old Woman and a 62-year-old Man With Drains

Michael F. McGee, MD
and Brian C. George, MD

Mrs. Blackwell is 78-year-old woman who underwent a pancreaticoduodenectomy (Whipple procedure) 3 days ago. After the team sees the patient during morning rounds, your senior resident instructs you to remove the left-sided Jackson-Pratt (JP) drain. You confirm that the left-sided drain output has fallen to 10 cm³/day, and the drain amylase levels are normal. Later, as you are collecting the necessary supplies, you are paged by the nurse of Mr. Whitepoor, a 62-year-old man who underwent percutaneous image-guided drainage catheter placement by interventional radiology (IR) yesterday. The nurses report he is leaking large amounts of brown fluid from around his drain. You decide to first investigate Mr. Whitepoor's drain issue.

1. **What are the principles of drain management and how do you manage a leaking drain?**
2. **When should a drain be removed?**
3. **What bedside supplies are necessary to remove a drain?**
4. **What are the steps to remove a Penrose drain?**
5. **What are the steps to remove a closed-suction drain (eg, a JP drain attached to a suction bulb)?**
6. **How should an image-guided percutaneous drainage catheter be removed?**

DRAINS

In the broadest sense, drains can be classified as active or passive. JP, Hemovac, and Blake drains are each attached to a suction apparatus and use active suction. When attached to a bulb, these drains form a closed system that applies negative pressure to the drain allowing suction-assisted evacuation of the target fluid. Some drains contain additional channels that allow sumping (ie, atmospheric venting) or combined irrigation–suction capabilities. In contrast, Penrose, Malecot, and Pezzer drains are passive drains reliant on gravity drainage, intra-abdominal pressure gradients, or capillary phenomena to drain fluid collections. Image-guided percutaneous drainage catheters can be either active or passive gravity drains depending on the collection apparatus used.

Answers

1. Drains require maintenance; therefore, knowledge of drain principles is essential for the surgical house officer. Narrow-bore closed drainage systems are prone to

clogging from fibrinous exudates and clots and may become ineffective in the postoperative period. Drainage from around the drain site usually indicates a clogged drain rather than too large a skin aperture and should be treated with drain patency maneuvers rather than skin sutures or dressing reinforcement. Drain systems with elastic tubing can be "stripped" by carefully milking drain debris into the suction bulb thereby assuring continued drain patency. It should be noted that drain stripping is not a universally accepted practice as some surgeons fear high suction pressures can be harmful to the structures adjacent to the drain. Some drains, including sumping multichannel systems, allow for continuous or intermittent bolus irrigation (ie, flushing) of sterile saline to ensure drain patency. For example, scheduled, routine flushing is often performed for drains placed by IR.

2. The decision to remove a drain is irreversible; therefore, you must be sure of your actions. If uncertain about drain removal, confer with your senior resident or attending. Removing the wrong drain can put the patient at risk of needing a procedure to replace it.

   There are some general guidelines regarding the timing of drain removal. Routinely placed intra-abdominal drains (like pelvic drains during routine pelvic dissection or perianastomotic JP during pancreaticoduodenectomy) are generally removed in the early postoperative period provided drainage is minimal and there is no evidence of leak or abscess. For intra-abdominal abscesses, the decision to remove a drain rests largely on the etiology of the abscess and the surgeon's preference. Drains placed to control a septic source are managed on a more individualized basis. Evidence of succus, bile, or amylase-rich fluid in a drain is worrisome for leak and typically precludes early removal of the drain.

3. Regardless of the gravity of the procedure, surgeons must first ensure the correct supplies and instruments are gathered prior to commencing. Typically, a pair of suture removal scissors (generally part of a suture removal "kit"), dry sterile gauze, and tape are needed to remove most drain types at the bedside. A disposable impermeable sheet (eg, "Chux") can also be helpful by limiting linen soilage and improving your standing with nursing.

   After collecting the supplies, ensure that the patient is lying down and that the bed is raised to an appropriate height. The patient should be positioned so the drain site is easily accessed. The physician should be positioned on the side of the patient that provides the best access to the drain. A garbage can, if not already close at hand, should be positioned nearby.

4. Simple passive abdominal drains (eg, Malecot and Penrose drains) can simply be removed by cutting the securing suture (if used) and gently applying constant pressure until the drain slides out. Resistance may indicate an occult securing suture and merits investigation. The wound can be covered with dry gauze and typically is allowed to heal secondarily. Persistent leakage from the drain tract is expected until the wound epithelializes.

5. Closed-suction systems should be opened to the atmosphere prior to removal. Opening the drainage system eliminates suction and is thought to minimize the likelihood of intra-abdominal tissue injury when the drain is removed.

6. Image-guided percutaneous drains are typically referred to as "pigtail" catheters due to the coiled configuration of the catheter tip and require special consideration during removal. Some brands of pigtail catheters are "nonlocking" and will uncoil automatically when pulled. Other types of "locking" catheters contain an embedded wire or suture within the catheter that is drawn and secured to lock the catheter into a rigid coiled configuration. Removal of locking pigtail drains requires the deployment suture to be found and released prior to removal. Releasing the embedded suture in a locking catheter allows the drain to uncoil into a straight configuration for atraumatic removal. To avoid premature removal and confusion between locking and unlocking drain systems (and out of courtesy), any image-guided drain removal must first be discussed with the interventional radiologist.

TIPS TO REMEMBER

- Drain removal is irreversible. Be doubly certain the correct drain is being removed at the appropriate time.
- Just because a drainage tube is in place does not guarantee it is working. Follow drain outputs and check for patency each day.
- Any image-guided percutaneous drain should be managed in consultation with the IR team.

COMPREHENSION QUESTIONS

1. Three days following an uneventful pancreaticoduodenectomy, you evaluate a patient for persistent drainage around a JP site. The patient's gown is soaked in serous fluid and 8 large gauze pads overlying the drain are saturated. This should best be handled by which of the following?
> A. Tightening the skin aperture around the drain site with an encircling skin stitch
> B. Carefully stripping the drain tube to remove clot and fibrin
> C. Applying additional pressure dressings to the drain site
> D. Beginning diuresis to manage ascites leak

2. You are asked to remove a pigtail catheter placed by IR 6 days ago. While pulling the drain, you encounter resistance and patient discomfort. This should be handled by which of the following?
> A. Opening the gravity collection bag to atmospheric pressure
> B. Obtaining a sinogram through the tube

C. Carefully applying more tension when removing
D. Checking the catheter for a locking suture

Answers

1. **B**. Fluid follows the path of least resistance. Carefully stripping the drain (or flushing, if possible) will ensure a low-resistance path through the system and should fix this problem. Generally, extra skin sutures will not fix the leakage and will be painful for the patient. Note that while the patient may have ascites, ascites is not the problem—collecting it is.

2. **D**. Many pigtail catheters are locked into a coiled position and require release of the locking suture prior to removal. While venting a drain during removal is generally a good principle, resistance encountered during drain removal is an ominous sign and merits a call for help. A sinogram will not be helpful in diagnosing this problem.

A 58-year-old Woman Who had a Drain Pulled by the Resident in Error

Peter Angelos, MD, PhD, FACS and Debra A. DaRosa, PhD

You are on the Endocrine surgery service and have been involved in the care of a 58-year-old woman who had an enucleation of an insulinoma from the head of her pancreas a week ago. At the time of that procedure, 1 drain was left anterior to the head of the pancreas and one drain was left posterior to the head of the pancreas. One of those drains, the posterior one, has actually had very little output over the last 48 hours and your chief resident has asked that you go pull that drain. You have been appropriately instructed in how to remove an abdominal drain, and you proceed to remove the drain. However, after doing so, much to your horror, you realize that although you were asked to remove the posterior drain, in fact, because of some confusion on your part as to which drain was which, you have removed the anterior drain. You realize this after the patient began complaining of abdominal discomfort and spiked a fever 12 hours after the drain removal. The attending and senior surgical residents are in the operating room and you have discussed this with them and they have explained that it is now necessary for this patient to have a CT scan.

1. Should the patient be told that an error occurred?

2. How would you address this error with the patient?

3. How might a resident contend emotionally with having made an error?

4. How might you address an error made by a colleague?

ERRORS

Answers

1. According to the Institute of Medicine's *To Error is Human* report, an error is defined as either the failure of a planned action to be completed as intended (ie, an error of execution) or the use of a wrong plan to achieve an aim (ie, error of planning). As noted in the report, medical errors are one of the leading causes of death in the United States. Medical errors may rank as high as the fifth leading cause of overall death in the United States, exceeding the number of deaths that occur from motor vehicle accidents, breast cancer, and AIDS combined. In the years since the IOM report was published, research has revealed that errors are a growing problem. Since all medical and surgical care is provided by humans and humans are fallible, we know that errors will occur. Patients also know that errors can occur even with the best of intentions to avoid them. An honest

discussion of what happened and how it happened is essential. Years ago, many physicians felt that to admit an error would be tantamount to inviting a lawsuit. In fact, the preponderance of data suggests that honest and prompt disclosure of errors is an important factor in reducing malpractice suits. More importantly, however, honest and prompt disclosure of errors is essential for the honest and ethical relationship between a patient and his or her physicians.

2. As noted above, prompt and frank disclosure of errors is essential. The resident should decide with the attending surgeon if the resident should go alone to discuss this with the patient (if the attending surgeon will be unavailable for a prolonged period of time) or whether the attending and resident should go together. A quiet setting is important for such communication. The resident and/or attending should sit down with the patient to apologize and frankly explain what happened, why it happened, and what impact it will have on the patient's future condition. The patient should be given the opportunity to ask questions and get the level of detail of information that he or she feels is needed and is comfortable with. The resident and/or attending should also be prepared to offer to the patient what will be done in the future to prevent the same error from happening to another patient.

   Most hospitals have a Risk Management office or division with representatives skilled in helping physicians and surgeons communicate with patients about errors. There may be policies and procedures in place to ensure that error disclosure and corresponding apologies are communicated appropriately and completely to the patient.

3. It can be difficult for residents or any health care providers knowing they harmed a patient. Individuals may respond differently and have various approaches for how to come to terms with having compromised a patient's outcome, even with the best of intentions. Common emotions include guilt, fear, anger, loss of self-confidence, shame, and embarrassment. Wu and colleagues identified two ways to cope with errors: a problem-focused and an emotion-focused approach. The former involves coping through a focus on the situation or variables that led to the error. The outcome is to promote change to prevent it from happening again. The latter is focusing on emotional distress with the aim to achieve psychological well-being through either formal counseling or dialoguing with mature minds who have "been there" and who can help a resident see different perspectives on the problem. The aim is to not push the feelings aside or internalize them to the degree that they are not dealt with at all. Those who cope by accepting responsibility for their mistakes are more likely to reflect on how to make constructive changes to their practices.

4. Should a fellow resident open up to you about having made a mistake, it is important to encourage a description of what happened, and to begin by accepting this assessment and not minimizing the importance of the mistake. Disclosing one's own experience of mistakes or "near misses" can reduce the

peer's sense of isolation. It is helpful to ask about and acknowledge the emotional impact of the mistake and discuss how the colleague is coping. Residents should make it feel safe to talk about mistakes as it is critical to creating a culture of mutual support and an environment with a patient safety focus.

TIPS TO REMEMBER

- Studies show that disclosure may help patients get treatment to offset the results of an error, may award them fair compensation, and may help restore trust in the health care provider. Thus, the honest, forthright disclosure of an error, including an apology, is an important component of an ethically attuned patient safety agenda.

- Residents should consult with their attendings or senior residents once an error is made or noticed. The attending may call for a consult with the Risk Management unit within the hospital. Your hospital may have policies and procedures in place for disclosing error information to patients.

- It is natural to have some emotional distress or reaction when dealing with an error. Coping mechanisms vary by individual, but honest and direct communication may be the best antidote.

COMPREHENSION QUESTIONS

1. Not disclosing an error to a patient can result in which of the following?
    A. Possible litigation
    B. Limiting opportunities for systems and process improvement
    C. Distrustful relationship between patient and provider
    D. All of the above

2. There is a difference between error "reporting" and error "disclosure."
    A. True
    B. False

3. What barriers exist that thwart error reporting and disclosure?
    A. Fear of blame
    B. Confusion as to what really "counts" as an error
    C. Poor match of administrative response to errors with severity of errors
    D. Burden of effort (paperwork, time, etc)
    E. All of the above

Answers

1. **D.** All of the above. Any of these and other ethical consequences can occur when physicians choose not to report or disclose errors.

2. **A**. True. A *report* of a health care error is an account of the mistake that conveys details of the occurrence, at times implicating health care providers, patients, or family members in error events. Both clinicians and patients can detect and report errors. Each report of a health care error can be communicated through established and informal systems existing in hospitals (internal) and outside organizations (external), and may be written (eg, electronic or paper) or verbal, voluntary or mandatory (policy driven). The core value supporting reporting is nonmaleficence: do no harm, or prevent the recurrence of errors. Error *disclosure* occurs when a health care provider shares with patients and significant others the actual error. Both provide opportunities to reduce the effects of errors and prevent the likelihood of future errors by, in effect, warning others about the potential risk of harm.

3. **E**. All of the above. Research as to why health care providers do not report or disclose errors includes fear, misunderstanding, administrative/organizational report process burdens, and the response anticipated from hospital leadership.

A Resident Who Is Unsure About How to Remove a Chest Tube

Peter Angelos, MD, PhD, FACS
and Debra A. DaRosa, PhD

It is early July. As the first-year surgical resident on the thoracic surgery service, you are asked by the senior resident to remove the chest tube on a patient who recently had a pulmonary resection. You have been on the service for a few days and you have seen the problems that can occur if a chest tube is pulled without appropriate management—namely, the patient may have an air leak into the pleural space requiring replacement of another chest tube. Although you have seen one chest tube removed, you are uncertain of the appropriate steps to take to ensure that the patient does not have a pneumothorax as a result of the chest tube removal.

1. **How should you manage your lack of comfort with this procedure?**

2. **Who would be the appropriate person to speak to in order to ensure that patient safety is maintained while you gain the experience that is required to proceed?**

3. **Should you tell the patient of your lack of experience?**

4. **How should you answer if the patient asks you, "How many times have you done this before?"**

5. **When describing the procedure to your patient, is your level of experience important for the patient's informed consent?**

OVER YOUR HEAD

Answers

1. When answering this question, it is critical to distinguish between *feelings* of inadequacy and the actual lack of training or experience with a procedure. It is not uncommon for surgical residents to have some concern about doing procedures with which they have little experience. Unfortunately, early in the first year of residency, many procedures fall into the category of "things I have little experience with." Being self-critical is important for the resident to determine if he or she has been adequately trained in all of the steps of the procedure and has seen it done by others. Lack of such minimal training in a procedure is a clear reason to ask for help from a senior resident or an attending.

2. Although there is a tendency for surgical residents to sometimes be hesitant to ask for help, doing so should never be seen as a "sign of weakness." As a physician, a surgical resident has a responsibility to do everything possible to

ensure the safety of the patient. If the resident has not been fully trained in a procedure, to proceed to do it on a patient without adequate training and/ or supervision should be viewed as unethical. In some cases, surgical skills are formally taught and competency is assessed formally. However, in many cases, the individual resident is the only one who can assess whether he or she has the training needed to carry out the procedure. A more senior surgical resident or fellow or a faculty member should be asked for help in learning how to do a procedure before it is done on a patient. Depending on the skill in question, you can also ask for help from experienced nurses, physician assistants, or other health providers who are usually happy to teach, assist, or guide you.

3. It is often challenging for surgical trainees to determine whether conveying information to a patient is helpful to the patient or rather a source of additional concern. If a resident is expressing uncertainty to a patient but is not prepared to get help if the patient requests it, then the uncertainty only causes doubt in the patient. There is no single answer to whether every patient needs to know the first time you do everything. Depending on the procedure and the risks as well as the alternatives available to the patient, the surgical resident should determine whether informed consent for the procedure should require disclosure of the level of experience.

4. In contrast to question #3 above, patients should be given truthful answers to direct questions. In an effort to alleviate patient concerns, however, the resident should be prepared to follow up the answer with the explanation of what preparation and training has occurred prior to the resident actually doing the procedure.

5. Similar to the answer to question #3 above, the answer is dependent on the nature of the procedure, the level of risk to the patient, and the alternatives available to the patient. A rule of thumb to use is for the resident to honestly answer the following question, "If I were the patient, would I want to know this information?" If the answer is "Yes," it becomes difficult to explain why a resident would not offer that information to his or her patient.

TIPS TO REMEMBER

- If you feel your lack of experience or knowledge might jeopardize the patient, it is your moral responsibility to ask for help rather than attempting the skill alone.
- It is not a sign of weakness to ask for help, but rather a sign of responsible self-awareness and placement of a priority on patient safety.
- Be honest with a patient when he or she directly asks about your experience with performing the skill.

● There is no one correct answer in determining whether a resident should disclose "this is my first time doing this procedure" to the patient. The decision to disclose this information should take into account the procedure and the risks as well as the alternatives available to the patient.

COMPREHENSION QUESTION

1. Which of the following statements are false? (Choose all that apply.)
    A. Senior residents do not require supervision when performing bedside procedures.
    B. The appropriate degree of delegation is important to patient safety.
    C. The attending surgeon is ultimately responsible for the patient's safety.
    D. It is at times uncomfortable to ask for help or oversight when performing a skill for the first time on an actual patient.
    E. A resident who demonstrates proficiency of a skill in the simulation laboratory is capable of performing that skill on an actual patient.

Answer

1. **A and E.** While senior residents require less direction than junior residents, they must also be supervised—especially for procedures with which they are unfamiliar. Accurately performing a skill in the simulation laboratory may demonstrate proficiency in a controlled environment, but performing the skill on an actual patient requires supervision to ensure positive learning transfer. Some skills may require multiple direct observation type supervision because of the skill's complexity or difficulty due to patient anatomy or circumstances.

A Surgical Intern in a Moral Dilemma

Peter Angelos, MD, PhD, FACS
and Debra A. DaRosa, PhD

You have been on the surgical oncology service for the past 2 weeks. During that time, you have been involved in the care of a 45-year-old gentleman who has had a pancreaticoduodenectomy performed for pancreatic carcinoma. The patient has had a number of complications associated with leaks from his operation and has required percutaneous drainage. His pathology report has come back that shows positive nodes as well as a positive margin. Based on this information, you know that his overall prognosis is poor. The patient has confided in you his desire not to have his life artificially prolonged unnecessarily. Nevertheless, as he has deteriorated and required intubation and pressors for his sepsis, his family has proceeded with a very aggressive course of treatment in accordance with the recommendations of the surgical attending. You believe that perhaps the patient's wishes have been discounted by the family and the attending surgeon.

1. **How should you approach this issue?**
2. **Who would be the appropriate person with whom to raise your concerns?**
3. **Do you believe your primary allegiance is to the service or to the patient for whom you have participated in care?**
4. **If you believe that the care being rendered is contrary to the patient's wishes, when is it appropriate to withdraw from this patient's case?**

MORALITY IN THE SURGICAL INTERN

Answers

1. As a junior member of the surgical team caring for the patient, it can be easy to lose track of the fact that the resident actually has a relationship with the patient and, as a result, responsibilities to the patient. The complicating factor, however, is that your relationship with your patient is not in isolation, but rather is present because of the relationship that the patient has with the attending surgeon. In an elective situation such as this, the patient has made the choice to have the attending surgeon operate on him. The relationship between the attending surgeon and the patient certainly arose prior to the relationship between the resident and the patient. As a result, the issues that are concerning you may have already been addressed preoperatively with the patient or postoperatively with the patient's family.

2. For the reasons noted above relating to the relationship between the attending surgeon and the patient, as a resident, you should communicate your concerns to the attending surgeon. This is best done as a private discussion between you

and the attending surgeon and not in the presence of the other members of the team or in front of the family. Although frank discussions and a vigorous debate of alternative approaches to a complex patient's care should occur in any teaching environment, ethical issues may be particularly emotionally charged for all involved and are best done privately. In such a context, the resident's concerns can clearly be expressed as being focused on the patient's interests and not misinterpreted as being a challenge to the attending surgeon's ethics or judgment.

3. For the reasons noted in question #1, the relationship between the resident and patient must always be seen in the broader context of the relationship between the attending surgeon and the patient. For the reasons noted in question #2 above, the discussion between resident and attending surgeon about sensitive issues such as what is in the patient's best interests should be done in private. You must not forget that your ability to effectively function as part of the surgical team and render good patient care is predicated on your ability not only to be proactive in rendering patient care but also to ensure ongoing communication and understanding between you and your attending supervisor, and the other health care professionals on the team.

4. No one should be expected to carry out what he or she perceives as an immoral or unethical action, no matter what "orders" might have been given. Certainly, in a situation such as described above, a difference of opinion about what a patient "would have wanted" is often so subjective that it would not normally be the sort of major issue for which a resident would withdraw from participating in the patient's care. However, when faced with a clear and significant breach of ethics (eg, if the resident were to feel that going along with the attending surgeon would lead to significant harm to the patient), then the resident should respectfully withdraw from the patient's care. Furthermore, if a resident perceives any health care provider is a danger to the patient or himself or herself, the resident should report it to the program director or other trusted individual positioned in an educational leadership role.

TIPS TO REMEMBER

- The attending surgeon and patient established a relationship prior to the resident–patient relationship. Therefore, resident concerns or disagreements in patient care should be communicated in private to the attending.
- If a resident has a major moral conflict with some aspect of a patient's care that cannot be resolved even after communicating with an attending, the resident should respectfully withdraw from the patient's care.
- Residents should communicate concerns or ethical conflicts with their program director, a trusted mentor, or other member of the educational leadership team.

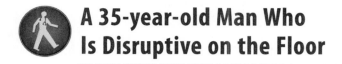

A 35-year-old Man Who
Is Disruptive on the Floor

Xavier Jimenez, MD and
Shamim H. Nejad, MD

Mr. Downey is a 35-year-old gentleman with a history of heroin dependence, alcohol abuse, and cocaine abuse, transferred from the county jail and admitted for observation after deliberately ingesting a razor blade in order to prevent being transferred to prison. He had a similar episode two months prior to this admission in which the razor blade was removed via EGD in the emergency room. On this presentation, however, he declined an EGD, demanding instead that he be operated upon. As there was no indication of an acute abdomen, he was instead admitted for observation with the plan for him to pass the razor blade on his own, and to surgically intervene only if he developed signs of peritonitis or perforation. In the emergency department, all vitals and laboratory results are unremarkable. The patient's last use of heroin, alcohol, and cocaine was approximately six months ago, prior to his incarceration.

On admission, the patient is accompanied by two guards and is shackled at all times. On the floor he begins demanding clonazepam for the treatment of his anxiety disorder and hydromorphone intravenously for acute pain complaints. His affect ranges from irritable to angry to bouts of tearfulness. He intermittently swears at nursing staff as well as at you and your senior resident. Whenever his requests are denied or perceived to not be met, he begins to kick his bedside stand, yell, or bang his head on the bed or the floor until he is restrained by his guards and hospital security. On the second hospital day, an abdominal KUB shows the presence of not only the razor blade but also two batteries that the patient apparently ingested from the television remote in his room. When asked why he ingested the batteries, the patient again states his fear of returning to jail and his strong desire to avoid going back to prison "at all costs." He then blames the surgical team for not treating his pain and anxiety causing him to "act out," and threatens that if "no one listens" to him, he will do it again.

1. **What diagnoses might this patient have that would explain this behavior?**

2. **What communication techniques would you use in approaching this patient?**

DIFFICULT PATIENTS

All patients bring aspects of themselves into clinical encounters—and so do you. A distinction can be made between healthy or adaptive traits and dysfunctional or maladaptive traits. *Adaptive traits* include sound judgment, adequate frustration tolerance, delayed gratification, an ability to cooperate, and emotional control, whereas Mr. Downey exhibits a number of *maladaptive traits*. He experiences emotion dysregulation, moving quickly from irritability to anger to sadness. He also shows low frustration tolerance and an inability to delay gratification, as evidenced by his outbursts when not given what he requests. In addition, he overtly attacks and devalues members of the clinical team, with little, if any, regard for their concerns. His history of polysubstance dependence and requests for numerous medications also suggest generally poor coping mechanisms for managing stress or pain. Globally, Mr. Downey lacks impulse control, sound judgment, and insight into his maladaptive traits.

Clinicians also carry aspects of their own identities and personalities into clinical encounters, and at times they can feel strong emotional reactions to their patients. This is particularly the case in difficult patients, especially those who devalue others or malinger symptoms. As such, Mr. Downey likely inspires negative feelings in clinicians involved with him, including discomfort, fear, anxiety, or anger. This can lead to avoidance or neglect of the patient by the clinician, contributing further to the patient's emotional and behavioral outbursts, which in turn leads to ever-more clinician resentment. In an effort to break this cycle, it is important to identify these reactions, and to discuss them openly with team members and supervisors.

Psychiatry can be consulted to assist in management with difficult patients. For instance, certain symptoms may be amenable to pharmacological management. Mr. Downey exhibits a labile mood and poor impulse control, suggesting the possible role for a dopamine antagonist if his outbursts cannot be otherwise managed. In the event of severe agitation or violence, patients may benefit from a dopamine antagonist as needed for behavioral control. This may reduce the incidence of agitation and violence along with decreasing the need for physical restraints. Benzodiazepines may need to be used in conjunction with dopamine antagonists to control extrapyramidal side effects and to potentiate the antipsychotic's effect, but must be used with caution in any patient with a history of substance abuse, as Mr. Downey has. Ultimately, very close or constant observation may be necessary in order to prevent further ingestion of items that will prolong his stay. This is particularly important as a patient improves medically and surgically as disposition out of a structured setting, such as a hospital, causes some patients to regress psychologically with resulting behavioral dysregulation. Other indications for consulting psychiatry include instances in which a patient may lack the capacity to accept or refuse treatments based on poor judgment or insight, as well as general breakdowns in communication or cooperation with the treatment team.

Answers

1. It is important to rule out any conditions (medical and psychiatric) that contribute to maladaptive expressions or behaviors. This includes mood disorders (eg, bipolar illness), anxiety disorders (eg, PTSD), psychotic disorders, delirium, factitious disorder, malingering, or substance-induced states. When traits appear in

the absence of other conditions and are pervasive, fixed, and severely maladaptive, it is important to seriously consider a personality disorder, although generally it requires a longitudinal history of this behavior before labeling a difficult patient with this kind of diagnosis. Personality disorders must be diagnosed with caution, as once a patient is labeled as such, it may make it difficult for the surgical team to treat the patient objectively without their own emotions interfering. Table 54-1 describes the various personality disorders. Mr. Downey has normal laboratory values and vitals, has not recently used mood-altering substances, is otherwise physically healthy, and has been admitted in the past for similar reasons. He very well might, therefore, have a personality disorder. However, he is clearly attempting to obtain secondary gain (remaining out of prison) by his behavior, and so malingering would be high on the differential list in this case too.

Given his maladaptive traits (lack of remorse for others, poor impulse control, emotional dysregulation, limited coping, etc), a history of incarceration, and the deliberate creation of medical problems with specific aims, Mr. Downey most likely is demonstrating malingering. He may also fit within Cluster "B" pathology and may fit the diagnosis of antisocial personality disorder.

2. Communicating with Mr. Downey may be difficult, but there are general techniques that can be used. First and foremost, a united, clear, and consistent

Table 54-1. Personality Disorder Diagnoses

Cluster A ("MAD" and "WEIRD"): odd, poor sense of reality with distorted thinking	
Paranoid personality d/o	Excessively suspicious, holds grudges, distrusts
Schizoid personality d/o	Disengaged, apathetic, uninterested in interaction
Schizotypal personality d/o	Eccentric, odd, holding strange or magical beliefs
Cluster B ("BAD" and "WILD"): labile, unstable, impulsive, and behaviorally difficult	
Histrionic personality d/o	Theatrical, exaggerated, flirtatious, seductive
Antisocial personality d/o	Lacking remorse, associated with criminality
Borderline personality d/o	Moody, self-injurious, impulsive, unstable relations
Narcissistic personality d/o	Grandiose sense of self, judgmental, dismissive
Cluster C ("SAD" and "WORRIED"): passive, preoccupied, anxious, and afraid	
Avoidant personality d/o	Excessively shy, feels awkward, afraid of rejection
Dependent personality d/o	Passive, lacking self-confidence, relying on others
Obsessive–compulsive personality d/o	Perfectionistic, rigid, preoccupied with detail

In considering personality disorder diagnoses, it is helpful to classify patients according to 1 of the following 3 clusters: "MAD-BAD-SAD" and/or "WEIRD-WILD-WORRIED."

message must be utilized when communicating with all difficult patients. Although most common in borderline personality disorder, all patients are capable of unintentionally *splitting* treatment teams so as to cause disagreements and difficulties that lead to disrupted care and poor outcomes. In addition, it is paramount that certain boundaries be clearly defined and maintained with all patients utilizing maladaptive traits.

A common technique equally useful for difficult, demanding, hostile, or dependent patients is scheduling specific, time-limited sessions that are entirely and solely treatment based (eg, seeing hospitalized patients twice at 8 AM and 1 PM daily for 15 minutes each, going over very specific treatment agendas). Informing the patient of the schedule up front and then enforcing it is crucial. One will need to cater the content of these sessions depending on the person's traits. For example, obsessive–compulsive personalities often dwell on details and minutiae; it may be helpful to enlist them in keeping track of their own recovery (vital signs, labs, medication regimen) while keeping them informed when small fluctuations and insignificant changes are not to be worried about to minimize anxiety.

Considerable anxiety, worry, and stress related to medical conditions, immobility, loss of function, or pain are each very real experiences. *Empathizing* with such an experience can be challenging due to a patient's toxic demeanor and attitude but also very powerful in creating an alliance. The principal mechanism of empathy is *validation* or acknowledgment of a patient's concerns. Empathy is a direct recognition of what the patient is experiencing and reflection of it back in a clear, simple, and nonjudgmental language. In Mr. Downey's example, one might recognize his concerns and confirm them with empathic statements (eg, "It must be terrifying to think about going to prison.") rather than with less empathic questions (eg, "What are you so worried about?"). Additionally, one may attempt to *normalize* concerns expressed by a patient ("Your reaction to a prison sentence is natural."), paving the road to a shared understanding. A patient who is validated in this manner may sense genuine concern and engage in a more cooperative dialogue, leading to shared clinical goals. Finally, depending on the patient's values, it is important to identify others who may assist in enhancing communication, including but not limited to family members, friends, intimate partners, social work, or clergy. In some instances, consultation with a psychiatric service may be indicated.

TIPS TO REMEMBER

- Personality disorders are organized in clusters according to general attributes (mnemonics of "BAD-MAD-SAD" and "WEIRD-WILD-WORRIED").
- Psychiatric consultation can assist in the management of difficult patients, especially in cases of severe aggression, behavioral outbursts, breakdowns in communication, or poor judgment suggesting a lack of decision-making

capacity. It should be said, however, that simply disagreeing with the surgical team does not mean a patient lacks decision-making capacity!

- Empathic validation and normalization packaged in statements (rather than questions) can increase the therapeutic alliance when working with difficult patients.

- Splitting should be reduced with unified and consistent messages. Specific and focused sessions can be useful when working with hostile, demanding, or dependent patients.

- Awareness of clinician feelings and reactions to difficult patients can prevent worsening in communication and cooperation with such patients.

COMPREHENSION QUESTIONS

1. Mr. J is a 44-year-old man who requires imminent below-the-knee amputation. He refuses on numerous accounts, reporting doctors cannot be trusted and that he generally shuns medical advice. On exam, he is oriented to time and space, reveals a flattened affect, and communicates various inaccurate thoughts, including that the infection will heal on its own. He wishes to be discharged. What is the next course of action?
>   A. Respect his autonomy and discharge the patient with oral antibiotics.
>   B. Consult psychiatry to evaluate for a psychotic disorder and capacity for decision making.
>   C. Override the patient's autonomy and operate emergently.
>   D. Treat empirically with antipsychotic medications.

2. A 31-year-old woman is admitted to the ICU for close observation after reportedly ingesting an entire bottle of acetaminophen as well as causing self-inflicted burns to her arms with her gas stove. These occurred in a fit of rage after her boyfriend of three months announced he would leave her. Her psychiatric history includes brief trials with antidepressants but no current treatment. She has seen literally dozens of psychiatrists. She has been admitted to psychiatric services over a dozen times since the age of 18, but she denies any serious suicide attempts. She was diagnosed with a personality disorder at age 19. Which of the following best characterizes this patient's recurrent behaviors?
>   A. Paranoid personality disorder
>   B. Antisocial personality disorder
>   C. Borderline personality disorder
>   D. Dependent personality disorder

3. Mrs. K, a 56-year-old retired nurse with no significant medical history, is sent to the ED by her outpatient surgeon who performed an unremarkable elective hernia repair three weeks prior. Postoperatively, she has healed poorly with numerous

bouts of fever, night sweats, and fatigue. She has not responded to trials of anti-biotics, and her surgeon is perplexed. On admission, blood cultures are drawn, revealing a gram-negative bacteremia. Her surgical site is erythematous and grossly infected. She is given IV antibiotics, but after numerous days in the hospital, a nursing assistant witnesses Ms. K rubbing something vigorously into her wound site. On confrontation she breaks down but cannot explain her behavior and is very ashamed. She begins to describe numerous difficulties at home, including a tumultuous divorce, an unruly son who was recently arrested, and chronic financial struggles including potential bankruptcy. Which of the following statements would you use in approaching Mrs. K at this point?

A. "Why are you infecting yourself?"
B. "It makes perfect sense that you are overwhelmed."
C. "Maybe you don't need to be in the hospital."
D. "You don't seem to want to be better."

Answers

1. **B.** Mr. J is refusing a presumably lifesaving intervention, and it is important to establish whether he has the capacity to refuse treatment. It is unclear at this point if he is simply uneducated about his disease, is afraid of doctors because he or a family member has had a bad experience in the past, has a psychotic illness, or is under the influence of a substance. Clarification of diagnosis, decision capacity, and whether dopamine antagonist medication is indicated may result from consultation with a psychiatrist. Although patient autonomy is an important value to uphold, discharging this patient prematurely may cause significant harm or even death.

2. **C.** This patient exhibits mood dysregulation, intense interpersonal relationships, impulsivity, a history of self-injury, and suicidal behavior in the absence of other psychiatric or medical explanations. She has had a long history or psychiatric contact and psychiatric hospitalizations since age 18, giving one a very longitudinal history, and she tells you she has been diagnosed with a personality disorder. The maladaptive traits discussed here are present in Cluster B ("BAD AND WILD") personality disorders, with borderline personality disorder being the most likely diagnosis.

3. **B.** Patients with suspicious symptoms (in this case, symptoms of a likely factitious disorder) can become very defensive when confronted, and may continue problematic behaviors if not empathically validated at some level. Mrs. K would benefit from normalization of her feelings, but not of her behavior. Gentle confrontation of her emotional difficulties can pave the way for a therapeutic alliance. Psychiatry consultation should be obtained on most suspected cases and perhaps a referral to social work for psychosocial support would be helpful.

Section IV.
Handling Patients in Clinic

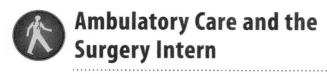

Ambulatory Care and the Surgery Intern

John Maa, MD, FACS

OVERVIEW AND EXPECTATIONS

As a surgeon, running an outpatient clinic effectively is critical to patient flow, patient safety, and patient satisfaction. In the United States, typically 15 to 20 minutes are allocated for an outpatient visit. Patients are often double booked. Recognize that in some Asian countries, outpatient clinic visits are only 3 minutes long. Clearly, much of the key work in clinic visits can be completed in a very short amount of time, but it requires a very focused discussion.

Recognize the possible destinations for patients after being seen by you in clinic. The majority will return home. Some will need urgent admission, possibly through the emergency room, or as direct admissions. A few will require urgent surgery. Others will be sent to a different specialty or primary care clinic as a result of your evaluation, to have an elusive diagnosis made by being seen in a different specialty clinic. For these patients, what you can do to be most helpful is to expedite that evaluation by a different consultant, perhaps by calling him or her directly. You will realize that a few patients have been sent to the wrong clinic; they may be quite frustrated and refunding their insurance copayments for the visit might be indicated. Some patients will have traveled long distances to be seen, and may be tired or anxious. Some patients are most appropriately seen by the chief resident because of the complexity of their chief complaints, whereas others are suitable for junior residents or interns. In some clinics, interns are assigned primarily to perform history and physical examinations within 30 days of surgery for patients who have already received a diagnosis and treatment plan. Performing examinations and reviewing final lab and x-rays are critical roles you can play. You can demonstrate your value if you identify key elements that may have been overlooked by the attending in the preoperative assessment (carotid bruit, abnormal EKG, incomplete preoperative consults).

PREOPERATIVE AND POSTOPERATIVE CLINIC VISITS

Clinic patients will fall into 1 of the following 2 phases: (1) preoperative and (2) postoperative.

Postoperative visits are relatively straightforward. A clinic schedule should be configured to allow a mix of preoperative and postoperative patients, with the easier postoperative visits an opportunity for the clinician to catch up on the schedule.

The key things to do in a postoperative visit are:

A. To review the surgical incisions for possible infections, hematomas, seromas, lymphoceles, or incisional hernias.

B. To check the pathology report and ensure that further treatment plans (particularly for cancer diagnoses) and referrals (ie, oncology) are in place.

C. To ensure adequate pain medication refills, work notes, and disability paperwork are complete.

D. To answer the final questions from the patient, with further instructions about activity level (no heavy lifting after hernia repair, bathing and the care of steri-strips, symptoms about which to be vigilant).

E. To transfer the patient back to the care of the primary care physician. Recall that the global period in surgery often allows patients to be seen for up to 90 days after surgery at no cost to the patient. New appointments to see the patient back should be made liberally available if there is uncertainty about wound healing and recovery.

Preoperative patients can be most complex. As you begin speaking to the patient, recall that you are essentially being asked to answer this focused question: does the patient require surgery for the surgical condition that is proposed? You are being asked for an expert opinion, as a consultant, and must thus answer at the level of an attending, not as a trainee. Most likely, restating the chief complaint in the patient's own words is most helpful to frame the discussion and presentation to the attending. At times, you will encounter patients who don't even know why they were referred by their other doctor to the surgery clinic. In such cases, you should carefully review all primary sources of data, which may include the medical record, paperwork in the patient's possession, recent radiology reports, or verbal communications with other family members.

As clinicians gain greater expertise, they often learn to focus on abnormalities as the subtle clues to find the true diagnosis. Ultimately, to complete your assessment expeditiously, think of yourself as a detective. Focus on the question at hand, and direct all of your questions, review of the vital signs, and physical examination toward this main point. There is no need to address chronic medical conditions that are under the care of other treating physicians and unrelated to the surgical question at hand.

Once the decision to operate is made, the next important question becomes how to perform the procedure safely. Deciding what incision to use will depend on the past surgical history and evaluation of the previous surgical scars, so your evaluation and presentation to the attending should focus on these findings. If available, all of the previous operative notes should be requested and reviewed. Read all sources of primary information, and beware of chart lore. Don't make assumptions about information, particularly anything that is critical to the decision to operate. Review of the complete medication list is necessary to determine which medications should be discontinued preoperatively (pay special attention to antiplatelet medications such as Plavix and aspirin and anticoagulants such as warfarin). The general health of the patient is assessed through the past medical history. Advising smoking cessation is also wise, especially for some orthopedic and plastic surgery procedures where active smoking may be a contraindication to elective surgery. Some patients will require joint procedures with other services (plastics, vascular) and coordinating surgery across specialists is a task you can delegate to the clinic staff.

TIME MANAGEMENT

1. *Keep the clinic flowing smoothly.* Most often, the number of examination rooms is the rate-limiting step in clinic throughput. Sometimes, this means sending a patient to the laboratory or radiology to free up clinic space temporarily while you collect more information that may assist in making the diagnosis or a decision about the need for admission to the hospital. If a patient needs to be admitted, the best strategy is for the patient to be moved out of the examination area and back to the waiting area or hospital admitting to await the availability of an inpatient bed. If a patient is particularly complex, move on to another patient, and sometimes a solution for the challenging patient will enter your mind as you are speaking to the second patient.

2. *Focus the conversation with the patient.* After a brief open-ended question such as "How are you feeling?" or "What may I do for you?," redirect the patient if the response is tangential. For example, the question "What brought you here today?" may yield the reply "an ambulance," or lead to a lengthy discussion of the difficulty in finding a parking space in the garage. Politely and professionally constrain extraneous conversations, and try to focus on the medical condition and the relevant history for which the patient has been referred. Before a lengthy discussion of the risks of surgery or plans for future care, it is most often helpful to bring interested family members who might be in the waiting room into the examination room, so that you don't find yourself repeating a 10-minute explanation again to another family member.

3. *Delegate appropriately.* You are a limited resource, so don't spend excessive time doing things you don't need to do. Defer prescription refills to the primary care provider, and involve the clinic staff to assist you with administrative matters such as obtaining insurance authorizations, HIPAA clearances, and completing disability paperwork or work requests. Some preoperative questions, such as the precise timing for discontinuation of anticoagulants, use of oral antihypertensives the morning of surgery, and fasting for breakfast, will be addressed by the anesthesiologist and preoperative staff. In some clinics, clinical decision aids and educational materials (handouts or videos) can be given to patients in the waiting room or as they wait in the examination room to be seen, to better prepare and focus the ensuing discussion once the doctor arrives. At times, a formal review of radiologic imaging from a different hospital will be needed, and speaking to a radiologist by telephone will be insufficient to make a clinical decision. One solution is to ask a member of the clinic staff to hand carry the films or CD to the radiology department for interpretation. Ultimately it may require having the patient return to clinic, or speaking to him or her later by telephone once the x-rays have been formally read, to make the final decision whether surgery is necessary.

PROFESSIONALISM

1. Arrive in clinic on time and try to stay on schedule. Delays only compound as the clinic progresses, as more time is spent hearing the subsequent complaints of frustrated patients who have been waiting prolonged periods. This can be minimized by starting clinic promptly.
2. Wear professional attire. In general, wearing surgical scrubs to clinic is discouraged. One's attire, grooming, and overall appearance can leave a lasting impression on the patient and family (both positive and negative).
3. Refrain from being excessively critical of other clinicians or referring providers. Try not to criticize the care delivered by other physicians based on allegations or hearsay, without confirming the facts. Be objective and truthful in your assessment.

COUNSELING THE PATIENT

1. You may be in the uncomfortable situation of caring for an unhappy patient. Don't speculate, and be willing to say "I don't know." Be certain to notify the attending promptly if this situation arises. At times you will be contacted by patient relations or risk management, and in those situations be completely honest, objective, and accurate in your description of the events and reports of the medical record.
2. Don't make pronouncements about prognosis or treatment too early, as the condition may be more complex than you realize. Use caution when making statements that may impact family perceptions and travel plans.
3. Don't try to oversimplify a complex situation, and don't try to place certainty on an uncertain situation. This is a first chance to meet with the patient, and it may take future repeat visits to make an accurate diagnosis and come to a final decision. Don't make guarantees or promises to patients that you can't fulfill. Sometimes you will encounter unrealistic patient expectations about the outcome or plan, which may sometimes be the result of information that has been inaccurately conveyed by the primary care provider, who may also have unrealistic expectations. You will have to handle these difficult situations delicately.

At times, referring doctors may have intentionally misstated the reason for referral to gain access to your clinic, so you sometimes have to question the diagnosis that is written on the referral sheet.

OTHER FINAL WORDS OF ADVICE FOR THE EFFICIENT INTERN

1. Dictate or write notes as you go. You may forget key information later on if you leave dictations until the end of clinic.

2. An effective intern uses time to call consults and to check labs if the opportunity to present a patient to the attending is delayed. Similarly, the time waiting to present to an attending can be well spent in self-directed reading about the clinical questions relevant to the patients you are seeing in clinic.

3. For effective time management, defer questions about insurance authorizations and hospital bills to the appropriate institutional offices.

4. Don't assume anything about what you are told or jump to conclusions. Some of the worst outcomes in patient care are a result of communication breakdowns, particularly in caring for complex patients.

5. Avoid performing procedures in clinic, which can consume significant amounts of time and clinic rooms.

6. To promote safety and quality in delivering care, beware of truncation and communication failures, errors propagated in sign-out, or chart lore.

A 55-year-old Man Who Was Struck by a Beer Truck and Needs a CT Scan

Haytham M.A. Kaafarani, MD, MPH, Brian C. George, MD, and Hasan B. Alam, MD

Mr. Gossman is a 55-year-old gentleman who was marching in a bagpipe band when he was struck by a beer truck. On arrival to the emergency department he is complaining of abdominal pain. He is hemodynamically stable with diffuse abdominal tenderness. The remainder of his exam is unremarkable.

Based on your evaluation you believe that it is safe to proceed with a CT scan.

1. **Who should you talk to before ordering the CT?**

2. **Should this patient get oral contrast and/or intravenous (IV) contrast?**

3. **After the CT is completed, is there anything that you do before reviewing the film with radiology?**

4. **What window should you use to look for free air?**

5. **In this patient, what does a fluid collection of 40 Hounsfield units (HU) most likely represent?**

ORDERING AND INTERPRETING A CT SCAN OF THE ABDOMEN: THE BASICS

As an intern in general surgery, you will often be asked to "pull up" the CT of the abdomen. Although no one expects you to become the expert on reading abdominal CTs in your first year of residency, your ability to understand the basics of ordering and interpreting a CT can help save a patient's life.

Answers

1. Knowing when (and whether) to order a CT scan is an important skill to acquire during your internship.

    The two rules of thumb are:

    A. Do not order a CT without talking to your senior resident first. This rule is not made to simply create unneeded hierarchy. Your senior resident might know some operative details that are essential to understand how your patient is doing, and the resident might have a lower or higher threshold for ordering an abdominal CT based on intraoperative details or findings.

    B. Always ask yourself how the CT will change your management. This second rule is a general one that you should apply every time you are ordering any test on your patient. No test, especially radiological, comes without a price. An unneeded abdominal CT results in unwarranted patient exposure to radiation, and cumulative radiation exposure is well known to increase the risk of malignancies in the long run. In the short term, a trip to the CT for patients with lines and tubes is a big burden for the nurses, and is not without its own risks: a chest tube might get dislodged, or the patient might be agitated thus requiring some conscious sedation, a further risk. So, always ask yourself "what will I find on the scan (or any test) that will change my current management?"

2. You answer your pager and hear: "Dr. Smith, radiology is on the line asking what kind of contrast you want for the CT scan you just ordered?" The answer is not that complicated if you remember four simple rules:

A. If your patient has intact kidneys and normal creatinine, IV contrast is almost always helpful. If your patient has acute or chronic renal failure, think twice before you order IV contrast. IV contrast is nephrotoxic, especially in elderly diabetic patients. If you suspect free air, a noncontrast CT (ie, without IV or PO contrast) will give you the answer. Otherwise, IV contrast, in general, allows better tissue and organ visualization.

B. If you need to evaluate the anatomy of the GI tract or are looking for an anastomotic leak, PO contrast will help a lot. PO contrast delineates intraluminal anatomy. Observing contrast within the appendiceal lumen is one of the radiological signs that almost "rules out" acute appendicitis. A tachycardic gastric bypass patient may have a leak. On the CT images, extravasation of the PO contrast out of the gastric pouch or the jejunojejunostomy is an essential finding to diagnose this complication.

C. If the pathology you're looking for is in the colon, a per rectum (PR) contrast can be helpful. Talk to your senior resident and radiologist about it. PR contrast can help diagnose a low rectal anastomotic leak, a colonic stricture, a colonic mass, or even acute appendicitis.

D. If the pathology you're looking for is intravascular, a different IV contrast dose and protocol are indicated. For the diagnosis of mesenteric ischemia, IV contrast is essential. Similarly, if you suspect a portal vein or a mesenteric venous problem, there is no direct IV access to the mesenteric venous circulation so you need to obtain much later images (different radiological protocol). The dose, timing, and protocol of IV contrast needed to visualize the arterial or venous system are very different; talk to the radiologist—he or she is your friend, and make sure he or she understands what you're suspecting.

3. Don't wait for the radiology report. *Look at the images yourself,* and then go and review the images with the radiologist. If you are disciplined about trying to first read the films on your own, your ability to read CTs will improve rapidly.

4 and 5. Questions #4 and 5 are best answered as part of a general, systematic strategy on how to approach a CT scan, which will be discussed below.

Opening the Images

A. Orientating yourself. Always start reading the abdominal CT from cranial to caudal, and look at the structures from the most anterior to the most posterior, looking at axial or transverse images. Therefore, structures on the left side of the screen are right-sided structures (eg, liver, inferior vena cava), while structures on the right side of the screen are left-sided structures (eg, spleen).

B. Choosing the right "window." The "window" is the amount of contrast and brightness with which you display the CT image data on the monitor. Most systems have presets such as "abdominal," "lung," and "bone" (to name but a few). If you're looking for free air, the lung window is better. If you need to evaluate the spine or the pelvis (following injury), make sure you choose the bone window. You may look through the images multiple times, each time with a different window.

C. The HU. The HU system is designed to standardize the density reading across different CT machines. By definition, water has 0 HU. Bone has the maximum density among all body tissues (up to 1000 HU). Proteinaceous fluid (including fresh blood) has 20 to 45 HU, and organized hematomas (ie, clots) have 45 to 70 HU.

D. Systematic reading. It does not matter in which order you read an abdominal CT, as long as you always read it in the same systematic fashion. This reduces the chances that you miss something. We suggest the following systematic steps to read an abdominal CT, but one should be free to derive his or her own system for reading images:

i. Check the abdominal wall:

- Look for any hernias or any irregularities in the abdominal wall.
- Look for any thickening of the abdominal wall layers or any bubbles of air that could be concerning, in the right clinical scenario, for necrotizing skin and soft tissue infections (see Figure 56-1).

ii. Look for free air:

- An easy trick is to look for free air using the "lung window" (see Figure 56-2).
- Free air can be normal in the immediate postoperative phase (up to 1 week), but is otherwise often an indication for emergent surgical intervention.

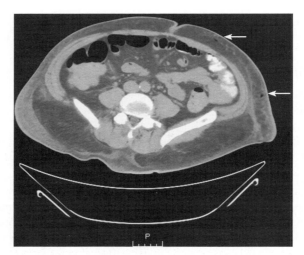

Figure 56-1. CT abdomen revealing abnormal air within the abdominal wall. In the right clinical scenario, this finding is suspicious for a necrotizing skin and soft tissue infection.

    iii. Look for free fluid and intra-abdominal fluid collections:

    • Free fluid in the abdomen is an abnormal finding and can be seen anywhere in the abdominal cavity (see Figure 56-3).

    • It most commonly represents blood, pus, ascites, or enteric contents.

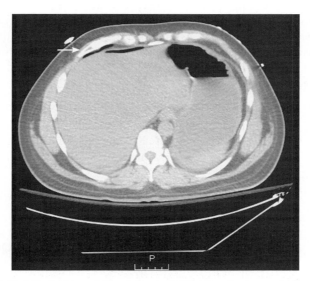

Figure 56-2. Quickly looking at the abdominal CT using the lung window helps better visualization of any abnormal free air versus intraluminal air in the peritoneal cavity.

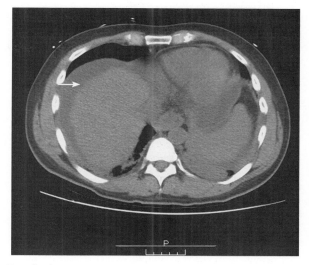

Figure 56-3. Free fluid.

- An intra-abdominal fluid collection could be a benign/malignant tumor or an intra-abdominal abscess (see Figure 56-4).

iv. Look for tubes and drains:

- Follow all Jackson-Pratt, radiology-placed, gastrostomy, nasogastric, and nasoenteric tubes to make sure their intra-abdominal tip positions are where they are supposed to be.

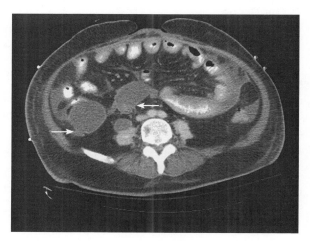

Figure 56-4. Two intra-abdominal fluid collections, suspicious for abscesses.

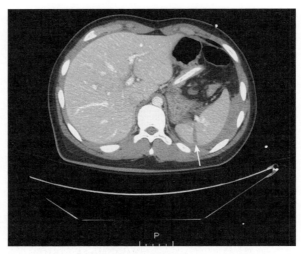

Figure 56-5. Splenic laceration caused by a motor vehicle crash.

    v. Check the liver and biliary tree:
- Look for any irregularities in the liver parenchyma, or any air in the biliary tree.
- Look for subcapsular hematomas or liver lacerations in trauma (see Figure 56-5), and for liver nodules in a patient with a history of malignancy.
- Look for gallbladder thickening or intracholecystic stones or polyps.

    vi. Check the spleen:
- Check for lacerations (eg, trauma), enlargement (malignancy, hypersplenism), or abnormal fluid collections (eg, liver abscess or cyst) (see Figure 56-6).

    vii. Check the pancreas.

    viii. Check for tumors, inflammation, ductal dilatation, and/or intraductal stones (see Figure 56-7). Check the kidneys for hydronephrosis, lacerations, or pericapsular hematoma (see Figure 56-8).

    ix. Follow the stomach and small bowel:
- PO contrast allows better definition.
- Look for "transition points" in suspected bowel obstruction.
- Look for mesenteric thickening, bowel wall thickening, and/or intestinal pneumatosis (see Figure 56-9).

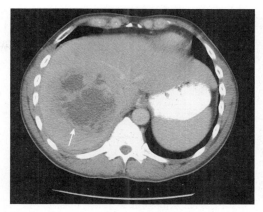

Figure 56-6. Liver fluid collection suspicious for liver abscess.

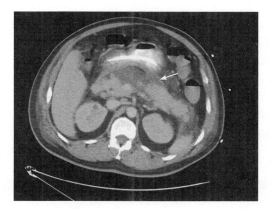

Figure 56-7. Severe pancreatic inflammation.

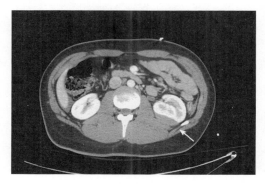

Figure 56-8. Left kidney hematoma caused by a motor vehicle crash.

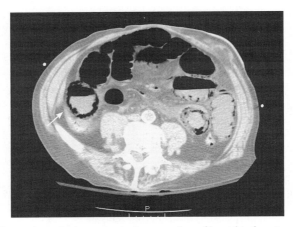

Figure 56-9. Severe intestinal pneumatosis suggestive of bowel ischemia.

x. Check the colon, appendix, and rectum:

- Follow the colon.
- Look for a thickened appendix and for absence of contrast (appendicitis) (see Figure 56-10).
- Look for diverticulosis versus diverticulitis.
- Look for masses or lymphadenopathy.

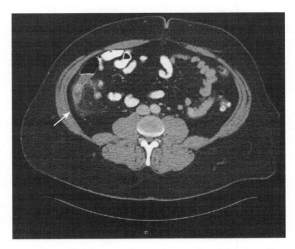

Figure 56-10. Acute appendicitis: note the periappendiceal fat stranding.

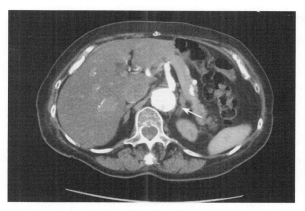

Figure 56-11. Celiac artery at its origin from the aorta.

xi. Check the aorta and its branches:
- Follow the aorta from the diaphragm level, identifying sequentially the celiac artery, the superior mesenteric artery, the renal arteries, the inferior mesenteric artery, and the aortic bifurcation (see Figure 56-11).
- Look for intraluminal filling defects or abrupt cutoffs, especially when mesenteric ischemia is suspected.

xii. Check the inferior vena cava:
- Look for filling defects (eg, thrombus).

xiii. Check the pelvic bones and spinal vertebrae:
- The bone window is helpful for assessing the pelvis and the spine for fractures, especially in the trauma setting.

CONCLUSION

Learning when to order abdominal CTs and how to interpret its images is a skill that you will learn over many years of your surgical training and beyond. However, knowing the basics and developing a systematic way to read a CT are essential tools to maximize your learning, especially in the first few years of residency. Building on the information in this chapter requires continued practice reading the CT images that you should do every time you order this type of study.

COMPREHENSION QUESTION

1. Which window choice helps you see pneumoperitoneum the best?
   A. Lung
   B. Abdomen
   C. Bone
   D. Mediastinum

Answer

1. **A.** If you are looking for free air, in this case in the peritoneum, the lung window is the best choice.

A 60-year-old Man With Postoperative Wound Complications

Michael W. Wandling, MD and Mamta Swaroop, MD, FACS

Mr. Smith is a 60-year-old man who recently underwent an elective open right hemicolectomy for an adenocarcinoma of the ascending colon. The case and postoperative course were unremarkable and he was discharged home on postoperative day number 4. The following day, however, he called your clinic to report subjective fevers, some increased discomfort around his incision, and new drainage from the wound. You instructed him to come to your clinic.

When he arrives, his vitals signs are T 101.4, HR 92, BP 135/85, RR 15, and O₂ 99% on RA. His abdominal exam is significant for a stapled midline laparotomy incision with new-onset erythema that extends approximately 3 to 4 cm laterally and inferiorly from the inferior one third of the wound. A small amount of yellow-tinged thin fluid is coming from between several of the staples. There is also a significant amount of this fluid on the dressing. Palpation reveals mildly increased superficial tenderness surrounding the inferior one third of the wound with no fluctuance or crepitus. There is no rebound tenderness and no guarding. The remainder of the physical exam is normal. You send some blood work, which reveals a white blood cell count of 11,400 cells/mm³.

1. If you know that this patient's surgical incision was classified as "clean-contaminated," what is the probability that he would develop a wound infection?

2. Name two other factors, besides the level of intraoperative contamination, which can modify the risk of surgical site infection (SSI)?

3. Is this most likely a hematoma, seroma, or wound infection? Why?

4. Should you order any imaging?

5. If this turns out to be an infection, should you open the wound?

6. If this turns out to be a seroma or hematoma, should you open the wound?

7. What is the most likely pathogen that caused this problem?

POSTOPERATIVE WOUND COMPLICATIONS

Answers

1. Wound classification is based on the degree of wound contamination. Consider the difference in exposure to bacterial load between an incision made for an inguinal hernia repair and an exploratory laparotomy for a penetrating abdominal trauma with numerous small bowel and colon injuries. In the former, proper

sterile technique should essentially eliminate bacterial contamination from the surgical site. In the latter, however, bacterial contamination of the incision site secondary to gross spillage of stool into the abdomen is virtually inevitable, making the risk of postoperative wound infection considerably higher.

Wound classification is an important concept for any surgeon to understand, as it often drives clinical decision making. For example, wound classification is fundamental in deciding how or even if to close a wound at the end of a case. Additionally, classifying wounds based on their degree of contamination provides a mechanism for postoperative wound infection risk stratification. Such a tool makes it possible to maintain appropriate levels of suspicion for wound infection when evaluating a postoperative patient with a fever, leukocytosis, or peri-incisional erythema. For a description of the wound classification system most commonly used, see Table 57-1.

Table 57-1. Wound Classification and Surgical Site Infection Risk

Wound Classification	Definition	Examples	Surgical Site Infection Risk
Clean	Sterile procedure with no entrance into the GI tract, GU tract, or respiratory tract	Hernia repair, mastectomy, thyroidectomy, AAA repair	1%-3%
Clean-contaminated	Procedure with only minor breaks in sterility with controlled entry into the GI tract, GU tract, or respiratory tract with no significant contamination	Cholecystectomy, appendectomy, small bowel resection, colon resection	5%-8%
Contaminated	Procedure with poor sterility secondary to gross spillage from GI tract, GU tract, or respiratory tract or presence of foreign debris	Cholecystectomy with bile spillage, appendectomy for perforated appendicitis, small bowel or colon resection in setting of perforation	20%-25%
Dirty/infected	Procedure involving contamination by established infectious processes	Abscess drainage, debridement of necrotizing soft tissue infections	30%-40%

2. While the degree of contamination is one of the determining factors, it should be noted that there are multiple other factors that can influence the rate of SSIs. These include the use of preoperative antibiotics, maintaining normothermia, maintaining euglycemia, patient factors such as immunocompromise, and modifications to surgical technique that can be made to reduce contamination. As an intern, the first two items deserve special attention as they are sometimes solely your responsibility. Hyperglycemia is also often under your purview, but complicated enough that it gets its own chapter.

Preoperative Antibiotics

Even in a clean case a skin incision obligatorily exposes vulnerable subcutaneous tissues to a bacterial challenge. Bugs love it if you inevitably sprinkle these subdermal spaces with pockets of the patient's blood—essentially blood agar incubated at 37°C. Your goal, therefore, is to synchronize the antibiotic "peak" with the skin incision. Preoperative antibiotics should be infused during the 1-hour window prior to the skin incision and every 3 to 4 hours (2-3 antibiotic half-lives) during longer procedures.

Normothermia

Trauma surgeons are exquisitely sensitive to the link between hypothermia and bleeding (the coagulation cascade is impaired by hypothermia). However, there are also antiseptic advantages to normothermia (or even hyperthermia—this is why we get a fever with infection). If you wheel your patient into the recovery room/PACU following a bowel resection, with a temperature of only 2° below normal (34.5°C), the chances of a wound infection double. Maintain your patient's core temperature above 36.5°C.

3. A seroma is a collection of liquefied fat, serum, and lymphatic fluid located underneath a surgical incision. These typically present with pressure, discomfort, and sometimes drainage of clear fluid from a well-circumscribed area of swelling around a surgical incision. Seromas most frequently develop following procedures that require elevation of skin flaps and transection of lymphatic channels.

A hematoma is an abnormal collection of blood and/or clot in a wound and is one of the most common wound complications seen in surgical patients. Most hematomas are caused by incomplete intraoperative hemostasis. Hematomas manifest differently based on their size, location, and underlying etiology. Generally, hematomas present as swelling and/or pain in the area of an incision. Discoloration of the wound edges and sometimes blood leaking through the incision may also be seen. It is essential to look for signs of hematoma expansion, particularly in the neck, where rapid expansion can lead to airway compromise.

Although both seromas and hematomas are risk factors for the development of postoperative wound infection (and they may in fact be associated with very similar signs), they are not themselves infections. SSIs are the result of contamination of the surgical site with microorganisms and are marked by a clinical presentation with features different from seromas and hematomas. Special attention must be paid to the presence of crepitus or pain out of proportion with other physical exam findings, as these are ominous signs of necrotizing soft tissue infection. If this diagnosis is missed, it can become fatal within hours. See Chapter 45 on this topic for more information.

This patient most likely does have a wound infection given his elevated temperature as well as the constellation of other signs and symptoms. While pain, drainage, and erythema are individually nonspecific, in combination they are suggestive of infection. His leukocytosis must be evaluated in the context of his previous lab values, and if it is higher than his discharge white count, it too would suggest infection.

4. Fundamental to the understanding of SSIs—and knowing the indications for imaging—is recognizing the depth of infection. SSIs are categorized into three groups: superficial incisional SSIs, deep incisional SSIs, and organ/space SSIs. Superficial incisional SSIs involve the skin, while deep incisional SSIs involve the fascia and muscle layers. Organ/space SSIs involve the organs or spaces that were opened up during the procedure. These include infections such as intra-abdominal abscess, hepatic abscess, and mediastinitis. This classification scheme is depicted in Figure 57-1.

Superficial incisional SSIs typically develop 3 to 6 days after surgery, but this may vary. Symptoms often include erythema, tenderness, edema, and purulent drainage from the wound. Unlike seromas and hematomas, a patient with a wound infection may also have a low-grade fever and/or a leukocytosis, similar to the patient in this case. On exam, the wound may be soft or fluctuant. Surgical site pain that worsens or fails to resolve within 7 to 10 days of surgery is a subtle, but important marker for occult infection.

Deep incisional and organ/space SSIs tend to become apparent later in the postoperative course. These may remain occult or present with symptoms that mimic superficial SSIs, which can delay diagnosis and lead to significant complications. Deep incisional SSIs typically present with pain that extends beyond what would be expected from a surgical wound and beyond any margin of superficial erythema. Symptoms of organ/space SSIs are typically related to involved organ systems. Examples include diarrhea, prolonged or recurrent return of ileus after an operation, or pain on rectal exam.

The diagnosis of superficial postoperative wound complications is primarily made by physical exam as described above. The diagnosis of deep wound complications is more difficult, as their signs and symptoms are often less clear. In cases where there is suspicion for wound complication but no definitive

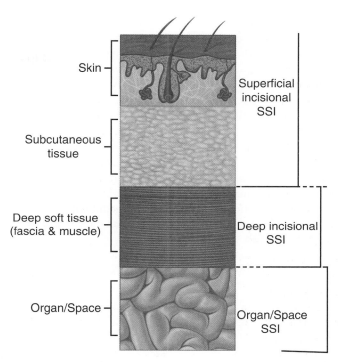

Figure 57-1. Cross-section of abdominal wall depicting the anatomy and classification of surgical site infections. (Reproduced, with permission, from Hoffman BL, Schorge JO, Schaffer JI, et al. *Williams Gynecology*. 2nd ed. New York: McGraw-Hill; 2012. Figure 3-21.)

diagnosis, imaging studies can be obtained. However, as with any studies, they should only be obtained if the result could alter clinical decision making.

Ultrasonography is a noninvasive, inexpensive, and often readily available tool for assessing subcutaneous wound complications. Ultrasound may be useful in identifying subcutaneous fluid collections in need of drainage in patients where physical exam is difficult (ie, in the obese). CT scans are rarely indicated in the evaluation of superficial or deep incisional SSIs, with the notable exception of when there is suspicion that the SSI is actually a manifestation of an underlying organ/space infection.

Although clinical presentation and physical exam can point toward organ/space SSIs, the diagnosis is often unclear. CT scan is often the most useful modality for identifying organ/space infections. Like in incisional SSIs, obtaining an imaging study should only be done if the results of the study would drive management (ie, identifying an intra-abdominal abscess that would subsequently be drained). When considering obtaining a postoperative CT scan, it is important to take into consideration the timing of the study. In the days following surgery, it is common for fluid to be present within the abdomen. Abscesses do not typically form until approximately postoperative days 5 to 7. Thus, a CT scan on postoperative day 3 is unlikely to provide useful information, as differentiating between normal postoperative fluid and an early abscess is often not possible. However, should concern for organ/space complications arise on postoperative day 5 or later, a CT scan is far more likely to provide useful information.

The type of CT scan is also important. Oral and intravenous contrasts make for an ideal radiographic evaluation of the abdomen for a source of postoperative organ/space SSIs. Oral contrast helps delineate the anatomy of the gastrointestinal tract. Additionally, extravasation of oral contrast into the abdomen is diagnostic of a leak. Intravenous contrast optimizes visualization of vascular structures and can identify a source of active bleeding. It can also help identify abscesses, which demonstrate peripheral rim enhancement when this type of contrast is administered.

A suspicion of leak may necessitate a dynamic study, such as a small bowel follow-through or a gastrographin enema. While CT scans are not the gold standard for determination of an anastomotic leak, they are frequently used due to their accessibility and comfort for patients.

For this patient, the exam and time course support the diagnosis of a superficial incisional SSI. Ultrasound is a viable imaging modality, although it is most useful when it is not already clear where to open the wound to drain the fluid. If this was later in the patient's course and/or there were any other indications that this might be an organ/space SSI, then CT would instead be indicated.

5. The most important principle in the management of suspected postoperative wound infections is to open the wound over the area of infection. Opening an infected wound makes several things possible. First, it allows for evacuation and persistent drainage of purulent, microorganism-laden fluid. This alone markedly decreases the bacterial load within an infected wound. Opening an infected wound also permits local wound exploration with a cotton-tipped applicator. Wound exploration makes it possible to identify and debride any nonviable tissue and assess the integrity of the underlying fascia. Debriding nonviable tissue is an important component of managing wound infections because dead tissue provides an ideal site for bacterial proliferation that is not readily penetrated by host defense mechanisms. Assessing fascial integrity is important because wound infection is a risk factor for fascial dehiscence. Additionally, fascial compromise may also be indicative of a more deeply rooted infectious process such as an intra-abdominal abscess that may require more significant intervention. Any persistent, heavy drainage of serous fluid should raise suspicion of fascial dehiscence, as this serous fluid may very well be peritoneal fluid. This essentially always warrants more extensive evaluation and having a senior resident involved is paramount.

Generally speaking, infected wounds that have been opened should remain open and be allowed to heal by secondary intention. This allows for frequent wet-to-dry dressing changes, continuous drainage from the wound, and prevention of purulent fluid reaccumulation. Along the same lines, the suprafascial portion of surgical wounds at a particularly high risk for infection may be preemptively left open in order to decrease the likelihood that a postoperative wound infection will develop. Although healing by secondary intention generates a significant wound care need for a prolonged period of time, it is often an essential component of postoperative wound infection management and is the standard approach.

If there is widespread cellulitis or signs of systemic infection, the use of empiric intravenous antibiotics should be strongly considered. Empiric antibiotics should target the microorganisms most likely responsible for the infection, yet not be so narrow as to miss other less likely but still potential pathogens. If broad-spectrum antibiotics are initiated, it is important to obtain a culture and Gram stain of the wound prior to the initiation of antibiotic therapy so that coverage can be tailored to the sensitivities as soon as they become available.

6. Seroma formation can lead to delays in healing and increase the risk of wound infection. The best method for managing seromas is prevention. This can be done by leaving closed-suction drains in surgical wounds at particular risk for seroma formation. By placing drains in the at-risk wounds, serous fluid passes into the drain, where it travels to a suction device (ie, a bulb). Drawing this fluid out of the body prevents its accumulation in the potential space created through tissue resection, thus preventing seroma formation. It is important that these drains are not pulled prematurely, as a seroma may subsequently develop. Applying pressure dressings to at-risk wounds is another technique to decrease the likelihood of seroma formation. This works by compressing damaged lymphatic channels and minimizing leakage of lymphatic fluid.

Once a seroma has formed, there are several management options available. If the seroma is small and not infected, one can simply observe it and wait for reabsorption. Another option is aspirating with a needle and a syringe. The benefit to the latter is that this is both diagnostic and therapeutic. Aspiration should be done under sterile conditions in order to avoid introducing any pathogens into an uninfected fluid collection. Aspiration may be repeated, but after several aspirations, the wound should be reopened and allowed to heal by secondary intention. If drainage is heavy, it may be necessary to take the patient to the operating room to explore the wound and ligate any leaking lymphatic channels. As with any superficial wound infection, when seromas become infected they should be reopened and allowed to heal by secondary intention. An example you are likely to encounter on a vascular surgery rotation, a seroma that develops following a dissection of the groin and subsequently becomes infected.

Table 57-2. The Most Common Inciting Pathogens for Wound Infections Based on Wound Classification

Wound Type	Common Pathogens
Clean surgical wounds	*Staphylococcus aureus*
	Enterobacteriaceae
	Group A streptococci
Dirty surgical wounds[a]	*S. aureus*
	Enterobacteriaceae
	Anaerobes
Trauma wounds	*Clostridium*
	Enterobacteriaceae
	Pseudomonas aeruginosa
Burn wounds	*P. aeruginosa*
	S. aureus
	Enterobacteriaceae
	Candida albicans

[a]Etiology determined by origin of contaminating pathogen.

The management of postoperative wound hematomas is similar to seromas. Small hematomas can be observed and will likely reabsorb. Larger hematomas may need sterile aspiration. If they recur or show signs of expansion, the patient may need to be taken back to the operating room to look for any ongoing bleeding. Importantly, decisions regarding observing or draining seromas and hematomas should always involve discussions with senior members of the surgical team.

7. In general, clean cases are associated with infections due to skin flora. Infections after a clean-contaminated case can be due to both skin flora and the flora associated with the viscera on which you operated. Contaminated and dirty wounds are almost always infected by pathogens from the source of contamination. In this patient the most likely culprit is *Staphylococcus aureus*. See Table 57-2 for an abbreviated list of the most common pathogens for different types of wounds.

TIPS TO REMEMBER

● Wounds are classified into four major groups: clean, clean-contaminated, contaminated, and dirty/infected—each with a progressively higher risk of SSI.

● The presence of a seroma or hematoma increases the risk for developing postoperative wound infections.

- Ultrasound may be useful in identifying or characterizing superficial or deep incisional SSIs. CT may be useful in identifying organ/space SSIs.
- The key to managing postoperative wound infections is to assess the wound, consider initiating antibiotics, and consider opening the wound to permit drainage of infected fluid.
- When persistent drainage of serous fluid from an abdominal wound is appreciated, fascial dehiscence must be considered. This warrants evaluation by a senior member of the surgical team.

COMPREHENSION QUESTIONS

1. An exploratory laparotomy is performed for a gunshot wound to the abdomen. The patient is found to have an enterotomy with spillage of fecal contents. What is the class of the wound?
    A. Clean
    B. Clean-contaminated
    C. Contaminated
    D. Dirty/infected

2. Which of the following are risk factors for the development of postoperative wound infections?
    A. Seromas
    B. Hematomas
    C. Gross spillage of GI tract contents during surgery
    D. B and C
    E. A, B, and C

3. A patient who underwent a laparoscopic appendectomy for perforated appendicitis presents to the ED on POD #8 with abdominal pain, distention, and no bowel movements or flatus for 2 days. He had been having normal bowel movements since POD #2. He has had no nausea or vomiting. He continues to have lingering RLQ abdominal pain and is found to have a mild leukocytosis. This presentation is most consistent with which of the following?
    A. A normal postoperative course
    B. Adhesive small bowel obstruction
    C. Urinary tract infection
    D. Organ/space SSI
    E. Stump appendicitis

Answers

1. C. Contaminated surgical wounds are defined as those resulting from a case where there is poor sterility secondary to gross spillage from the GI tract, GU

tract, or respiratory tract or by the presence of foreign debris—and without an established infection. Although this patient has fecal contamination, it is an acute process and is unlikely to have resulted in surrounding soft tissue infection or abscess formation.

2. **E.** Seromas, hematomas, and contaminated wounds are all risk factors for postoperative wound infection. Patients with contaminated wounds have a 20% to 25% risk for developing a postoperative wound infection.

3. **D.** Organ/space SSIs involve organs or spaces that were opened at the time of surgery. In perforated appendicitis, patients are at a particularly high risk for SSIs, given the local (or sometimes even diffuse) contamination of the normally sterile peritoneal cavity. An abscess is the likely diagnosis, manifested by recurrent ileus, abdominal tenderness, and a leukocytosis. Adhesive SBO is less likely than organ/space infections as it often takes weeks for adhesions to develop. Focal RLQ tenderness is not characteristic of UTIs. Stump appendicitis is the case in which residual appendix tissue remains unresected and becomes inflamed. Although this is possible, it is very rare and quite unlikely.

SUGGESTED READINGS

Ryan KJ, Ray CG, Sherris JC. *Sherris Medical Microbiology*. 5th ed. New York: McGraw Hill Medical; 2010. <http://www.accessmedicine.com/resourceTOC.aspx?resourceID=656>.
Sabiston DC, Townsend CM. *Sabiston Textbook of Surgery: the Biological Basis of Modern Surgical Practice*. 18th ed. Philadelphia: Saunders/Elsevier; 2008.

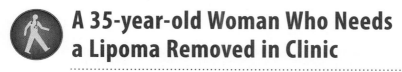

A 35-year-old Woman Who Needs a Lipoma Removed in Clinic

Roy Phitayakorn, MD, MHPE (MEd)

A 35-year-old woman presents to general surgery resident clinic with a 3 × 4 cm soft tissue mass on her upper back that she would like to have removed. She states that the mass has been there for several years, but recently started growing after she hit that portion of her back on a door. The mass is soft and mobile and pictured in Figure 58-1. Her lymph nodes are all normal and the mass feels like a lipoma.

1. **What are the 2 main classes of local anesthetics?**
2. **What is the mechanism of action of local anesthetics?**
3. **Where in the body is local anesthetic mixed with epinephrine contraindicated?**
4. **What is the most serious risk of using local anesthetics?**
5. **Name 2 things you can do to minimize the pain associated with injection of local anesthetics.**
6. **How many distinct skin injections are required for a small field block?**

LOCAL ANESTHETICS

Answers

1. Local anesthetics can be separated into 2 distinct groups called amides or esters based on their chemical structures. All anesthetics that end in "-caine" and contain the letter i in the prefix are amide agents. An easy way to remember this for the ABSITE is that the word amide also has an "i" in it. So, for example, lidocaine is an amide and cetacaine is an ester. Esters have the advantage of being faster acting. The disadvantages of ester anesthetics are that they have a shorter shelf life and cannot be combined with epinephrine.

2. Remember from your preclinical years that pain signals are transmitted via action potentials along the peripheral nerves. Local anesthetics act by reversibly blocking these nerve impulses by disrupting cell membrane permeability to sodium during an action potential. The basic pharmacokinetics of common local anesthetics is illustrated in Table 58-1. The 2 most common local anesthetics general surgery residents use are lidocaine (Xylocaine®) and bupivacaine (Marcaine®). Both take several minutes to take effect after injection and last anywhere from several hours in the case of lidocaine to many hours for bupivacaine.

   The most important detail to remember when using these agents is to keep track of the total amount of anesthetic given. This is especially important when

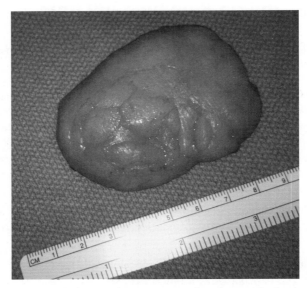

Figure 58-1. A picture of a lipoma that was removed in clinic under local anesthetic.

you may be suturing by yourself in the emergency department on a patient with multiple lacerations. If you think you will need a lot of local anesthetic due to multiple lacerations, then the 1% concentration of lidocaine (10 mg/mL) or 0.5% bupivacaine (5 mg/mL) is a convenient choice. For an average patient with no hepatic impairment, up to 4.5 mg/kg of lidocaine or 2.5 mg/kg of bupivacaine can be given during the procedure.

3. Epinephrine is combined with these anesthetics in various concentrations and helps to promote vasoconstriction of nearby vessels. This provides several benefits including lower required dosages of anesthetic, prolonged duration of action, and improved control of local bleeding. Local anesthetic with epinephrine is contraindicated in areas of the body with end arterioles. These

Table 58-1. Common Local Anesthetics

Agent	Brand Name	Class	Available Concentration (%)	Duration of Action
Procaine	Novocaine	Ester	0.5-1	15-90 min
Tetracaine	Prontocaine	Ester	0.25	2-3 h
Lidocaine	Xylocaine	Amide	0.5-2	1-4 h
Bupivacaine	Marcaine	Amide	0.125-0.25	4-16 h

anatomical areas are easily remembered by the rhyme "No epinephrine in the fingers, nose, toes, ear lobes, and 'hose.'"

4. There are several problems that you may encounter when using local anesthetics. One problem is systemic toxicity, which frequently manifests first as central nervous system–type symptoms such as confusion, dizziness, tinnitus, somnolence, and possible seizures. These symptoms can eventually progress if unrecognized to cardiovascular collapse, ventricular arrhythmias, and asystole due to a direct blocking effect on cardiac and vascular smooth muscle. Treatment is mainly supportive until the anesthetic has been metabolized. Pregnant patients are a special case in terms of local anesthetics as pregnancy reduces the risk of toxicity, but much higher dosages of the local anesthetics are required to achieve effective anesthesia. The mechanism for this tolerance is not clearly understood.

5. There are 5 things you can do to minimize the pain of injection: buffering, medications for anxiety, use a small needle, inject slowly, and wound pretreatment.

   Buffering: Local anesthetic is an acidic solution and therefore creates a burning sensation when you inject it into the skin. Anyone who has not experienced the feeling of lidocaine should definitely try it before one tells a patient "This won't hurt a bit." There are several proven techniques to reduce the pain of injection. One technique is to use sodium bicarbonate, which buffers the acidic solution so that it does not burn as much. Generally, you use the bicarbonate in a 1:10 ratio for 1% lidocaine and 2:10 for 2% lidocaine. It used to be believed that buffering lidocaine increased the rate of infection in contaminated wounds, but this was found to be untrue in experimental models. However, the use of bicarbonate does decrease the shelf life of lidocaine considerably so you should generally use whatever you mix. Also, when you ask for lidocaine from the inpatient pharmacy, it may have been stored in a refrigerator to preserve shelf life. It is important to warm the solution to body temperature if possible as cold lidocaine is more painful for the patient on injection than room-temperature lidocaine.

   Medications for anxiety: Another important technique to minimize pain associated with local anesthetics is to remember the old cliché that "perception is reality" and that local anesthetics do not do anything for patient anxiety. If the patient is particularly anxious, he or she may benefit from a preprocedure injection of opioids or anxiolytics before you inject the anesthetic as a way to decrease overall receptiveness to pain. Common choices are fentanyl or morphine and Ativan or Versed. Fentanyl and Versed work faster if you are ready to start the procedure, but may be more difficult to obtain quickly.

   Use a small needle: Although it is quicker to draw up the lidocaine using an 18- or 20-gauge needle, you should inject with the smallest needle possible. Nothing stimulates anxiety like watching someone approach you with a large needle.

Inject slowly: You should also strive to inject the local anesthetic slowly into the skin as this allows the tissue to slowly expand and decreases pain. A good rule of thumb is 1 mL of local anesthetic over 5 seconds of time. You should also try to inject local anesthetic through areas of the skin that are already anesthetized.

Wound pretreatment: The last technique to minimize pain is the most complicated and is in the broad category of wound pretreatment. One type of wound pretreatment is distraction. Mechanical distraction is a very interesting, but poorly understood phenomenon. Likely the mechanism is that your peripheral nerves can only carry so much sensory information at a given time. A good use of this technique is when you need to start peripheral IVs. If you take your skin and pinch it hard, you will notice after you let go that the area is slightly numb. Similarly, stretching the skin around a wound while injecting local anesthetic seems to decrease the perception of pain. Psychological distraction works on the belief that anxiety may play a large role in the perception of pain, especially in children. Therefore, for adult patients, try to engage them in conversation to keep them occupied. For pediatric patients, try to use child life specialists if possible to provide age-appropriate distracters such as blowing bubbles, music, or videos.

Another form of wound pretreatment is thermal anesthesia. A clean piece of ice or ice pack on top of a wound for at least 10 seconds is very effective at decreasing pain. A chemical version is ethyl chloride (also called Pain-eze®), as it functions to cool the skin and thus decrease pain perception. If you do use ethyl chloride, you have to be very careful to spray only for a few seconds as prolonged exposure to ethyl chloride can cause frostbite on the skin.

The last common form of wound pretreatment is EMLA cream, which is predominantly used in the pediatric population. EMLA stands for eutectic mixture of local anesthetics. As the chemistry majors who are reading this may remember, a eutectic mixture is a mixture of 2 substances that has a melting point lower than either substance by itself. In EMLA cream, the crystalline bases of lidocaine and prilocaine are combined to produce a liquid at room temperature. The cream is applied to an area and covered with occlusive dressing. Onset time is 15 minutes, but requires 1 hour to penetrate the first 3 mm of skin. One common fear is toxicity, but the literature suggests that systemic toxicity is very unlikely. Generally you should use enough so that you still see residual cream when you remove the occlusive dressing.

6. A useful technique when removing soft tissue masses such as a lipoma or an epidermoid inclusion cyst is illustrated in Figure 58-2. First, inject anesthetic at 2 points across the mass from each other. Once these areas are anesthetized,

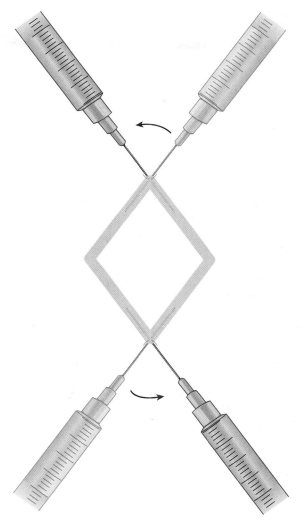

Figure 58-2. The field block technique.

inject local anesthetic through these points to form a rectangle around the mass. Remember, the goal is to inject the local anesthetic into the deep dermis (*not* the subcutaneous fat or the epidermis) to block the sensory plexus. This technique is called a field block and essentially completely disrupts the ability to send any pain signals out of the area where you will be dissecting, and yet only requires 2 skin injections.

TIPS TO REMEMBER

- Lidocaine and bupivacaine are the most commonly used local anesthetics for general surgery problems.
- Local anesthetics can lead to toxicity if given in incorrect dosages.
- There are several steps that can be used to minimize the pain associated with local anesthetics including mixing in sodium bicarbonate, anxiolytics, and wound pretreatment techniques.

COMPREHENSION QUESTIONS

1. What is the mechanism of action of local anesthetics?
      A. Temporary inhibition of sodium channels along cellular membranes
      B. Reduced calcium uptake into the sarcoplasmic reticulum
      C. Decreased extracellular magnesium concentrations
      D. Depletion of intracellular chloride stores

2. You are about to suture a very large laceration in a 75-kg man with normal liver function. How much 1% lidocaine can you safely inject without worrying about toxicity?
      A. 30 mL
      B. 40 mL
      C. 50 mL
      D. 60 mL

3. Which of the following skin layers should you be aiming for when injecting local anesthetic?
      A. Epidermis.
      B. Dermis.
      C. Subcutaneous tissue.
      D. All skin layers should be anesthetized.

Answers

1. **A.** Local anesthetics act by reversibly blocking nerve impulses by disrupting cell membrane permeability to sodium during an action potential.

2. **A.** For an average patient with no hepatic impairment, up to 4.5 mg/kg of lidocaine can be given during the procedure. Therefore, this patient can receive around 330 mg of lidocaine total. A 1% concentration of lidocaine has a concentration of 10 mg/mL so this patient can receive around 30 mL without worrying about toxicity.

3. **B.** When injecting local anesthetics, the goal is to inject the local anesthetic into the deep dermis to block the sensory plexus.

A 52-year-old Woman With a Suspected Congenital Coagulopathy

Jahan Mohebali, MD

Ms. Smith is a 52-year-old female who presents to your office for a possible laparoscopic sigmoid colectomy. She states that she has no significant medical history other than diverticulitis. Her only previous surgery was a wisdom tooth extraction at the age of 21. She notes that the procedure was uneventful; however, she continued to have significant oozing from her gums for approximately 24 hours. On review of systems, she notes that she has always bruised quite easily as long as she can remember. Further questioning reveals that she may have also had menorrhagia, although this was never formally diagnosed. Her laboratory data reveal a normal complete blood count. Her coagulation panel is notable for a mildly elevated partial thromboplastin time (PTT) and a prolonged bleeding time.

1. **What is the single best predictor of an inherited disorder of coagulation?**
2. **What are the two major categories of coagulation abnormalities and what symptoms are associated with each?**
3. **What is the standard workup when an inherited coagulopathy is suspected?**
4. **Which laboratory tests will distinguish a platelet disorder from a problem with coagulation factors?**

CONGENITAL COAGULOPATHY

In order to understand congenital coagulation disorders, one must begin by briefly reviewing the steps of normal hemostasis (see Figure 59-1). Although it is not essential to memorize every step of the cascade, one must understand that there is an intrinsic pathway that is initiated by exposure of blood to collagen as may happen with endothelial damage and an extrinsic pathway that is initiated with exposure to tissue factor. These pathways converge with the activation of factor X and formation of the tenase complex, which initiates the final common pathway by converting prothrombin to thrombin, and finally fibrinogen to fibrin. It is also important to note that platelets not only are involved in forming the initial hemostatic plug but also serve as the surface on which the tenase complex assembles.

Answers

1. The single best predictor is the preoperative history and physical exam. Careful history taking is usually more revealing than preoperative coagulation studies.

    The preoperative hematologic history should focus on whether or not the patient has ever experienced a previous episode of abnormal bleeding. If the

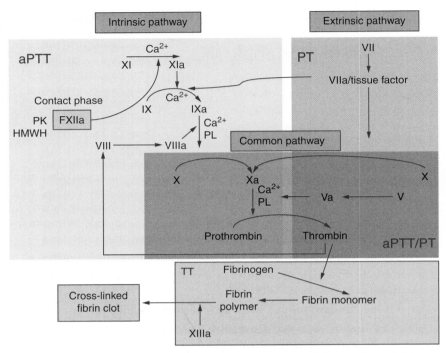

Figure 59-1. Coagulation cascade and laboratory assessment of clotting factor deficiency. (Reproduced, with permission, from Longo DL, Fauci AS, Kasper DL, Hauser SL, Jameson JL, Loscalzo J. *Harrison's Principles of Internal Medicine.* 18th ed. New York: McGraw-Hill Education; 2012. Figure 116.1. <www.accessmedicine.com>. Copyright © The McGraw-Hill Companies, Inc. All rights reserved.)

patient has had a previous operation, he or she should be questioned regarding any complications related to bleeding or poor hemostasis intraoperatively or in the postoperative period. If the patient has not undergone a previous surgical procedure, the history should focus on prolonged or abnormal bleeding related to trauma, previous episodes of mucosal bleeding or epistaxis, a history of menorrhagia in women, extensive bleeding after dental procedures, or a history of subcutaneous, intramuscular, or intra-articular hemorrhage.

2. Most congenital coagulopathies are the result of an abnormality related to platelets, to coagulation factors, or, occasionally, to both. Whenever a disorder of hemostasis is suspected, an attempt should be made to determine which of these is the culprit. Bleeding related to thrombocytopenia or decreased platelet function is typically manifested as mucosal bleeding, epistaxis, prolonged bleeding after tooth extraction, and menorrhagia (in women). Bleeding as a result of coagulation factor abnormalities is more likely to present as major

Table 59-1. Comparison of Signs Associated With Each Type of Coagulation Disorder

Platelet Disorder	Coagulation Factor Deficiencies
Mucosal bleeding	Major bleeding following minor trauma:
Epistaxis	
Prolonged bleeding after tooth extraction	Subcutaneous
	Intramuscular
Menorrhagia	Intra-articular

subcutaneous, intramuscular, and, classically, intra-articular hemorrhage following minor trauma (see Table 59-1).

Platelet disorders

The most commonly encountered inherited coagulopathy is von Willebrand disease (vWD). This disorder should be thought of as a functional platelet disorder. The prevalence of vWD has been reported to be as high as 1 in 100 in some populations. The second and third most commonly encountered hereditary coagulopathies are factor VIII deficiency resulting in hemophilia A with a prevalence of roughly 1 in 10,000 and factor IX deficiency resulting in hemophilia B with a prevalence of roughly 1 in 100,000.

von Willebrand factor (vWF) is a multimeric protein contained within vascular endothelial cells and in plasma that facilitates the binding of platelets to subendothelial collagen through Gp1b receptors. It also serves as a stabilizer of factor VIII, which is why patients with vWD may also have some degree of factor VIII deficiency. As previously mentioned, because vWD is a functional platelet disorder, these patients will typically have a history of mucosal bleeding, significant bleeding after dental procedures, epistaxis, and menorrhagia (in women). In fact, patients with the most severe form (type 3) may actually suffer from hemarthroses because of their factor VIII deficiency.

Other less common congenital platelet disorders may include thrombocytopenia from splenic sequestration as a result of a multitude of congenital storage and hematopoietic disorders, and other functional platelet disorders. Glanzmann thrombasthenia and Bernard-Soulier syndrome are two other inherited functional platelet disorders that result in bleeding despite a normal platelet count (see Figure 59-2).

Coagulation factor deficiencies

Hemophilia A and hemophilia B resulting from factor VIII and factor IX deficiency, respectively, are considered to be the second and third most common hereditary bleeding diatheses. Both diseases are inherited on the X chromosome

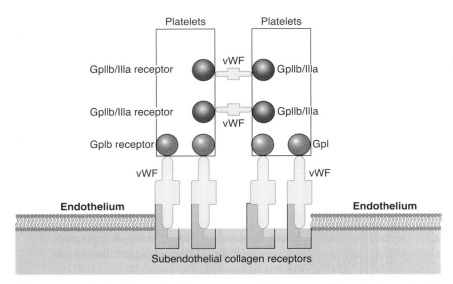

Figure 59-2. Platelet adhesion and aggregation. GpIb receptors allow platelets to bind to the collagen in the subendothelium with the help of vWF. These are the receptors affected in Bernard-Soulier syndrome. GpIIa/IIIb receptors allow platelets to bind to one another with the help of fibrinogen and are decreased in Glanzmann thrombasthenia.

and because they are coagulation factor abnormalities, patients will typically present with subcutaneous, intramuscular, or intra-articular hemorrhage following minor trauma. The degree of bleeding depends on the level of factor present in plasma. It is important to remember that factor VIII is the only coagulation factor that is not synthesized in the liver. Mild deficiencies in factor VIII can be treated with cryoprecipitate that contains high concentrations of the factor, or with desmopressin (DDAVP) that increases release of vWF and factor VIII from the endothelium. In most cases, however, deficiencies in factor VIII or IX are treated with the administration of factor concentrates. In general, factor levels need to be maintained at a minimum of 50% of normal in the intraoperative and postoperative periods until wound healing is complete in order to prevent complications related to hemorrhage. Other congenital factor deficiencies exist, but these are exceedingly rare and beyond the scope of this chapter.

3. When a congenital coagulopathy is suspected, workup should proceed as follows:

A. Step 1—History and physical exam. Begin with a full history and physical exam focusing on any bleeding complications associated with previous operations, or a history of abnormal bleeding. It is important to remember that acquired causes of coagulopathy are more prevalent than congenital causes and the history and physical exam should be used to look for these diseases as well.

B. Step 2—Obtain a medication list. A full list of antiplatelet and antithrombotic medications taken by the patient should be obtained, and the patient should be asked about other medications that may interfere with platelet function such as aspirin, NSAIDs, fish oil, or H2 blockers.

C. Step 3—Screen for acquired causes of coagulopathy such as organ dysfunction. Liver disease may result in a coagulopathy as a result of poor synthetic function, and uremia secondary to renal failure results in abnormal platelet function by interfering with the action of both GpIIb/IIIa and GpIb receptors. The physical exam should not only look for evidence of abnormal hemostasis and hematopoiesis such as petechiae, hematomas, lymphadenopathy, and splenomegaly but also screen for stigmata of advanced liver and renal disease.

D. Step 4—If indicated, obtain appropriate laboratory studies. If there is ongoing concern for a bleeding diathesis, a complete blood count and prothrombin time (PT), international normalized ratio (INR), and PTT should be obtained. If there is concern for a platelet disorder despite a normal platelet count, a bleeding time assay and ristocetin cofactor assay should be obtained.

4. In order to interpret laboratory data in the workup of congenital coagulopathies, one must understand which tests are representative of each part of the normal hemostasis pathway (see Figure 59-2).

Laboratory evaluation of platelet disorders

Platelet disorders can be evaluated with a complete blood count and bleeding time. If the complete blood count does not demonstrate thrombocytopenia and there is ongoing concern for a platelet disorder, a bleeding time assay can be obtained. To determine the bleeding time, a 9 mm long × 1 mm deep incision is made on the forearm and a blood pressure cuff is inflated to 40 mm Hg to create back pressure. Blood is blotted away every 30 seconds from the incision until bleeding stops. Although this test is extremely sensitive for picking up functional platelet disorders, it is quite difficult to standardize and is therefore not commonly used.

If there is suspicion for vWD, a ristocetin cofactor assay can be obtained. When added to normal blood, ristocetin will cause vWF to bind the GpIb receptor on platelets. In vWD, addition of ristocetin will not result in platelet clumping. It should be reiterated that vWD will result in a factor VIII deficiency and, therefore, some degree of PTT prolongation.

Table 59-2 shows the most common lab abnormalities associated with each of the above-mentioned bleeding diatheses.

Laboratory evaluation of factor deficiencies

PT: In general, the PT will be prolonged when there are low levels of factors in the extrinsic pathway and everything downstream of it, that is, VII, X, and

Table 59-2. Common Lab Abnormalities Associated With Bleeding Diatheses

Disorder	PT	PTT	Bleeding Time	Platelet Count
Hemophilia A	Unchanged	⇑	Unchanged	Unchanged
Hemophilia B	Unchanged	⇑	Unchanged	Unchanged
vWD	Unchanged	⇑	⇑	Unchanged
Glanzmann thrombasthenia	Unchanged	Unchanged	⇑	Unchanged
Bernard-Soulier syndrome	Unchanged	Unchanged	⇑	Unchanged
Splenic sequestration	Unchanged	Unchanged	⇑	⇓

V, prothrombin, and fibrinogen. The INR is a standardized measurement of the PT and is used to monitor anticoagulation therapy.

PTT: The PTT is representative of the function of the intrinsic pathway and everything downstream of it, that is, factors VIII, IX, XI, XII, X, V, prothrombin, and fibrinogen. Therefore, hemophilia A and B are associated with a prolonged PTT.

Clearly, both the PT and PTT are affected by factors in the final common pathway and therefore any abnormality of the tenase complex and downstream of it will result in an elevation of both the PT and PTT.

A prolonged PT in the setting of a normal PTT ensures that the abnormality lies within the extrinsic pathway, upstream of the final common pathway. Only factor VII deficiency can cause this pattern of lab values.

Likewise, a prolonged PTT, but normal PT, implies that the abnormality lies within the intrinsic pathway, upstream of the final common pathway. This pattern will be seen with deficiency of factor VIII, IX, XI, or XII.

TIPS TO REMEMBER

- The best screening test for a congenital coagulopathy is the preoperative history and physical exam.
- Bleeding disorders may be a result of abnormalities of platelets, coagulation factors, or both.
  - Platelet disorders typically present with mucosal bleeding, epistaxis, prolonged bleeding after tooth extraction, and occasionally menorrhagia (in women).

■ Coagulation factor disorders typically present with more severe bleeding such as intramuscular and intra-articular hemorrhage.

● A prolonged PT with a normal PTT suggests a problem in the extrinsic pathway (ie, factor VII deficiency). A prolonged PTT with a normal PT suggests a problem in the intrinsic pathway. If both the PT and PTT are prolonged, the problem must affect the final common pathway.

● Bleeding time is prolonged in functional platelet disorders, but the test is not used very often because of difficulty in its standardization.

● The three most common congenital coagulopathies are vWD (~1 in 100), hemophilia A (~1 in 10,000), and hemophilia B (1 in 100,000).

COMPREHENSION QUESTIONS

1. A 25-year-old male presents to your clinic for preoperative evaluation prior to repair of a right inguinal hernia. Your history and physical exam reveals a previous history of two episodes of intra-articular hemorrhage. If the patient has a congenital coagulopathy, he may have any one of the following diseases except which one?

A. Hemophilia A
B. Hemophilia B
C. Splenic sequestration

2. What is the most important step in screening for the presence of a congenital coagulopathy?

A. Obtaining a complete blood count
B. Checking PT, INR, and PTT
C. Obtaining a ristocetin cofactor assay
D. Performing a thorough history and physical exam

3. Administration of desmopressin (DDAVP) will help to correct all of the following congenital coagulopathies to some degree except which one?

A. vWD
B. Hemophilia A
C. Hemophilia B

4. A preoperative history reveals previous episodes of epistaxis and prolonged bleeding after wisdom tooth extraction. The patient is likely to have any of the following congenital coagulopathies except which one?

A. Bernard-Soulier syndrome
B. Factor VII deficiency
C. Glanzmann thrombasthenia
D. vWD

Answers

1. **C.** A history of intra-articular hemorrhage suggests a problem with the coagulation cascade. This means either hemophilia A or B. Splenic sequestration, on the other hand, is a platelet disorder and rarely results in intra-articular hemorrhage.

2. **D.** A thorough history and physical exam should be used for screening in order to avoid unnecessary testing.

3. **C.** Desmopressin or DDAVP administration results in release of factor VIII and vWF from the endothelium (remember that factor VIII is the only factor that is not produced in the liver). Factor IX is synthesized in the liver and, therefore, DDAVP will have no efficacy in hemophilia B.

4. **B.** The symptoms described suggest a platelet disorder such as A, C, or D.

Bibliography

The following is a list of high-yield papers that you will hear referenced frequently. If you were only going to read 11 articles, these should be where you start.

Dellinger RP, Levy MM, Carlet JM, et al. Surviving Sepsis Campaign: international guidelines for management of severe sepsis and septic shock: 2008. *Intensive Care Med*. 2008;34(1):17–60.

Duncan JE, Quietmeyer CM. Bowel preparation: current status. *Clin Colon Rectal Surg*. 2009;22(1):14.

Graham AS, Ozment C, Tegtmeyer K, Lai S, Braner DA. Videos in clinical medicine. Central venous catheterization. *N Engl J Med*. 2007;356(21):e21.

Marik PE, Vasu T, Hirani A, Pachinburavan M. Stress ulcer prophylaxis in the new millennium: a systematic review and meta-analysis. *Crit Care Med*. 2010;38(11):2222.

McGee S, Abernethy WB III, Simel DL. Is this patient hypovolemic? *JAMA*. 1999;281(11):1022–1029.

Moore FA, Moore EE. Initial Management of Life Threatening Trauma. ACS Surgery: Principles and Practice. <http://129.49.170.167/Volumes/ACSCD+July+2010/ACSCD/pdf/ACS0701.pdf>; 2005.

Napolitano LM, Kurek S, Luchette FA, et al. Clinical practice guideline: red blood cell transfusion in adult trauma and critical care. *Crit Care Med*. 2009;37(12):3124.

Nelson RL, Glenny AM, Song F. Antimicrobial prophylaxis for colorectal surgery. *Cochrane Database Syst Rev*. 2009;(1):CD001181. <http://onlinelibrary.wiley.com/doi/10.1002/14651858.CD001181.pub3/pdf/standard>.

Ochoa JB, Caba D. Advances in surgical nutrition. *Surg Clin North Am*. 2006;86(6):1483.

Rivers E, Nguyen B, Havstad S, et al. Early goal-directed therapy in the treatment of severe sepsis and septic shock. *N Engl J Med*. 2001;345(19):1368–1377.

Smith-Bindman R. Is computed tomography safe? *N Engl J Med*. 2010;363(1):1–4.

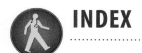

INDEX

Page numbers followed by *f* or *t* indicate figures or tables, respectively.